European Observatory on Health Care Systems Series

Edited by Josep Figueras, Martin McKee, Elias Mossialos and Richard B. Saltman

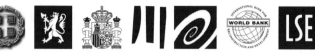

Funding health care: options for Europe

Edited by

Elias Mossialos, Anna Dixon, Josep Figueras and Joe Kutzin

D0101051

Open University Press

Buckingham · Philadelphia

Open University Press
Celtic Court
22 Ballmoor
Buckingham
MK18 1XW

email: enquiries@openup.co.uk
world wide web: www.openup.co.uk

and

325 Chestnut Street
Philadelphia, PA 19106, USA

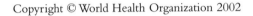
First Published 2002
Reprinted 2002

A catalogue record of this book is available from the British Library

ISBN   0 335 20924 6 (pb) / 0 335 20925 4 (hb)

Library of Congress Cataloging-in-Publication Data
Funding health care: options for Europe / edited by Elias Mossialos . . . [*et al.*].
    p. cm. — European Observatory on Health Care Systems series)
    Includes bibliographical references and index.
    ISBN 0-335-20925-4 (hb) — ISBN 0-335-20924-6 (pb)
    1. Medical care–Europe–Finance. 2. Medicine–Europe–Finance. 3. Federal
aid to medical care research–Europe. 4. Medical care–Economic aspects–
Europe. I. Mossialos, Elias. II. European Observatory on Health Care Systems
series

R852 .F86 2002
338.4′33621′094—dc21   2001036111

Typeset by Graphicraft Limited, Hong Kong
Printed and bound in Great Britain by Biddles Ltd, www.biddles.co.uk

Contents

List of figures, tables and boxes

List of contributors

Sara Bennett is Lecturer in Health Economics and Financing at the London School of Hygiene & Tropical Medicine, United Kingdom, currently based in Tbilisi, Georgia.

Reinhard Busse is Associate Professor for Epidemiology, Social Medicine and Health Systems Research at Medizinische Hochschule in Hannover, Germany, and is Head of the Madrid hub of the European Observatory on Health Care Systems.

Anna Dixon is Research Officer at the European Observatory on Health Care Systems and Lecturer in European Health Policy at the London School of Economics and Political Science, United Kingdom.

Robert Evans is Professor of Economics at the University of British Columbia Centre for Health Services and Policy Research in Vancouver, Canada.

Josep Figueras is Head of the Secretariat and Research Director of the European Observatory on Health Care Systems and Head of the European Centre for Health Policy, WHO Regional Office for Europe in Copenhagen, Denmark.

Melitta Jakab is Health Economist in the Human Development Network at the World Bank.

Martin Knapp is Co-director of LSE Health and Social Care at the London School of Economics and Political Science, United Kingdom.

Joe Kutzin is Senior Resident Adviser for the WHO Regional Office for Europe at the Ministry of Health of Kyrgyzstan in Bishkek.

Maureen Lewis is Sector Manager for Human Development Economics at the World Bank, Washington, DC.

Alan Maynard is Professor of Health Economics and Co-Director of the York Health Policy Group at the University of York, United Kingdom.

Anne Mills is Professor of Health Economics and Policy in the Health Economics and Financing Programme, Department of Public Health and Policy at the London School of Hygiene & Tropical Medicine, United Kingdom.

Elias Mossialos is Research Director of the European Observatory on Health Care Systems and Brian Abel-Smith Reader in Health Policy in the Department of Social Policy at the London School of Economics and Political Science, United Kingdom and Co-Director of LSE Health and Social Care.

Charles Normand is Professor of Health Policy at the London School of Hygiene & Tropical Medicine, United Kingdom.

Alexander S. Preker is Chief Economist for Health, Nutrition and Population at the World Bank, Washington, DC.

Nigel Rice is Senior Research Fellow at the Centre of Health Economics at the University of York, United Kingdom.

Ray Robinson is Professor of Health Policy at LSE Health and Social Care at the London School of Economics and Political Science, United Kingdom, and a Senior Research Fellow of the European Observatory on Health Care Systems.

Becky Sandhu is Economic Adviser on Social Care Policy at the Department of Health for England.

Markus Schneider is Director of BASYS (Beratungsgesellschaft für angewandte Systemforschung) in Augsburg, Germany.

Peter C. Smith is Professor of Economics at the Centre of Health Economics and the Department of Economics at the University of York, United Kingdom.

Sarah M.S. Thomson is Research Officer at the European Observatory on Health Care Systems based at the London School of Economics and Political Science, United Kingdom.

Raphael Wittenberg is Research Officer at LSE Health and Social Care at the London School of Economics and Political Science, United Kingdom, and Economic Adviser at the Department of Health for England.

Series editors' introduction

European national policy-makers broadly agree on the core objectives that their health care systems should pursue. The list is strikingly straightforward: universal access for all citizens, effective care for better health outcomes, efficient use of resources, high-quality services and responsiveness to patient concerns. It is a formula that resonates across the political spectrum and which, in various, sometimes inventive configurations, has played a role in most recent European national election campaigns.

Yet this clear consensus can only be observed at the abstract policy level. Once decision-makers seek to translate their objectives into the nuts and bolts of health system organization, common principles rapidly devolve into divergent, occasionally contradictory, approaches. This is, of course, not a new phenomenon in the health sector. Different nations, with different histories, cultures and political experiences, have long since constructed quite different institutional arrangements for funding and delivering health care services.

The diversity of health system configurations that has developed in response to broadly common objectives leads quite naturally to questions about the advantages and disadvantages inherent in different arrangements, and which approach is 'better' or even 'best' given a particular context and set of policy priorities. These concerns have intensified over the last decade as policy-makers have sought to improve health system performance through what has become a European-wide wave of health system reforms. The search for comparative advantage has triggered – in health policy as in clinical medicine – increased attention to its knowledge base, and to the possibility of overcoming at least part of existing institutional divergence through more evidence-based health policy-making.

The volumes published in the European Observatory series are intended to provide precisely this kind of cross-national health policy analysis. Drawing on an extensive network of experts and policy-makers working in a variety of academic and administrative capacities, these studies seek to synthesize the available evidence on key health sector topics using a systematic methodology. Each volume explores the conceptual background, outcomes and lessons learned about the development of more equitable, more efficient and more effective health care systems in Europe. With this focus, the series seeks to contribute to the evolution of a more evidence-based approach to policy formulation in the health sector. While remaining sensitive to cultural, social and normative differences among countries, the studies explore a range of policy alternatives available for future decision-making. By examining closely both the advantages and disadvantages of different policy approaches, these volumes fulfil a central mandate of the Observatory: to serve as a bridge between pure academic research and the needs of policy-makers, and to stimulate the development of strategic responses suited to the real political world in which health sector reform must be implemented.

The European Observatory on Health Care Systems is a partnership that brings together three international agencies, three national governments, two research institutions and an international non-governmental organization. The partners are as follows: the World Health Organization Regional Office for Europe, which provides the Observatory secretariat; the governments of Greece, Norway and Spain; the European Investment Bank; the Open Society Institute; the World Bank; the London School of Hygiene & Tropical Medicine and the London School of Economics and Political Science.

In addition to the analytical and cross-national comparative studies published in this Open University Press series, the Observatory produces Health Care Systems in Transition Profiles (HiTs) for the countries of Europe, the Observatory Summer School and the *Euro Observer* newsletter. Further information about Observatory publications and activities can be found on its web site at www.observatory.dk.

Josep Figueras, Martin McKee, Elias Mossialos and Richard B. Saltman

Foreword

At a time when expectations of health care systems are rising, yet costs challenge sustainability, governments face the central question: 'How should our health care be funded?'

WHO wants to ensure that public health decision-making is increasingly based on the evidence of what works and what does not, within a particular socioeconomic, political and cultural context.

There is a growing body of evidence about the impact of different funding methods. This book explores the ways of raising revenue, and the implications of choosing each mechanism or a mix of several. The different mechanisms are judged by various criteria, one of which is their impact on equity. How far do we want the burden of payment to fall most heavily on the poor or the sick? The evidence indicates that in raising revenue, market mechanisms have limitations. Privatization may involve a loss of equity and access: private health insurance is highly regressive and user charges are a blunt policy instrument.

The European Observatory on Health Care Systems serves an important role in WHO by charting the process of change in European health care systems, providing analysis and information, and disseminating evidence to policy-makers. In producing this study, the Observatory has drawn on the conceptual skills of academics and consultants, as well as the practical experience of policy-makers, to offer insights on effective health policy-making, and to help make the decisions easier and better informed. Improving mechanisms to raise the funds needed to provide decent health care is valuable to everyone.

Marc Danzon
WHO Regional Director for Europe

Acknowledgements

This volume is one in a series of books undertaken by the European Observatory on Health Care Systems. We are very grateful to our authors, who responded promptly both in producing and later amending their chapters in the light of ongoing discussions.

We particularly appreciate the detailed and very constructive comments of our reviewers, Phillip Berman, Luca Brusati, Antonio Duran, Julian Le Grand, Martin McKee, Ray Robinson, Richard B. Saltman and Herbert Zöllner. Additional material for the overview was provided by Peter Lutz, Stefan Gress, Agnes Couffinhal and Regina Riphahn. We should also like to thank the Observatory partners for their review of, and input to, successive versions of the manuscript.

We also thank all our colleagues in the Observatory. Our special thanks go to Anna Maresso, who patiently processed and formatted successive versions of the chapters, to Jeffrey Lazarus, Jenn Cain and Phyllis Dahl for managing the manuscript delivery and production, to Suszy Lessof for coordinating the studies and to Myriam Andersen for administrative support. We are also grateful to David Breuer for copy-editing the manuscript.

Finally, we are especially grateful to the Veneto Region Department of Health, which provided financial support to the authors' workshop in Venice in December 1999. Particular thanks go to Luigi Bertinato, Patricia Mason, Filippo Palumbo and Franco Toniolo for organizing the workshop. In addition, we would like to express our gratitude to Marino Cortese, President of the Querini Stampalia Foundation, and Dora De Diana for their collaboration in hosting the meeting at the Foundation's museum. Special thanks to John Appleby,

Fons Berten, Rene Christensen, Martin Dlouhy, Julian Forder, Peter Gaal, George Gotsadze, Unto Häkkinen, Lise Rochaix, Laura Rose, Igor Sheiman, Francesco Taroni and Akaki Zoidze for their useful comments on early drafts presented in Venice.

Elias Mossialos, Anna Dixon, Josep Figueras and Joe Kutzin

chapter one

Funding health care: an introduction

Elias Mossialos and Anna Dixon

Why a book on funding health care?

Sustainable health care systems are built on reliable access to human, capital and consumable resources. Securing these inputs requires financial resources to pay for investment in buildings and equipment, to compensate health service staff for their time and to pay for drugs and other consumables. How these financial resources are generated and managed – the process of collecting revenue and pooling funds – raises important issues for policy-makers and planners faced with the challenge of designing systems of funding that meet specific objectives related to social policy, politics and economics.

Most countries feel constant pressure because expenditure is increasing and resources are scarce. Policy-makers have three options: containing costs, increasing funding for health services or both. Concern about an expenditure crisis in health care has led to the introduction of major changes in how health care is organized and financed. Cost containment has been driving health policy discussions in industrialized countries since the 1970s (Mossialos and Le Grand 1999). However, if budgets are to balance, sufficient revenue has to be generated. Since large-scale public borrowing is no longer considered to be sound economic policy in many countries, concern currently focuses on revenue policies – how to fund health care on a sustainable basis.

What approach does the book adopt?

This book explores the options available to decision-makers to raise revenue, especially the implications of choosing one funding mechanism over another or, more usually, a particular mix of funding sources. The book builds on a substantial body of literature already published on funding health care (Appleby

1992; Wagstaff *et al.* 1993, 1999; Schieber 1997; Barer *et al.* 1998; van Doorslaer *et al.* 1999). A distinctive feature of this book is that it:

- combines theory and empirical evidence;
- provides up-to-date analysis of recent experience of funding health care in western Europe, central and eastern Europe (CEE) and the former Soviet Union (FSU);
- brings together issues related to the funding of both health care and long-term care; and
- goes beyond funding mechanisms and examines the relationship between funding and resource allocation.

The chapters examine the relative merits and public policy implications of the main methods of funding health care.[1] This book does not provide blueprints or prescribe particular models, but critically analyses the growing body of evidence on the effects of different funding methods. The book offers both a theoretical perspective and empirical evidence from across Europe, together with examples drawn from other industrialized and less-developed countries. This book covers developments up to autumn 2000.

Analytical approaches to health care funding

This section presents and discusses several frameworks that have been developed to facilitate an analysis of health care funding. These are reflected in the discussion and analysis presented in the chapters.

The health care triangle

The provision and financing of health care can be simplified as an exchange or transfer of resources: the providers transfer health care resources to patients and patients or third parties transfer financial resources to the providers (Figure 1.1). The simplest form of transaction for a good or service is direct payment. The consumer (the first party) pays the provider (the second party) directly in return

Figure 1.1 The health care triangle

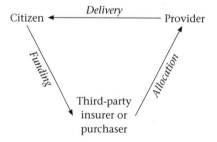

Source: adapted from Reinhardt (1990)

for the good or service. Health care systems have developed in which a third party offers protection to a population against the financial risk of falling ill. The third party may be a public or private body.[2] The development of the third-party payment mechanism in health care results in part from the uncertainty of ill health; it allows risks to be shared. However, it is also a means to achieve interpersonal redistribution.[3] To finance health care services, the third party must collect revenue directly or indirectly from the population it protects (this may cover the whole population or a subgroup of the population such as those who are employed). This revenue is then used to reimburse the patient or the provider.

The financing equation

The total of all revenue must be equal to all expenditure, which should be equal to the incomes plus profits of those working within the system. The following equation, devised by Evans (1998), which assumes no deficits, illustrates these elements. It posits that revenue – the sum of taxation (TF), compulsory or social insurance contributions (SI), out-of-pocket payments and user charges (UC), and voluntary or private insurance premiums (PI) – is equal to expenditure – the result of the price (P) times the quantity (Q) of goods and services. These, in turn, must be equal to the income of those who provide health care services – the quantity and mix of inputs (W) times the price of those inputs (Z).

$$TF + SI + UC + PI = P \times Q = W \times Z$$

This book explores the implications of adopting different mixes of revenue in the first part of the equation. Few systems in Europe have single sources of revenue. Most rely on a mix of taxation, social insurance contributions, out-of-pocket payments and private insurance premiums.[4] External sources, such as donations from non-governmental organizations, transfers from donor agencies and loans from international banks, also contribute significantly in some countries, especially low- and middle-income countries. These are also considered where relevant. We also explore how revenue sources may affect the price and quantity of goods and services ($P \times Q$) and the mix of inputs ($W \times Z$).

Revenue collection, fund pooling and purchasing

The health care system can be broken down into functional components, as shown in Figure 1.2: revenue collection, fund pooling and the purchasing and provision of health care. Functions can be integrated and separated in various combinations, even within the same country. In some cases, the functions are integrated within a single organizational entity; in others, one entity may collect and pool the funds while other bodies purchase and provide the services (Kutzin 2001). Resources are then allocated between these different entities.

Figure 1.2 Functions of health care systems

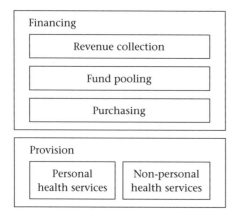

Source: adapted from Murray and Frenk (2000)

Revenue collection

The process of revenue collection is specifically concerned with who pays, the type of payment made and who collects it. Figure 1.3 illustrates the diversity of sources of funding, contribution mechanisms and collection agents and how these might interrelate. Funds derive primarily from the population (individuals and corporate entities). The funding mechanisms include taxation, social insurance contributions, private insurance premiums, individual savings, out-of-pocket payments and loans, grants and donations. Collection agents can be private for-profit, private not-for-profit or public. The status of the insurers affects their motivation and incentives – that is, whether they act in the interests of shareholders or members.

Taxes can be levied on individuals, households and firms (direct taxes) or on transactions and commodities (indirect taxes). Direct and indirect taxes can be levied at the national, regional or local levels. Indirect taxes can be general, such as a value-added tax, or applied to specific goods, such as an excise tax. Some social or compulsory insurance contributions are, in fact, a payroll tax collected by government. Here we distinguish between taxes, which are collected by government, and compulsory insurance contributions, which are normally collected by an independent or semi-independent agent. Taxes can be general or hypothecated – that is, earmarked for a specific area of expenditure.

Social health insurance contributions are usually related to income and shared between the employees and employers. Contributions may also be collected from self-employed people, for whom contributions are calculated based on declarations of income or profit (this income may be underdeclared in some countries). Contributions on behalf of elderly, unemployed or disabled people may be collected from designated pension, unemployment or sickness funds, respectively, or paid for from taxes. Social health insurance revenue is generally earmarked for health and collected by a separate fund.

Figure 1.3 Examples of funding sources, contribution mechanisms and collection agents

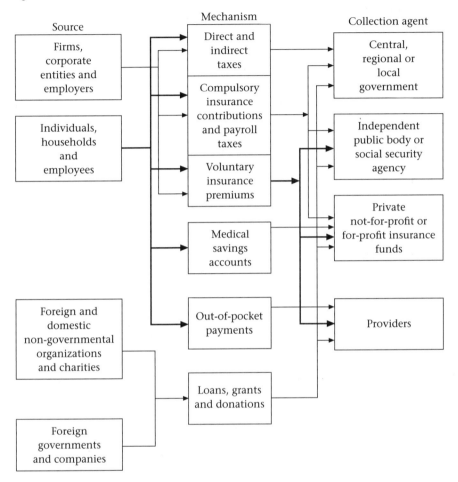

Source: adapted from Kutzin (2001)

Private health insurance premiums are paid by an individual, shared between the employees and the employer or paid wholly by the employer. Premiums can be: individually risk rated, based on an assessment of the probability of an individual requiring health care; community rated, based on an estimate of the risks across a geographically defined population; or group rated, based on an estimate of the risks across all employees in a single firm. The agents collecting private health insurance premiums can be independent private bodies, such as private for-profit insurance companies or private not-for-profit insurance companies and funds. Government may subsidize the cost of private health insurance using tax credits or tax relief.

Medical savings accounts are individual savings accounts into which people are either required to, or given incentives to, deposit money. The money must be spent on personal medical expenses. Medical savings accounts are usually combined with high-deductible catastrophic health insurance.

Patients may be required to pay part or all of the costs of some types of care in the form of user charges. These charges may be levied as a co-payment (a flat-rate payment for each service), co-insurance (a percentage of the total cost of the service) or a deductible (a ceiling up to which the patient is liable after which the insurer covers the remaining cost). The collection agent is usually the provider, such as a physician, hospital or pharmacist.

Fund pooling

Revenue collection must be distinguished from fund pooling, as some forms of revenue collection do not enable financial risks to be shared between contributors, such as medical savings accounts and out-of-pocket payments. Kutzin (2001) defined fund pooling as the 'accumulation of prepaid health care revenues on behalf of a population'. The importance of fund pooling is that it facilitates the pooling of financial risk across the population or a defined subgroup.

If collection and pooling are integrated, the allocation from collection agent to pooling agent is internalized. Examples of this include social health insurance contributions collected by funds and retained by them and national, regional or local taxes that are collected and retained. If different agents carry out these functions, a mechanism is required to distribute resources from the collection agent to the pool. If there are multiple pools, allocation is increasingly being adjusted according to the risk profile of the population covered by each pool. This process is referred to as 'risk adjustment' and is analysed in Chapter 11. Risk adjustment in competitive social health insurance systems has developed mainly from a concern to prevent cream-skimming (van de Ven *et al.* 1994; Oliver 1999). Within tax-financed systems, risk-adjusted capitation methods developed from a concern to ensure equity of access by ensuring a fair allocation of resources to territorial health authorities based on the needs of the population. Irrespective of the source of funds, however, the underlying rationale for allocating based on risk-adjusted capitation is the same – to ensure that each pool (insurance fund or territorial health authority) has the 'correct' relative level of resources for the population for which it is responsible (Kutzin 2001).

Under private health insurance, funds are pooled between subscribers of the same insurance provider. The extent of risk pooling is limited, however, with actuarial premiums related to an individual's risk. If premiums are community rated, pooling is between high-risk and low-risk members in the same geographic area. Group rating allows pooling between employees of the same firm.

Medical savings accounts prevent pooling by keeping funds in individual accounts. Medical savings accounts are therefore usually supplemented with catastrophic insurance for very expensive treatments.

User charges are paid at the point of service and are therefore not a form of pooling.[5] The revenue generated by user charges is handled differently depending on how the system is designed. For example, the individual health care provider may retain the money as income. It may be retained at the level of a clinic or hospital and, together with other revenue, contribute to the cost of maintaining local service provision. If the user charges are surrendered to, or levied by, the insurer or government, they may be used to meet any gap between premium or tax revenue and expenditure.

Purchasing

Purchasing means 'the transfer of pooled resource to service providers on behalf of the population for which the funds were pooled' (Kutzin 2001). In some systems, separate agents purchase services (for example, Primary Care Trusts in England); in this case, the resources have to be allocated to the purchasers. Pursuing widely held objectives of equity and efficiency requires allocating resources according to health care need. As Chapter 11 demonstrates, capitation is the main method for calculating purchasers' budgets adopted in Europe. However, many health care systems continue to allocate resources based on political negotiation, historical precedent or the lowest bids.

Balancing revenue and expenditure

Although revenue is the main focus of this book, it is important to understand both sides of the balance sheet – expenditure and revenue. This section presents basic data to illustrate recent trends in health care expenditure, highlights methodological problems in measuring health care expenditure and examines the contributions of different sources of revenue to health care expenditure.

Health care expenditure trends in Europe

After rapidly increasing in the 1960s and early 1970s, welfare spending in the largest OECD (Organisation for Economic Co-operation and Development) countries levelled off (Glennerster 1997). During the 1970s, a combination of economic recession following the 1974 oil crisis and the growing burden of unemployment eroded the view that increased welfare spending was sustainable. This led to a view shared by the left and the right that the welfare state was in crisis. These fears were not realized; in fact, welfare state spending has stabilized in many countries. However, health care expenditure has continued to rise in real terms. This may intensify the conflict between the demand for, and the supply of, public revenue for health care, unless countries pursue deficit financing,[6] cut other areas of public expenditure, shift to private sources of revenue or increase efficiency.

International comparison of health expenditure data presents several methodological problems. These include defining the boundaries between health care and social care, standardizing definitions across countries, methods of data collection and organizational differences. Problems are also associated with measuring and reporting expenditure as a percentage of gross domestic

Table 1.1 Percentage mean annual growth rates of total health expenditure (public health expenditure in parentheses) in selected European countries based on national currency units at 1995 GDP prices,[a] 1980–85, 1985–90 and 1990–95

	1980–85	1985–90	1990–95
Austria	−1.2 (0.8)	4.7 (4.0)	6.2 (5.8)
Belgium	2.9 (2.5)	3.8 (5.6)	3.9 (3.9)
Czech Republic	NA	NA	8.4 (7.6)
Denmark	1.6 (1.1)	0.6 (−0.1)	2.4 (2.4)
Finland	6 (5.9)	6.1 (6.7)	−1.8 (−3.1)
France	4.2 (3.7)	4.1 (4.1)	3.8 (3.6)
Germany	1.9 (1.6)	2.2 (1.8)	7.7 (8.2)
Greece	NA	NA	3.2 (1.8)
Iceland	5.4 (5.1)	5.3 (5.2)	1.5 (1.0)
Ireland	1.3 (−0.2)	2.7 (1.6)	6.7 (7.0)
Italy	2 (1.2)	6.8 (7.1)	1.6 (−1.3)
Luxembourg	NA	8.7 (9.6)	6.2 (6.0)
Netherlands	0 (0.5)	4.8 (3.6)	3.6 (4.7)
Norway	2.7 (2.8)	1.5 (0.9)	3.4 (3.4)
Poland	NA	NA	4.5 (0.6)
Portugal	2.7 (−0.6)	7 (11.0)	6.5 (6.5)
Spain	2.2 (2.5)	8.9 (8.3)	2.7 (2.6)
Sweden	1.3 (0.8)	2.5 (2.4)	−1.2 (−2.3)
Switzerland	4 (3.6)	4.2 (4.9)	3.1 (4.2)
United Kingdom	NA	NA	5.1 (5.3)

[a] The GDP price deflator is used because data are available and because health care price deflators are biased towards pharmaceuticals. NA = not available.

Source: OECD (2000)

product (GDP), as estimates may vary and do not account for the informal sector in the economy or the informal sector in health care in southern European, CEE and FSU countries. Alternatives such as using exchange rate conversions and purchasing power parity in comparing per-capita expenditure on health have their own difficulties. For example, exchange rates fluctuate, and the prices in the basket of goods and services used to construct purchasing power parity are biased towards pharmaceuticals (Kanavos and Mossialos 1999). Expenditure data should thus be interpreted with some caution.

Nevertheless, data show that health care expenditure has continued to grow in real terms throughout the 1980s and 1990s in most European countries (Table 1.1). This was also the case with public health expenditure, especially in Germany, Ireland, the Netherlands, Switzerland and the United Kingdom, where public expenditure on health care grew faster than total expenditure. Private expenditure in these countries is mostly out-of-pocket payments rather than private health insurance.

During the 1990s, average total health expenditure as a percentage of GDP has stabilized in the European Union (EU) countries, CEE countries and FSU countries (Figure 1.4). Detailed data for the EU countries show that health care expenditure as a percentage of GDP stabilized in the latter part of the 1990s

Figure 1.4 Total expenditure on health care as a percentage of gross domestic product (GDP) in Europe as a whole (average for the European Region of WHO) and regional averages for the European Union (EU), the countries of central and eastern Europe (CEE) and the countries of the former Soviet Union (FSU), 1985–99

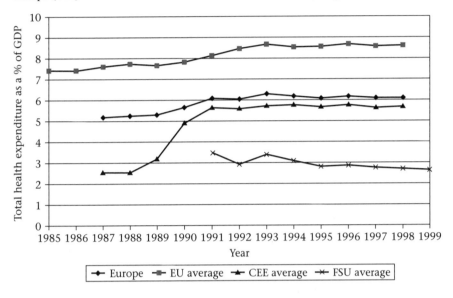

Source: WHO (2001)

and even declined in some countries (Table 1.2). However, GDP grew faster than health care expenditure between 1995 and 1998 in eight of the 15 current EU countries, and in Denmark, Greece, Portugal and Spain health care expenditure grew only slightly more than GDP. Thus, the stabilization of health care expenditure as a percentage of GDP in some EU countries may not reflect success in controlling growth in health care expenditure but rather economic growth. For example, health care expenditure in Ireland grew by 3.4 per cent from 1995 to 1998 and the economy grew by 8.8 per cent. In Finland and Sweden, health care expenditure actually declined. For Sweden, this is an artefact caused by shifting expenditure from health care budgets to social service budgets. Severe economic recession in Finland resulted in large-scale cuts in expenditure, especially public expenditure (OECD 2000). Health care expenditure in the FSU countries increased as a percentage of GDP in 1990; however, this reflects economic decline rather than real growth in expenditure on health.

Expenditure by source of revenue

Most systems in Europe rely on a mix of funding sources (Figure 1.5). Most funding is public expenditure from taxation and social health insurance, except in Azerbaijan, Georgia and Kyrgyzstan, where prepaid sources of revenue are

Table 1.2 Total health care expenditure (public health care expenditure in parentheses) as a percentage of GDP in EU countries, 1990–98

	1990	1991	1992	1993	1994	1995	1996	1997	1998
Austria	7.2	7.2	7.6	8.1	8.1	8.9	8.9	8.2	8.2
	(5.3)	(5.3)	(5.6)	(6.0)	(6.0)	(6.4)	(6.3)	(5.8)	(5.8)
Belgium	7.4	7.8	7.9	8.1	7.9	8.2	8.6	8.6	8.8
	(6.6)	(6.9)	(7.0)	(7.2)	(7.0)	(7.3)	(7.6)	(7.7)	(7.9)
Denmark	8.4	8.3	8.4	8.7	8.5	8.2	8.3	8.2	8.3
	(7.0)	(6.9)	(7.0)	(7.2)	(6.9)	(6.8)	(6.8)	(6.8)	(6.8)
Finland	7.9	9.0	9.1	8.3	7.8	7.5	7.7	7.3	6.9
	(6.4)	(7.3)	(7.3)	(6.3)	(5.9)	(5.7)	(5.8)	(5.5)	(5.3)
France	8.8	9.0	9.2	9.7	9.6	9.8	9.7	9.6	9.6
	(6.7)	(NA)	(NA)	(NA)	(NA)	(7.5)	(7.4)	(7.3)	(7.3)
Germany	8.7	9.1	9.7	9.7	9.8	10.2	10.6	10.5	10.6
	(6.7)	(7.1)	(7.6)	(7.5)	(7.6)	(8.0)	(8.3)	(8.0)	(7.9)
Greece	7.6	7.9	8.3	8.3	8.3	8.3	8.3	8.5	8.3
	(4.8)	(4.8)	(4.9)	(4.8)	(4.9)	(4.8)	(4.9)	(4.9)	(4.7)
Ireland	7.0	7.4	7.8	7.8	7.7	7.4	7.2	7.0	6.4
	(5.0)	(5.4)	(5.6)	(5.7)	(5.5)	(5.4)	(5.2)	(5.3)	(4.8)
Italy	8.1	8.4	8.5	8.6	8.4	8.0	8.1	8.4	8.4
	(6.3)	(6.6)	(6.5)	(6.3)	(5.9)	(5.4)	(5.5)	(5.7)	(5.7)
Luxembourg	6.6	6.5	6.6	6.7	6.5	6.3	6.4	6.0	5.9
	(6.1)	(6.0)	(6.1)	(6.2)	(6.0)	(5.8)	(5.9)	(5.5)	(5.4)
Netherlands	8.8	9.0	9.2	9.4	9.2	8.9	8.8	8.6	8.6
	(6.1)	(6.4)	(6.8)	(7.0)	(6.8)	(6.5)	(6.0)	(6.0)	(6.0)
Portugal	6.4	7.0	7.2	7.5	7.5	7.7	7.7	7.6	7.8
	(4.2)	(4.4)	(4.3)	(4.7)	(4.8)	(5.0)	(5.1)	(5.1)	(5.2)
Spain	6.9	7.0	7.4	7.6	7.4	7.0	7.1	7.0	7.1
	(5.4)	(5.5)	(5.8)	(6.0)	(5.9)	(5.5)	(5.5)	(5.4)	(5.4)
Sweden	8.8	8.7	8.8	8.9	8.6	8.4	8.7	8.5	8.4
	(7.9)	(7.6)	(7.7)	(7.7)	(7.3)	(7.2)	(7.4)	(7.2)	(7.0)
United Kingdom	6.0	6.4	6.9	6.9	7.0	7.0	7.0	6.7	6.7
	(5.1)	(5.4)	(5.9)	(6.0)	(5.9)	(5.9)	(5.9)	(5.6)	(5.6)

NA = not available

Source: OECD (2000)

minimal and most services are funded through out-of-pocket payments. Figure 1.5 shows the proportion of total health expenditure from social health insurance and taxation and the proportion from private sources (the distance from the diagonal) in selected western European countries; Figure 4.1 in Chapter 4 shows this for selected CEE and FSU countries. Taxation plays some role in funding health services in nearly all European countries. It is the predominant

Figure 1.5 Percentage of total health expenditure financed by taxation and by social health insurance in selected western European countries in 1998 or latest available year

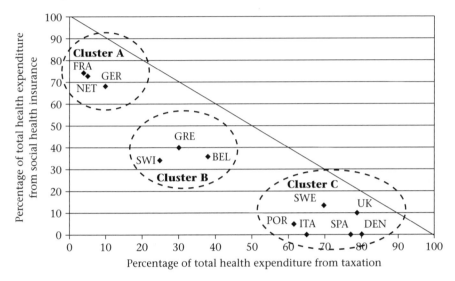

Key: BEL, Belgium; FRA, France; DEN, Denmark; GER, Germany; GRE, Greece; ITA, Italy; NET, Netherlands; POR, Portugal; SPA, Spain; SWE, Sweden; SWI, Switzerland; UK, United Kingdom.

Source: authors' estimates based on OECD (2000)

source of revenue in Albania, Denmark, Italy, Kazakhstan, Latvia, Romania, Poland, Portugal, Spain, Sweden and the United Kingdom. Social health insurance contributions are the predominant source in Croatia, the Czech Republic, Estonia, France, Germany, Hungary, the Netherlands, Slovakia and Slovenia. Belgium, Greece and Switzerland are dual systems with about equal proportions funded from taxation and social health insurance. Such aggregate data fail to distinguish between private health insurance expenditure and out-of-pocket payments. In all European countries, with the exception of France[7] and the Netherlands, out-of-pocket payments form a larger proportion of private health expenditure than private health insurance.

Factors affecting expenditure and revenue

Several explanations are offered as to why health care expenditure continues to grow, including the ageing population, the fact that health care is a labour-intensive or 'handicraft' industry, rapid innovation in technology, rising public expectations and the pressure of providers (Altman and Blendon 1979; Scitovsky 1984; Barer *et al.* 1987; Baumol 1993, 1995; McGrail *et al.* 2000). The true contribution of these factors to growth in health care expenditure continues to be debated. The increase in the ageing population may, however, lead to larger increases in expenditure on long-term care compared with acute health care. The options related to funding long-term care are discussed in Chapter 10.

Faced with rising health care expenditure, policy-makers may implement policies to contain expenditure growth. Containing costs is not, however, synonymous with increasing efficiency. They may also attempt to increase the technical efficiency of health care services to maximize the return on financial inputs. These issues are not within the scope of this book. Nevertheless, several factors may affect the ability to raise revenue and thus to maintain existing levels of funding or increase funding (where necessary).

The context in which a system of funding operates may determine its ability to function and to achieve the desired outcomes. A policy, even when based on evidence and experience, has more chance of achieving its objectives if the context in which it is to be implemented has been assessed (Walt 1998). External factors may affect the potential revenue supply or may affect the ability to realize the potential and convert the supply of revenue into actual revenue. Contextual factors that may have a direct effect on revenue collection and funding arrangements can be organized according to whether they are situational, structural, environmental or cultural (Leichter 1979).

Situational factors are transient events or impermanent factors that have a direct influence on policy-making. These factors might include major political events such as revolution in the FSU and CEE countries, reunification in Germany or the fall of dictatorships in Portugal and Spain. They might also include internal political changes, such as a new political party being elected or a new minister of health being appointed.

Structural factors are constant features such as the economic base, political institutions or demographic structure. Aspects of the economy and labour market that may affect revenue collection include the rate of economic growth, the size of the informal economy, the ratio of earned income (from labour) to capital income (from investment), labour force participation rates (of men and women), types of employment (part-time and contracted) and levels of unionization and capital mobility. Political structures and institutions can affect the functioning of the funding mechanism. Factors include: the stability of political institutions; the capacity of administrative bodies at the national, regional and local levels; levels of corruption and the will of political institutions to combat corruption within the administration; the composition of decision-making bodies; and the balance of power between central and regional authorities. Changes in the demographic structure – such as the age structure of the population, the dependency ratio (measured by the ratio of people aged 65 years or older and 14 years or younger to those 15–64 years old) and household structure (for example, the dissolution of extended family networks) – affect both the ability to raise revenue and the demand for health care and long-term care.

Environmental factors are events, structures and values that exist outside the boundaries of a political system but influence decisions within the system. Events such as war and civil strife (such as in Yugoslavia) profoundly affected – usually adversely – the ability to generate revenue. They also, in their aftermath, create opportunities to change the system of funding. European Union regulation affects how member countries fund health care, such as European

Commission directives to create a single market for non-life insurance (including private health insurance). Recent decisions of the European Court of Justice (such as the cases of Kohll and Decker), upholding the free movement of goods and the freedom to provide services, may have some implications for funding and reimbursement of drugs and ambulatory care in countries where patients' expenses are reimbursed rather than prepaid (Kanavos 2000; Kanavos and McKee 2000). Decisions of the World Trade Organization have the potential to influence revenue collection and fund-pooling arrangements globally (Price *et al.* 1999). Furthermore, developments in science, especially the ability to carry out accurate genetic tests, present new challenges for health care funding, particularly those involving actuarial insurance (Murthy *et al.* 2001). In the future, determining more accurately the genetic make-up of an individual and thus the risk of requiring health care treatment will become technically possible.

Cultural factors are the value commitments of groups within the community or the community as a whole. Examples of such factors include a belief in government and the rule of law, the status of professionals, ideological preferences, cultural belief in informal payments and gifts, and the perceptions of informal networks and decision-making processes.

The ability to collect taxes and contributions in some countries is severely restricted by the lack of trust in the state and government. Population beliefs about how much should be spent on health care, how health care should be funded and how much solidarity there should be between the rich and poor, the sick and healthy and the young and old frame policy discussions and shape public opinion on health care systems.

For example, a comparative survey of attitudes to funding health care showed that most respondents in all EU countries believe that the national government should ensure that health care is provided for all people irrespective of income. Most respondents in Greece, Ireland, Italy, Portugal, Spain, Sweden and the United Kingdom thought that the government should spend more on health (Mossialos 1998). Among the people who support increased government spending on health care, most thought it should be found by spending less on other things rather than raising taxes or health insurance contributions: 80 per cent or more in all EU countries except Sweden (66 per cent), Denmark (69 per cent) and the United Kingdom (58 per cent) (Mossialos 1998).

Together, these factors provide the context within which policymakers must establish sustainable funding systems for health care.

The advantages and disadvantages of different funding methods

As discussed above, most systems in Europe rely on a mix of funding sources. Although the choice is not usually one or another, but a combination of sources, analysing the main advantages and disadvantages of each mechanism for generating revenue remains important. This section draws heavily on Chapters 2, 3, 5, 6 and 7. The evidence for these arguments is synthesized and analysed in the concluding Chapter 12.

Taxation

Taxation is heterogeneous – that is, there are different sources (direct or indirect), different levels (national or local) and different types of taxation (general or hypothecated). All types of taxes have varying implications for equity and efficiency. Health care is predominantly funded from direct taxation in the United Kingdom. Hypothecated or earmarked income taxes for health contribute in France and Italy. At least part of the tax revenue from the sale of cigarettes has been earmarked for health care in Belgium and the United Kingdom. Regional or local taxes are the main source of revenue for health care in Bulgaria, Denmark, Finland, Norway, Sweden and, since 2000, in Italy. National taxes are the main source of revenue in Albania, Greece, Poland, Portugal, Spain and the United Kingdom. As discussed in the following subsections, tax revenue is also used to subsidize or make transfers to other funding systems.

Direct or indirect taxes

Direct taxes are taxes levied on individuals, households or firms and include, for example, personal income tax, corporate profit taxes and property taxes. Personal income taxes are usually progressive and redistribute income between rich and poor people. This requires a progressive system in which tax rates are higher for those with higher incomes.

Several institutional characteristics of direct taxation may create horizontal inequity (differential effects on people with the same income). For example:

- if income tax rates vary geographically;
- if some forms of income are exempt from income tax; and
- if some forms of expenditure are tax-deductible (such as mortgage interest payments, private health insurance premiums or out-of-pocket payments on health care).

(Van Doorslaer *et al.* 1999)

Direct taxes are administratively simple where formal records of earned income or profit income for companies are kept. Income is an easily identifiable source and tax can therefore be deducted at source, increasing compliance. If the informal economy is large, strong institutional capacity is required to reduce tax evasion.

Indirect taxes are taxes on transactions and commodities and include, for example, sales tax, value-added tax, excise taxes and import and export taxes. Hills (2000) argues that indirect taxes can be regressive because:

- people with higher incomes save more, and savings are not subject to indirect taxes;
- people with lower incomes spend proportionately more of their income on heavily taxed goods such as tobacco; and
- many indirect taxes are set as lump-sum amounts (for example, vehicle licenses).

Indirect taxation on goods and services is highly visible and therefore an easily identifiable source, especially when there is a large informal economy and widespread evasion of direct taxes. Differential rates of taxation, when applied to health-damaging goods, such as cigarettes and tobacco, may deter consumption, thus promoting health. If higher rates are applied to luxury goods and zero taxes to essential goods, they can also be progressive. Usually, however, indirect taxes are regressive, as the payments are related to consumption and not overall income.

National or local taxes

Several arguments have been put forward in favour of local taxation.

- *More transparency*: health care expenditure usually forms the bulk of local budgets and thus the link between the amount levied in local taxes and the amount to be spent on health care is more direct (it is not hypothecated but displays some of the features of hypothecation).
- *Improved accountability*: local politicians are closer to the electorate and decisions on spending money are therefore more apparent.
- *Responsiveness to local preference*: health care spending can be guided by local population needs.
- *Separation of health from competing national priorities*: health may be the main political priority at the local level, where fewer demands are competing for resources. This depends on the functions of local government and the extent of devolution.

There are also several counterarguments. The domination of health care spending in local budgets (up to 70 per cent of most county council budgets in Sweden) may generate inertia because local politicians are unwilling to risk change. Such circumstances arise because health services employ large sections of the population, creating strong pressure to maintain generous funding. Local taxes may also lead to horizontal inequity if different tax rates are applied in different regions. Moreover, the same tax rate may result in more (less) revenue for rich (poor) regions according to the wealth of different regions. Internal migration, especially of the young working population from rural to urban areas, may exacerbate regional inequity because the dependency ratio in rural areas is very high. Local taxation can be as progressive or regressive as national taxation in theory but is more limited in scope. It does not have the potential to redistribute across the whole of the income distribution within a country, only across the income distribution within a region.

National taxation allows trade-offs to be made between health and other public policies. Decisions about how much should be spent on the health sector in relation to other areas of public spending are made explicitly under tax-financed systems. At the national level, the trade-offs are with other spending or transfer programmes, tax or debt reduction. Allocations will reflect the relative negotiating power of the ministry of health vis-à-vis other ministries. The annual process of setting budgets and allocating resources to sectors or departments within government has traditionally found health (usually in the form of a ministry of health) lacking in authority in relation to the treasury or ministry of finance in most countries. Collecting taxes nationally has the advantage of economies of scale in administration. Devolving revenue collection to regions produces fewer economies of scale and thus higher costs.

General or hypothecated taxes

The main advantages of general tax funding are that:

- it draws on a broad revenue base – the range of tax mechanisms means that tax revenue can be drawn from a diversity of sources; and
- it allows trade-offs between health care and other areas of public expenditure – the spending priorities of the population (as reflected in the decisions of elected representatives) can be reflected when taxes are not earmarked or hypothecated.

Funding health care through general taxation also means that allocation to health care is subject to (annual) public spending negotiations. This politicizes the process but also gives democratic structures of accountability.

Hypothecated taxes are earmarked for health care and can be either direct or indirect taxes. A hypothecated income tax or health tax has several advantages over general taxation. For example, it may reduce resistance to taxation because it is more visible (Commission on Taxation and Citizenship 2000). Establishing genuine linkage between taxation and spending makes the funding of health care more transparent and responsive (Jones and Duncan 1995). One possible advantage of hypothecation is that it makes people feel more 'connected' to the tax system, which, in turn, may increase the pressure on providers to improve quality (Commission on Taxation and Citizenship 2000). Earmarked or hypothecated taxes may be less susceptible to political manipulation.

On the other hand, there are a number of potential disadvantages. Not all taxes that bear the name or appearance of a hypothecated tax are strictly earmarked in practice – the revenue may be merged together with other taxes (Wilkinson 1994). This weakens the connection between revenue and expenditure and consequently undermines the trust of the population. Hypothecation can also introduce rigidity into the budgetary process, in which expenditure is determined by the revenue generated and not by policy decisions. Revenue is, therefore, cyclical and is more susceptible to periods of boom and bust. Separating health care from other areas of public spending could lead to other calls to have earmarked budgets and prevent the integrated health policy now being more widely recognized as the key to improving population health (Mossialos et al. 2000). Hypothecation may be to the advantage of interest groups and professional lobbies that are able to exert a proprietary influence over the money.

Social health insurance

Social health insurance contributions are not related to risk, are levied on earned income and collected by a body at arm's length from government – otherwise it amounts to an earmarked payroll tax. Contributions are usually compulsory and shared between the employee and the employer. The collection agent can be a single national health insurance fund (such as in Croatia, Estonia, Hungary and Slovakia) or a single social insurance fund (Belgium). The collection function may be devolved to independent funds (France), local branches of a national fund (Romania), individual health insurance funds, either occupationally or geographically defined (Austria, Czech Republic, Germany, Lithuania and Switzerland), or an association of insurance funds (Luxembourg).

Social health insurance has two distinct variants in Europe: the established systems of social health insurance in western Europe following the Bismarck tradition, and the systems in the CEE countries newly established after the collapse of communism and Semashko-type systems.[8] The mature systems of western Europe have developed over a long time, and many of the organizational features and regulatory relationships are the result of a process of adaptation to changing circumstances. In CEE countries, the process of change has been more recent, radical and rapid. The predominant attraction of social health insurance for CEE countries was the independence of the insurer from government and perceived greater responsiveness to the patient or consumer. Independence was partly driven by ideological factors – the population mistrusted the state and no longer regarded it as a legitimate means of securing protection against risks such as ill health. In addition, decentralization and privatization have been strongly emphasized throughout the period of reform.

Problems with the governance, accountability and regulation of funds have meant that, in some countries in which the insurance funds were initially established as independent public bodies, the ministry of health or the ministry of finance is reasserting control. Other countries, such as Estonia and Poland, have taken a more cautious approach and have only recently made their insurance fund independent of government after their operational capacity had been developed sufficiently (Karski *et al.* 1999; Jesse and Schaefer 2000).

Social health insurance as a means of collecting revenue has several advantages in common with hypothecated taxes, discussed above. It is more transparent and, therefore, usually more acceptable to the public. In theory, social health insurance revenue is better protected from political interference, since budgetary and spending decisions are devolved to independent bodies. However, Preker *et al.* (Chapter 4) suggest that social health insurance may, in fact, be more politicized because independent agencies may be more vulnerable to capture by vested interest groups than the state would be.

Its advantage over risk-rated health insurance is that it is highly portable for insurees when moving jobs or moving in and out of the labour force (unless it is occupationally determined), coverage is continuous and contributions are independent of individual risk. Social health insurance creates a much larger risk pool than does private health insurance – the pool is at the level of the whole workforce or fund, rather than just the firm.

Social health insurance has disadvantages, however. Employers are usually required to contribute part of the cost of social insurance. This can result in higher labour costs and may reduce the international competitiveness of a country's economy. In some social health insurance systems, eligibility is based on employment or linked to contributions. This may limit the access of the non-employed population, including elderly and unemployed people and dependants, to health services. As the link between benefits and contributions remains strong, coverage also tends to be limited to curative and medical interventions and few, if any, public health interventions. Because social health insurance relies on a narrow revenue base dependent on the contributions of employed people, it may not generate sufficient revenue, especially in countries with low participation in the formal labour force. Furthermore, wage-related contributions do not account for an individual's or household's wealth or income generated through savings or investment. As the ratio of total income from capital income to earned income rises, wage-related contributions become less equitable. An increasing proportion of the workforce is self-employed or in multiple occupations, which also increases the difficulty of collecting social insurance contributions. If social insurance is not mandatory for the entire working population, it can create a perverse incentive for employers. Thus, they may offer (part-time) jobs that pay below the minimum threshold, outsource employment so that contractors are self-employed or create jobs in the shadow or unofficial sector (Schmahl 1998). These practices are common in CEE and FSU countries with newly established social health insurance schemes: employers, faced with an adverse economic climate, have tried to minimize labour costs by evading contributions to social health insurance.

Finally, certain advantages and disadvantages are associated with the specific organizational arrangements of the insurers; for example, a single fund versus multiple funds. There may or may not be competition between multiple funds. A single fund may produce low administration costs, ease regulation and make the risk pool universal. However, subscribers have no choice, and some conservative commentators fear inefficiency and a lack of consumer responsiveness. The population coverage of non-competing funds is usually defined by occupation or region. Occupational funds can tailor services to meet the needs of the workforce and may allow for services at work. Nevertheless, contribution rates may be higher than average, especially for hazardous occupations. If occupational insurance provides more benefits than would be available from another insurer, this may restrict labour market mobility. More importantly, perhaps, occupational funds serve overlapping geographical areas, duplicating administrative costs and limiting the total size of the risk pool. Conversely, regional funds are geographically distinct and cover the entire population of a territory, allowing for larger pools and spreading administrative functions over a larger base. Regional funds can also tailor services to meet the health needs of the local population. However, they also display some of the problems of local taxation in terms of regional inequity in wealth and income, employment and health risks. Unless mechanisms are established to redistribute between regional funds, this inequality in funding may result in unequal access to services.

Health reform proposals in the late 1980s and 1990s in Germany and the Netherlands sought to introduce competition between insurers in social health insurance systems. In theory, a system of competing public insurers offers enhanced choice and can reduce contribution rates and improve quality. However, there may be problems of cream-skimming or adverse selection, which could concentrate risks in certain funds and highly differentiate the contribution rates. Competition has not been motivated by an explicit desire to increase subscriber choice. The motivations behind attempts to introduce insurer competition in Germany and the Netherlands were specifically financial, including increasing the efficiency of insurers, reducing variation in contribution rates and reducing the level of contribution rates or at least reducing any increases. As statutory insurers are obliged to accept all applicants for insurance, competition between funds requires a mechanism for adjusting for risk to stop some insurers from bearing a disproportionate part of the risk or adopting covert forms of cream-skimming. Initial assessments do not show clearly the extent to which competition is working in practice. Few people exercise their right to change funds, but the number has been increasing since it has been authorized by legislation (Müller *et al.* 2000).

Finally, tax revenue is important in several social health insurance systems. Tax funds may be transferred to insurance funds to cover the contributions of the non-employed population, preventing the fragmentation of coverage. The non-employed population has the same entitlements as the working population and can access the same providers, thus solidarity is maintained across the population. It also prevents the duplication of administrative and purchasing functions.

Taxes may also cover the deficits of insurance funds. This can prevent public insurers from becoming insolvent and may also prevent year-on-year increases in contribution rates and thereby avoid increases in labour costs. On the other hand, if insurers do not carry the risk of deficit, they will have no incentive to contain costs or to operate efficiently.

Private health insurance

The early development of mutual and voluntary benefit associations in Europe and their subsequent emergence as consolidated national health insurance funds has left a residual role for private health insurance. Private health insurance can be classified as substitutive, supplementary or complementary (see Chapter 6 for a fuller discussion). Private health insurance can then be distinguished further according to how premiums are calculated (risk, group or community rated), how benefits are determined and the status of the insurance providers (for-profit or not-for-profit).

Substitutive insurance is an alternative to statutory insurance and is available to sections of the population who may be excluded from public cover or who are free to opt out of the public system. In Germany and the Netherlands, individuals with high incomes may purchase substitutive health insurance. As income is related to the risk of ill health, separation of public and private insurance according to income concentrates those with high risk in the public system. Those with lower incomes pay higher premiums to compensate for the higher risk and the lower average income of the subscribers. This undermines the redistributive effect of the funding arrangements and makes the combination of funding mechanisms regressive.

Where health insurance is supplementary, it may allow quicker access to services or increase the quality of 'hotel' facilities in the public sector. This can result in differential access between those with and those without private insurance.

Complementary health insurance offers full or partial cover for services that are excluded or not fully covered by the statutory health care system. Those policies which cover user charges nullify their effect on the utilization of services (van de Ven 1983). Moreover, complementary insurance is least affordable to those on the lowest incomes, so they often have to pay the charges. This leads to a disproportionate funding burden on poor people (Kutzin 1998). Other complementary policies enable access to services not available under the public insurance systems (a top-up policy). This can result in a two-tiered system of benefits.

Risk-rated premia are based on the actuarial calculations of the probability of an individual subscriber making a claim. This is the most common way of calculating premia in the individual private health insurance market. Where policies are purchased through an employer, premia are usually group-rated, that is, based on a calculation of the average risk of the employees in that firm. Finally, some insurance premia are community-rated, that is, based on the average risk of the population in a geographically defined area.

The agents collecting private health insurance premiums can be independent, private bodies such as private for-profit insurance companies (in most countries that have a private health insurance market) or private not-for-profit insurance companies and funds (in Belgium, Denmark, Finland, France, Germany, Ireland,[9] Italy, Luxembourg, Netherlands, Spain, Switzerland and the United Kingdom). Private health insurance may be subsidized in part by the state using tax credits or tax relief (in Austria, Ireland and Portugal). Germany and the Netherlands have limited tax relief that does not offer an incentive to purchase policies because relief is capped for all social security. Belgium, Denmark, Finland, France, Spain, Sweden and the United Kingdom do not offer tax relief on private health insurance.

Private long-term care insurance has been recommended as a means of protecting against the risk of dependence in old age. However, research suggests that this insurance is likely to be inefficient. The funnel of doubt (the area of uncertainty between the lowest and the highest values obtained in projections) about future formal and informal care needs is extremely large. Calculating actuarial premiums using existing data is difficult, as predicted and actual costs vary extensively (Burchardt et al. 1996). Insurers can be more discriminating as the age at which a person buys a policy increases. However, the ability to pool risks falls as the age of entry increases. This presents a problem for private health insurance, which operates most efficiently when the aggregate risks are well known but individual risks are not.

Transaction costs tend to be higher under private health insurance due to considerable administrative costs related to billing, contracting, utilization review and marketing.[10] Risk rating involves extensive administration to assess risk, set premiums, design complex benefit packages and review and pay or refuse claims. Systems of health care funded through private insurance do not generally control costs despite the introduction of aggressive managed-care techniques. Consumer information problems are also associated with defining benefits and setting premiums.

Taxation may be an important way of subsidizing private health insurance. Tax revenue can be used to target subsidies at poor or uninsured people to enable them to purchase health insurance. These could be in the form of vouchers or means-tested cash benefits or direct purchase by the state on behalf of the claimant. This aims to achieve wide coverage among low-income people and to rectify the problems of adverse selection in the market.

The main forms of tax-expenditure subsidy for the purchase of private health insurance are tax relief (premiums deducted from gross income before tax is charged) and tax credits (deducted from the tax liability of an individual or household). Tax-expenditure subsidies are often not recorded in national accounts and are therefore a covert form of public expenditure (see Chapter 2). They may have political advantages, especially in an environment in which increased public expenditure is not widely acceptable. However, tax-expenditure subsidies are both inequitable and an inefficient use of public money. First, they subsidize people with high incomes among whom private health insurance subscribers are concentrated. Second, the value of the tax relief is higher for taxpayers with higher marginal tax rates, making it regressive. Third, tax-expenditure subsidies are administratively complex and therefore generate higher transaction costs. Fourth, they affect the demand for private health insurance by distorting the price signals, resulting in excessive purchase of insurance. Finally, tax-expenditure subsidies may create additional opportunities for fraud and tax evasion. By promoting private health insurance, tax-expenditure subsidies shift the overall mix of funding sources in a more regressive direction.

Medical savings accounts

Although medical savings accounts have been extensively debated in the international literature (Hsiao 1995; Massaro and Wong 1995; Ham 1996; Saltman 1998; Scheffler and Yu 1998), they have only been implemented in practice in Singapore and to a limited extent in the United States (more recently in China). In this system, individuals contribute a proportion of their income regularly to their account. The money is then used for health care at the point of use. In Singapore, medical savings accounts are complemented by mandatory catastrophic insurance, for which a premium is paid. A public fund pays for the people with low incomes. In the United States, medical savings accounts must be combined with a high-deductible health plan that insures against catastrophic costs (General Accounting Office 1997). Hence, medical savings accounts must always be considered as part of a mix of funding mechanisms. In the absence of these complementary systems, medical savings accounts offer no catastrophic risk protection, because there is no pooling. As Maynard and Dixon (Chapter 5) stress, the particular savings culture and high GDP per capita in Singapore make it a special case. Such a scheme is unlikely to be feasible in other settings.

In the United States, the stated motivation for introducing medical savings accounts was to overcome the problems of moral hazard and adverse selection in the private health insurance market. By making patients fully aware of the cost of the health service, it was thought that they would become more price sensitive and therefore reduce demand for frivolous services and curb cost inflation. However, a lack of adequate consumer information has left patients unable to assess clinical quality, and providers therefore compete based on quality measures such as high-technology equipment. In addition, medical savings accounts were expected to offer people who are self-employed or working for a small employer, who otherwise find it difficult to afford individual private health insurance, an alternative way to pay for health care. However, the take-up has been lower than expected (Jefferson 1999).

Out-of-pocket payments

Out-of-pocket payments include all costs paid directly by the consumer, including direct payments, formal cost sharing and informal payments. Direct payments are for services not covered by any form of insurance (the purely private purchase of uncovered services). Other payments are for services included in the benefit package but not fully covered (e.g. formal cost-sharing) or for services that should be fully funded from pooled revenue but additional payment is demanded (e.g. informal payments in CEE and FSU countries in Chapter 8). Information on the extent of formal cost-sharing in selected European countries is provided in Tables 7.1 and 7.2 in Chapter 7 and on informal payments in CEE and FSU countries in Chapter 8.

Direct payments

Consumers pay the full cost of health care services not covered by the public system of insurance or to which access is limited (due to a lack of supply or long waiting times). These payments are usually made in the private sector: dentists, pharmacists for over-the-counter or de-listed drugs, physicians for private appointments or hospitals for private treatment, and laboratories or clinics for tests. Private expenditure on health care is tax-deductible in some countries, thus providing an incentive for patients to seek private care. In practice, such subsidies can be significant. For example, in Portugal, the government subsidy for private health expenditure is an estimated 4.8 per cent of direct tax revenue or 0.2–0.3 per cent of GDP (OECD 1998; Dixon and Mossialos 2000). Means testing for long-term care financing often means higher direct payments than for health care services.

Formal cost-sharing

Proponents of user charges claim that such charges reduce overall demand for services and raise revenue to expand health service provision. In fact, whether these two objectives are achieved depends on different assumptions about the elasticity of demand. Logically, if the first objective (reducing demand) is achieved, then the second (raising revenue) cannot be (Towse 1999). Thus, if increasing user charges reduces the utilization of health services, it will not increase aggregate revenue. The argument for raising revenue is based on the assumption that demand for health care is inelastic; that is, at the level of prices being charged to users, utilization will not fall enough to offset the increased revenue from higher user charges (Kutzin 1998).

A second assumption also needs to be satisfied if user charges are to work – that is, the cost of collection must be less than the revenue raised. Introducing user charges may involve additional administrative effort and costs (van de Ven 1983; Rice and Morrison 1994; Evans and Barer 1995), especially if complex exemption systems are in place or charges are nominal to preserve equity. The costs of implementing exemption schemes to protect the access (and incomes) of poorer people should not be underestimated. Experience from developing countries suggests that considerable administrative, informational, economic and political constraints need to be overcome (Abel-Smith 1994; Kutzin 1998).

It is argued that user charges may be introduced to raise supplementary revenue for the health system (Nolan and Economic and Social Research Institute 1988; Abel-Smith 1994; Chalkley and Robinson 1997; Kutzin 1998; Willman 1998). This is pertinent in certain circumstances; for example, when there is no functioning universal health care system, when government resources are inadequate to fund the health care system (see Chapters 4 and 9 for examples from low- and middle-income countries), or when citizens are not prepared to fund health services through increased taxes or contributions (see Chapter 7 for examples from western Europe).

Advocates of user charges maintain that the extra revenue raised could be targeted at poor people or to tackle inequality in the health care system. They could also be used to bridge the funding gap when public budgets are under pressure, ensuring that more expensive and important forms of treatment are more readily available (Willman 1998).

However, user charges often have undesirable effects on equity. They shift the funding burden away from population-based, risk-sharing arrangements – such as funding based on tax or social insurance – and towards payments by individuals and households (Creese 1991). The higher the proportion of user payments in the total mix of funding for health, the greater the relative share of the funding burden falling on poor people and people in poor health (Rice and Morrison 1994). In this way, user charges reduce solidarity in the health sector between healthy and unhealthy people (van de Ven 1983), because affluent (and healthier) people no longer subsidize poor (and sicker) people. Countries with limited tax capacity (general or payroll) have high private payments. Formalizing fees in this context does not necessarily erode solidarity because it never really existed. In many cases (especially the CEE and FSU countries), user fees may be a necessary evil and also a part of the process of setting priorities for public (or more precisely, pooled) spending.

Informal payments

Out-of-pocket payments are made in the public sector in some countries despite not being officially endorsed. These may range from ex-post gifts to 'thank' staff for care (for patients with chronic ailments, these may also have the nature of ex-ante payments) to large envelope payments given to the physician before treatment to secure their services. As these payments are covert, much of the 'evidence' in western Europe is anecdotal. However, experts acknowledge that such payments are widespread in Greece (Calltorp *et al.* 1994) and, to a lesser extent, in France (Bellanger and Mossé 2000). In general, more research and attention has focused on informal payments in CEE and FSU countries, where they have come to represent a large proportion of total health expenditure as other sources of revenue have collapsed (Ensor and Duran-Moreno 2002). These payments exist for several reasons:

- *Lack of financial resources in the public system.* Without payment, patients cannot obtain basic supplies such as the drugs or bandages required for treatment. Staff rely on payments to supplement their small or non-existent public salaries.
- *Lack of private services.* The private sector is not fully developed, so patients with money have fewer options to obtain services elsewhere. In western Europe, physicians may legally work across the public–private divide, shifting patients to their private practice. Treating patients for a 'private' payment in the public sector may arise where private practice does not exist.
- *Desire to exercise consumer leverage over providers.* No third party is involved in the transaction, which makes the provider accountable to the patient. This seems to be an important factor in the level of informal payments in southern Europe and may explain the lack of demand for private health insurance there (see Chapter 6).
- *Cultural tradition.* Southern European, CEE and FSU countries have a long tradition of informal payments that has persisted despite attempts in some countries to curb it.

Information on the extent and size of informal payments is limited because they are covert and, in some countries, illegal. Furthermore, a lack of transparency means that tapping this revenue is difficult for publicly funded systems. Converting informal payments into formalized cost-sharing arrangements requires compliance from the providers, who may lose substantial income (especially if income has to be declared for tax purposes) and public support. Securing these is not an easy task. Lewis (Chapter 8) sets out several different arrangements that could replace informal cost-sharing. Experience from other low-income countries (see Chapter 9) suggests that whether such initiatives can be implemented in practice depends on the ability of government to regulate providers and their willingness to set priorities or limit the services on offer. The ability to achieve improved efficiency and quality without jeopardizing equity critically depends on several policy measures. These encompass the skills and capacity of staff, the development of appropriate incentives and exemption systems and suitable information systems to support the accounting and auditing of such payments (Mills *et al.* 2001). Informal payments do, however, represent an important source of revenue in countries in which prepayment systems have collapsed (see Chapter 4), and phasing them out without developing suitable alternatives would probably be damaging.

Loans, grants and donations

Donations and grants from non-governmental organizations, transfers from donor agencies and loans from international banks account for a significant proportion of total revenue, especially in low- and middle-income countries. Most low-income countries rely heavily on external assistance to fund health care. In Africa, for example, donor assistance counts on average for almost 20 per cent of health care expenditure and, in several countries, more than 50 per cent (Schieber 1997). Unfortunately, no equivalent information is available for the central Asian republics, since some local grants bypass central government and go directly to regions (in Kazakhstan) or to non-governmental organizations (in Tajikistan). Similarly, there is no systematic listing of external donors.

The main concern is whether grants increase net expenditure in the health sector or substitute for government revenue. If revenue is not channelled through government, problems arise, such as inappropriate or uncoordinated aid programmes that can undermine the capacity of the national system.

There are problems with such a heavy reliance on external assistance, as it is susceptible to the changing priorities of the donors and cannot be relied on to ensure long-term financial sustainability. Foreign charitable donations are similar to foreign grants but usually have fewer or different conditions attached. Domestic charitable donations have an opportunity cost and, if there is tax relief, may have an economic cost (Schieber 1997).

Regardless of whether the loans are granted by foreign or domestic sources or taken by government or a private entity, the funds eventually have to be repaid and therefore impose a burden on future generations. The problems of debt in low-income countries are well publicized, and many countries are rightly seeking alternatives to relying on borrowed funds.

How is the book structured?

This introductory chapter has set out the rationale for the book. We have discussed some of the analytical approaches to funding health care, analysed expenditure trends and briefly touched on the factors affecting both expenditure and revenue to put into context the debate on how to fund health care on a sustainable basis. Finally, we have presented some of the advantages and disadvantages of the main methods of funding health care. These methods and how they are applied in different countries are analysed further in the following chapters.

Chapters 2 to 11 tackle specific topics relating to the main themes of the book. Some focus specifically on the method of revenue collection; others examine in depth the experience of funding health care in a specific region or sector. There are also chapters on the funding of long-term care and resource allocation.

In Chapter 2, Evans analyses taxation and its alternatives. Regardless of the dominant method of revenue collection, taxation plays a significant role in funding health care in many European countries.

Two chapters on social health insurance then follow. In Chapter 3, Normand and Busse explore how social health insurance has evolved and evaluate the variants existing in western Europe. They analyse why and how social health insurance differs from other models of health funding. In Chapter 4, Preker, Jakab and Schneider analyse the recent implementation of social health insurance in the CEE and FSU countries. The rapidity with which social health insurance has been introduced in this economic and social environment makes this an important area for closer evaluation.

Although private health insurance is not a dominant means of funding health care in Europe, the expansion of private health insurance continues to find some political and ideological resonance. In Chapter 5, Maynard and Dixon focus on the experience with private health insurance in Australia, Chile, Switzerland and the United States, where it has at one time or another been promoted (not always successfully) as a major source of revenue. In Chapter 6, Mossialos and Thomson consider the role of voluntary health insurance within the European Union, where it is only a supplementary source of revenue.

Two chapters focus on out-of-pocket payments. In Chapter 7, Robinson focuses on formal user charges, especially in western Europe, considering their contribution to revenue, impact on access and political reactions to them. Then, in Chapter 8, Lewis focuses on informal payments in selected CEE and FSU countries. She presents data on their size and scope and offers explanations as to why they have developed and persisted.

Chapter 9 (Mills and Bennett) is the last to deal directly with health care funding and focuses on the experience of low- and middle-income countries outside Europe. Mills and Bennett examine the relevance of experience from outside Europe with social health insurance, community-based health insurance and user charges to low- and middle-income countries within Europe.

Most chapters focus on health care, but what constitutes health care changes over time and varies between countries. Health and social care often overlap. In Chapter 10, Wittenberg, Sandhu and Knapp examine emerging concerns about how to fund long-term care for elderly people and how the funding arrangements often differ from those adopted in the health care sector.

Going beyond the funding of health – the collection of revenue and the pooling of funds – Rice and Smith (Chapter 11) focus on resource allocation. They analyse whether the method of funding and the method of resource allocation adopted are connected and describe the process by which resources are allocated in different European countries.

Finally, in Chapter 12, we synthesize and analyse the available evidence on the effects of different funding methods on several public policy objectives.

Notes

1 Funding health (that is, improvements in population health), as opposed to health care, may require allocating resources in other areas such as education, housing and the environment. Discussion on the allocation of funding to other spending priorities is not within the scope of this book.

2 A third-party insurance model with multiple insurers creates several problems resulting from information asymmetry between the insurers and the population, including adverse selection, moral hazard and risk selection. Information asymmetry refers to the unequal distribution of information between the insurer and the population. For example, the people seeking protection may have information regarding their risk status that is not available to, or concealed from, the insurer. Moral hazard occurs when the act of insurance increases the likelihood of the occurrence of the event being insured against. Consumer moral hazard may result in the subscriber using excessive services and provider moral hazard in the provider prescribing excessive treatment. Adverse selection occurs because an insurer cannot calculate accurately an actuarial premium and, therefore, charges an average premium. This is attractive to people with above-average risk and unattractive to people with below-average risk. Those with below-average risk may choose to forego insurance, leaving insurers to cover high-risk individuals and causing premiums to escalate continually. Risk selection, also called 'cream-skimming' or 'cherry-picking', refers to the process by which insurers charging a non-risk-related premium seek to encourage business from individuals with below-average risk or discourage or refuse insurance to individuals with above-average risk (OECD 1992).

3 The distribution of benefits in kind is often referred to by economists as the 'second best approach', the best being redistribution through the tax and benefit system.

4 In most European countries the decision to purchase private health insurance is voluntary. However in Switzerland and in Spain for civil servants who choose to opt out of the public scheme, it is compulsory to purchase private health insurance. This is also the case in some countries outside Europe. For the purposes of the general discussion in this chapter and Chapter 12 we employ the term 'private health insurance'. In Chapter 6, where the focus is on the European Union, the term 'voluntary health insurance' is used as this is the predominant form.

5 Health care providers may levy charges according to ability to pay, thus operating a system of informal pooling.

6 Deficit financing is not a realistic option for the EU countries that have joined the Economic and Monetary Union.

7 In France, the apparently low value of out-of-pocket payments reflects the fact that 85 per cent of the population has supplementary insurance to cover co-payments.

8 Nikolaj Semashko was Minister for Health of the Russian Republic from 1918 to 1930. He was a friend of Lenin and a physician. His name has been associated with the centrally planned and state-funded system of health care introduced in Soviet Russia, which was subsequently implemented in the Soviet Union and in most CEE countries.

9 The Voluntary Health Insurance Board is currently a quasi-public body with government retaining control through a majority share. However, the government share is planned to be sold, and the Voluntary Health Insurance Board will become an independent not-for-profit body.

10 It has been argued that 'hidden' transaction costs for the patient, such as long waiting times, may in fact be higher in publicly funded systems (Danzon and American Enterprise Institute for Public Policy Research 1994).

References

Abel-Smith, B. (1994) *An Introduction to Health: Policy, Planning, and Financing*. London: Longman.

Altman, S. and Blendon, R. (eds) (1979) *Medical Technology: The Culprit Behind Health Care Costs?* Washington, DC: Government Printing Office.

Appleby, J. (1992) *Financing Health Care in the 1990s*. Buckingham: Open University Press.

Barer, M., Evans, R., Hertzman, C. and Lomas, J. (1987) Aging and health care utilization: new evidence on old fallacies, *Social Science and Medicine*, 24(10): 851–62.

Barer, M., Getzen, T.E. and Stoddart, G.L. (1998) *Health, Health Care and Health Economics: Perspectives on Distribution*. Chichester: Wiley.

Baumol, W. (1993) Health care, education and the cost of disease: a looming crisis for public choice, *Public Choice*, 77: 17–28.

Baumol, W.J. (1995) *Health Care as a Handicraft Industry*. London: Office of Health Economics.

Bellanger, M. and Mossé, P. (2000) Contracting within a centralised health care system: the ongoing French experience. Paper presented to the First Meeting of the European Health Care Systems Discussion Group (EHCSDG), London, 14–15 September.

Burchardt, T., Hills, J. and Joseph Rowntree Foundation (1996) *Private Welfare Insurance and Social Security: Pushing the Boundaries*. York: York Publishing Services for the Joseph Rowntree Foundation.

Calltorp, J., Abel-Smith, B. and Ministry of Health and Social Welfare (1994) *Report on the Greek Health Services*. Athens: Pharmétrica.

Chalkley, M. and Robinson, R. (1997) *Theory and Evidence on Cost Sharing in Health Care: An Economic Perspective*. London: Office of Health Economics.

Commission on Taxation and Citizenship (2000) *Paying for Progress: A New Politics of Tax for Public Spending*. London: Fabian Society.

Creese, A. (1991) User charges for health care: a review of recent experience, *Health Policy and Planning*, 6(4): 309–19.

Danzon, P.M. and American Enterprise Institute for Public Policy Research (1994) *Global Budgets versus Competitive Cost-control Strategies*. Washington, DC: AEI Press.

Dixon, A. and Mossialos, E. (2000) Has the Portuguese NHS achieved its objectives of equity and efficiency?, *International Social Security Review*, 53(4): 49–78.

Ensor, T. and Duran-Moreno, A. (2002) Corruption as a challenge to effective regulation in the health sector, in R. Saltman, R. Busse and E. Mossialos (eds) *Regulating Entrepreneurial Behaviour in European Health Care Systems*. Buckingham: Open University Press.

Evans, R.G. (1998) Going for gold: the redistributive agenda behind market-based health care reform, in D. Chinitz, J. Cohen and C. Doron (eds) *Governments and Health Systems: Implications of Differing Involvements*. Chichester: Wiley.

Evans, R.G. and Barer, M.L. (1995) User fees for health care: why a bad ideas keeps coming back (or, what's health got to do with it?), *Canadian Journal of Aging*, 14(2): 360–90.

General Accounting Office (1997) *Medical Savings Accounts: Findings from Insurer Survey*. Washington, DC: US General Accounting Office.

Glennerster, H. (1997) *Paying for Welfare: Towards 2000*, 3rd edn. Englewood Cliffs, NJ: Prentice-Hall.

Ham, C. (1996) Learning from the Tigers: stakeholder health care, *Lancet*, 347: 951–3.

Hills, J. (2000) *Taxation for the Enabling State*, CASE Discussion Paper No. 41. London: Centre for Analysis of Social Exclusion, London School of Economics and Political Science.

Hsiao, W.C. (1995) Medical savings accounts: lessons from Singapore, *Health Affairs*, 7(4): 260–6.

Jefferson, R.T. (1999) Medical savings accounts: windfalls for the healthy, wealthy and wise, *Catholic University Law Review*, 48(3): 685–723.

Jesse, M. and Schaefer, O. (2000) *Health Care Systems in Transition: Estonia*. Copenhagen: European Observatory on Health Care Systems.

Jones, A. and Duncan, A. (1995) *Hypothecated Taxation: An Evaluation of Recent Proposals*. London: Office of Health Economics.

Kanavos, P. (2000) The single market for pharmaceuticals in the European Union in light of European Court of Justice rulings, *Pharmacoeconomics*, 18(6): 523–32.

Kanavos, P. and McKee, M. (2000) Cross-border issues in the provision of health services: are we moving towards a European health care policy?, *Journal of Health Services Research and Policy*, 5(4): 231–6.

Kanavos, P. and Mossialos, E. (1999) International comparisons of health care expenditures: what we know and what we do not know, *Journal of Health Services Research and Policy*, 4(2): 122–6.

Karski, J., Koronkiewicz, A. and Healy, J. (1999) *Health Care Systems in Transition: Poland*. Copenhagen: European Observatory on Health Care Systems.

Kutzin, J. (1998) The appropriate role for patient cost sharing, in R.B. Saltman, J. Figueras and C. Sakellarides (eds) *Critical Challenges for Health Care Reform in Europe*. Buckingham: Open University Press.

Kutzin, J. (2001) A descriptive framework for country-level analysis of health care financing arrangements, *Health Policy*, 56(3): 171–204.

Leichter, H.M. (1979) *A Comparative Approach to Policy Analysis: Health Care Policy in Four Nations*. Cambridge: Cambridge University Press.

Massaro, T.A. and Wong, Y-N. (1995) Positive experience with medical savings accounts in Singapore, *Health Affairs*, 14(2): 267–72, 277–9.

McGrail, K., Green, B., Barer, M.L. *et al.* (2000) Age, costs of acute and long-term care and proximity to death: evidence for 1987–88 and 1994–95 in British Columbia, *Age and Ageing*, 29(3): 249–53.

Mills, A., Bennett, S. and Russell, S. (2001) *The Challenge of Health Sector Reform: What Must Governments Do?* Hampshire: Palgrave.

Mossialos, E. (1998) *Citizens and Health Systems: Main Results from a Eurobarometer Survey*. Brussels: European Commission, Directorate-General for Employment, Industrial Relations and Social Affairs.

Mossialos, E. and Le Grand, J. (1999) *Health Care and Cost Containment in the European Union*. Aldershot: Ashgate.

Mossialos, E., Dixon, A. and McKee, M. (2000) Paying for the NHS, *British Medical Journal*, 320: 197–8.

Müller, R., Braun, B. and Gress, S. (2000) *Allokative und distributive Effekte von Wettbewerbselementen und Probleme ihrer Implementation in einem sozialen Gesundheitswesen am Beispiel der Erfahrungen in den Niederlanden* [*Allocative and Distributional Effect of Competition and Problems with its Implementation in a Social Health Care System: the Example of the Netherlands*]. Bremen: University of Bremen.

Murray, C.J. and Frenk, J. (2000) A framework for assessing the performance of health systems, *Bulletin of the World Health Organization*, 78(6): 717–31.

Murthy, A., Dixon, A. and Mossialos, E. (2001) Genetic testing and insurance: implications of the UK Genetics and Insurance Commission (GAIC) decision, *Journal of the Royal Society of Medicine*, 94(2): 57–60.

Nolan, B. and Economic and Social Research Institute (1988) *Financing the Health Care System*. Dublin: Economic and Social Research Institute.

OECD (1992) *The Reform of Health Care: A Comparative Analysis of Seven OECD Countries*. Paris: Organisation for Economic Co-operation and Development.

OECD (1998) *OECD Economics Surveys 1997–1998, Portugal*. Paris: Organisation for Economic Co-operation and Development.

OECD (2000) *OECD Health Data 2000: A Comparative Analysis of 29 Countries*. Paris: Organisation for Economic Co-operation and Development.

Oliver, A.J. (1999) *Risk Adjusting Health Care Resource Allocation: Theory and Practice in the United Kingdom, the Netherlands and Germany*. London: Office of Health Economics.

Price, D., Pollock, A.M. and Shaoul, J. (1999) How the World Trade Organization is shaping domestic policies in health care, *Lancet*, 354(9193): 1889–92.

Reinhardt, U.E. (1990) Economic relationships in health care, in *OECD Health Care Systems in Transition: The Search for Efficiency*. Paris: Organisation for Economic Co-operation and Development.

Rice, T. and Morrison, K.R. (1994) Patient cost sharing for medical services: a review of the literature and implications for health care reform, *Medical Care Review*, 51(3): 235–87.

Saltman, R.B. (1998) Medical savings accounts: a notably uninteresting policy idea, *European Journal of Public Health*, 8: 276–8.

Scheffler, R. and Yu, W. (1998) Medical savings accounts: a worthy experiment, *European Journal of Public Health*, 8: 274–8.

Schieber, G.J. (ed.) (1997) *Innovations in Health Care Financing: Proceedings of a World Bank Conference*, 10–11 March 1997. Washington, DC: World Bank.

Schmahl, W. (1998) Financing social security in Germany: proposals for changing its structure and some possible effects, in S.W. Black (ed.) *Globalization, Technological Change and Labor Markets*. Dordrecht: Kluwer Academic.

Scitovsky, A.A. (1984) 'The high cost of dying': what do the data show?, *Milbank Memorial Fund Quarterly*, 62(4): 591–608.

Towse, A. (1999) Could charging patients fill the cash gap in Europe's health care systems?, *Eurohealth*, 5(3): 27–9.

van de Ven, W.P.M.M. (1983) Effects of cost-sharing in health care, *Effective Health Care*, 1(1): 47–56.

van de Ven, W.P.M.M., van Vliet, R.C., van Barneveld, E.M. and Lamers, L.M. (1994) Risk-adjusted capitation: recent experiences in the Netherlands, *Health Affairs*, 13(5): 120–36.

van Doorslaer, E., Wagstaff, A., van der Burg, H. *et al.* (1999) The redistributive effect of health care finance in twelve OECD countries, *Journal of Health Economics*, 18(3): 291–314.

Wagstaff, A., Rutten, F. and van Doorslaer, E. (eds) (1993) *Equity in the Finance and Delivery of Health Care: An International Perspective*. Oxford: Oxford University Press.

Wagstaff, A., van Doorslaer, E., van der Burg, H. *et al.* (1999) Equity in the finance of health care: some further international comparisons, *Journal of Health Economics*, 18: 263–90.

Walt, G. (1998) Implementing health care reform: a framework for discussion, in R.B. Saltman, J. Figueras and C. Sakellarides (eds) *Critical Challenges for Health Care Reform in Europe*. Buckingham: Open University Press.

WHO (2001) *WHO European Health for All Database*. Copenhagen: WHO Regional Office for Europe.

Wilkinson, M. (1994) Paying for public spending: is there a role for earmarked taxes?, *Fiscal Studies*, 15(4): 119–35.

Willman, J. (1998) *A Better State of Health: A Prescription for the NHS*. London: Profile.

chapter two

Financing health care: taxation and the alternatives

Robert G. Evans[1]

Introduction

Modern health care systems cannot be financed from the out-of-pocket expenditure of patients. The mismatch between individual resources and health care needs dictates that the costs of individual care should largely be met from the pooled contributions of groups. In principle, these groups or third parties could take several forms, from extended families and voluntary associations, through commercial and social insurance programmes, up to the state at the national or regional level. In practice, however, the advantages of scale and the fundamental limitations of private insurance markets have led to the predominance of public institutions. In almost all industrialized countries, most health care is paid for either by governments, with funds raised from various forms of taxation, or by social insurance institutions, largely or wholly outside the commercial marketplace, which impose compulsory levies on all or most of the population.

All financing systems, whatever their structure, can be represented by a basic identity adapted from the fundamental income–expenditure identity of national income accounting. The total amount raised to pay for health care for a particular population, through whatever channels, must equal exactly the total amount spent on health care for that population, and that in turn must equal the total amount of income earned, in various forms, by those paid (directly or indirectly) for providing care. This identity of revenue, expenditure and income is not a theory but a logical necessity and is fundamental to understanding both the effects of, and the controversies over, all financing and funding systems. This can be expressed as follows:

$$TF + SI + UC + PI = P \times Q = W \times Z$$

where TF is the amount of revenue raised through tax financing, SI through social insurance, UC through private, out-of-pocket payments or user charges and PI through private insurance premiums. P and Q are vectors, listing the average prices (P) paid for and total quantities provided or used (Q) of each of the various forms of health care. W and Z are also vectors, standing for the amounts of different types of resources (Z) used in providing care and the rates of payment (W) of those resources. One element of Z, for example, could be nursing hours worked, and the corresponding element of W would be the average rate of reimbursement per hour worked. P and Q correspond to units of output such as physician visits, surgical procedures or drugs.

Tax-financed systems are those in which most health expenditure is derived from tax payments (TF > SI + UC + PI), or at least the tax-financed component is substantially larger than any other component. The various questions that one might raise about the behaviour and relative performance of different financing systems can be posed, at a very general level, in terms of the components of this identity relation. Do predominantly tax-financed systems differ more or less consistently from those drawing more heavily on other sources of financing on some or all of the most significant dimensions of system performance as reflected in the internal structure of the identity?

The question is complicated, however, by the fact that tax financing is not a standard process. In principle, the government pays for health care from a general revenue fund into which all taxes flow. Most countries have several levels of government, and the powers and responsibilities of each level vary considerably by country. The characteristics of tax financing vary according to the amount of involvement of different levels of government.

Another question is how best to assess the performance of different financing systems. There are many ways to categorize the dimensions of health systems performance, including the distribution of burden and benefits across the population, the allocation of resources to the health sector and among its various sub-sectors, and technical efficiency and responsiveness. Assessing the strengths and weaknesses of different financing systems under each dimension would be a monumental exercise, especially because much of the necessary data currently exist in fragmentary form, if at all. Moreover, system performance on several of these dimensions depends more on how providers are funded than on how payers raise revenue from the population. Providers are organized and paid in very different ways in Canada, Finland, Sweden and the United Kingdom, for example, although they all have tax-financed systems. This chapter, therefore, focuses primarily on the first dimension of performance, the distribution of burdens and benefits, for which considerable comparative information exists.

The distribution of the burdens and benefits of a health care system can be represented along three axes:

- Who pays – and what share?
- Who gets – what and when?
- Who gets paid – and how much?

I explore these in the first three sections. This is followed by a section on the potential of tax-financed systems versus other financing systems to control expenditure. Next, I explore the role of covert taxes. Finally, I discuss several policy implications.

Who pays – and what share?

The most clear-cut difference among alternative financing systems is how they apportion the total cost of health care among the national population. Tax financing includes this burden within the general tax system; in most high-income countries, tax liability is roughly proportional to income or mildly progressive (Wagstaff *et al.* 1999). People with higher income thus contribute, through tax financing, a share of their incomes that is the same as, or larger than, that contributed by lower-income people. Out-of-pocket payments, by contrast, whether co-payments or payments for private uninsured services (user charges, UC), are proportional to the use of care and not related to income. Accordingly, user charges for health care consist, on average, of a much larger share of the incomes of lower-income people.[2]

These generalizations are well illustrated in two North American studies, one in Manitoba, Canada (Mustard *et al.* 1998a,b) and one in the United States (Rasell *et al.* 1993, 1994). The Manitoba study is especially interesting, as it links individual-level administrative records from the universal public programmes covering hospital and physicians' services with census records of family incomes and estimated tax liability for much of the provincial population. The distribution of expenditure and of corresponding tax liability by income decile (scaled up to the whole provincial population of about 1 million) is displayed in Figures 2.1 to 2.4, with the small but expensive institutionalized population as a separate category.

Figure 2.1 shows the amount (in Canadian dollars) spent by the public plans on the care of people in each income decile in 1994; Figure 2.2 shows the estimated amount of tax contributed according to income decile; Figure 2.3 shows the difference, by income decile, between the total cost of care used and total taxes paid; and Figure 2.4 shows this gain or loss as a share of total family income. (Permanently institutionalized people have no significant income.)

The scale of the transfers is quite striking, especially from the top income bracket, making very clear that people in that group would benefit from lowering the tax-financed share and introducing some form of private payment. Since people with very low incomes are unlikely to be able to bear a substantial portion of the costs of their own care, any shift in financing from tax financing to private payment would transfer funds primarily from the middle to the upper deciles of the income distribution.

The Manitoba study focused only on the public, tax-financed programmes. In the United States, using survey data for non-institutionalized people only, Rasell *et al.* (1993, 1994) analysed the distribution by income decile of payments for a more comprehensive definition of health care through tax financing, user charges and private insurance. Their results are displayed in Figures 2.5 and 2.6; Figure 2.5 shows the pattern for the whole population and Figure 2.6 distinguishes households with heads 65 years or older and those

Figure 2.1 Expenditure (in millions of Canadian dollars) on publicly financed health care according to pretax income decile (10 is the highest income) in Manitoba, Canada, 1994

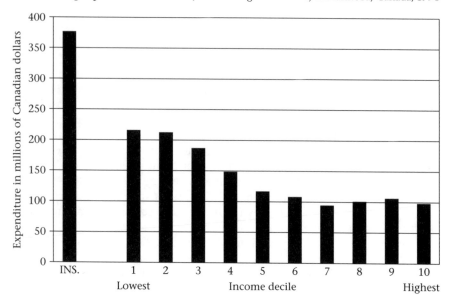

INS. = institutionalized population

Sources: adapted from Mustard *et al.* (1998a,b)

Figure 2.2 Tax contribution (in millions of Canadian dollars) to publicly financed health care according to pretax income decile (10 is the highest income) in Manitoba, Canada, 1994

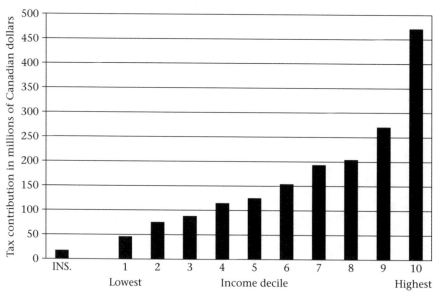

INS. = institutionalized population

Sources: adapted from Mustard *et al.* (1998a,b)

Figure 2.3 Net transfer (in millions of Canadian dollars) to (positive numbers) or from (negative numbers) each pretax income decile (10 is the highest income) from the public financing of health care in Manitoba, Canada, 1994

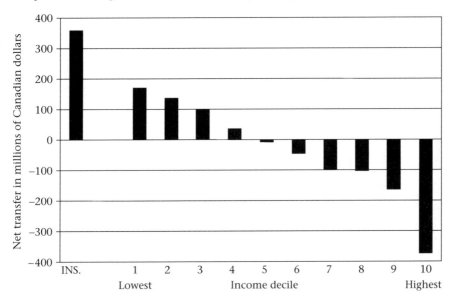

INS. = institutionalized population

Sources: adapted from Mustard *et al.* (1998a,b)

Figure 2.4 Net transfer to (positive percentages) or from (negative percentages) each pretax income decile (10 is the highest income) as a share of pretax income from the public financing of health care in Manitoba, Canada, 1994

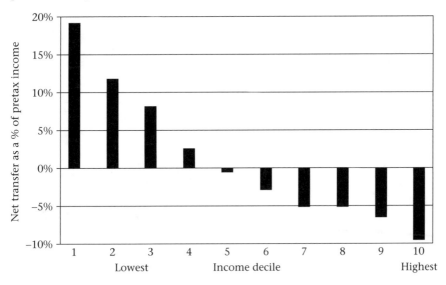

Sources: adapted from Mustard *et al.* (1998a,b)

Figure 2.5 Expenditure on health care in the United States as a percentage of pretax family income according to family income decile (10 is the highest income) and type of expenditure, 1987

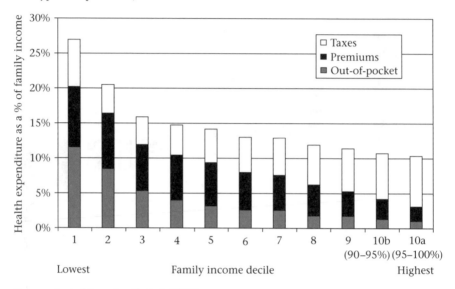

Source: adapted from Rasell *et al.* (1993)

Figure 2.6 Expenditure on health care in the United States as a percentage of pretax family income according to family income decile (10 is the highest income), type of expenditure and the age of the head of household 65 years or older (left column in each decile) versus younger than 65 years (right column in each decile), 1987

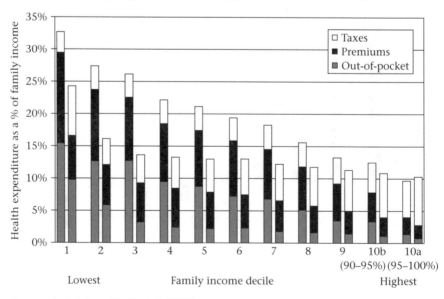

Source: adapted from Rasell *et al.* (1993)

under age 65 years. People 65 years or older are covered, for hospital and physicians' services, by Medicare, which is national, universal and tax-financed.

These findings emphasize the contrast between the progressivity of tax financing in the United States and the regressivity of both user charges and private insurance. (The similar pattern for both modes of private financing is what one would predict *a priori* in an efficient competitive insurance market.) These highly regressive components of the financing mix, widespread in the United States, overwhelm the progressivity of the tax-financed component and make the whole distribution highly regressive. Perhaps surprisingly, however, this pattern is found even among elderly people, who are covered by the universal tax-financed plan. The very substantial deductibles and co-payments built into the public programme, ostensibly to control overall costs, contribute to making the overall mix markedly regressive. Individuals can and do buy Medigap private coverage for these charges, as do people in France to cover the co-payments in the statutory health insurance scheme. But Medigap coverage, being private, is also regressive in its distribution of financing burden (premiums are based on risk status, not income), as in France.

Tax financing and user charges thus provide the clearest contrast in who pays. Tax financing places a heavier financial burden on those with higher incomes, whereas user charges place more on those with lower incomes. This fairly obvious difference motivates much of the policy controversy over alternative forms of financing, generating a permanent tension in every national health care system. In addition, tax financing detaches payment liability from the experience of ill health, or at least the use of care, whereas user charges link the two directly. Regardless of income, sick people will contribute relatively less and healthy people more under tax financing than under user charges. Financially, extending the scope of user charges is a wise strategy for the healthy and wealthy, and extending tax financing reduces the share of the burden borne by the unhealthy and unwealthy.

Where private insurance is widespread, as in the United States and Switzerland, it generates a highly regressive pattern of distribution similar to that of user-charge financing. Competition in private insurance markets forces insurers to adjust the premiums of enrollees according to their relative risk, which, in practice, means according to their past claims. Thus private insurance, like user charges, links individual contributions to illness experience rather than income; both are highly regressive compared with tax financing.

Social insurance, on the other hand, bases contributions on income, but the income base is not all-inclusive, and some systems place a ceiling on contributions. *A priori* one might expect social insurance systems to be more progressive than private financing, but less so than tax financing – an early finding of the ECuity Project (Wagstaff *et al.* 1993).

Tax financing is predominant among the northern countries, including Canada, Denmark, Finland, Sweden and the United Kingdom, and in southern Europe – Italy,[3] Spain and Portugal. Figure 2.7 presents summary estimates of the progressivity or regressivity of total health care funding in these and several other countries (excluding Canada), plotted against the percentage of health expenditure financed by taxes (Wagstaff *et al.* 1999). Unfortunately, the source data are now a decade or more old.

Figure 2.7 Estimates of the progressivity (Kakwani (1977) Progressivity Index) of total health care expenditure in 12 OECD countries in various years according to the percentage of health expenditure financed by taxation

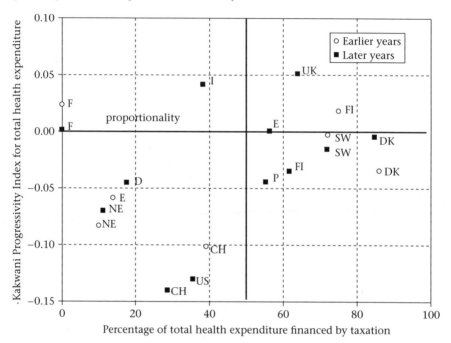

Key: DK, Denmark (1981, 1987); FI, Finland (1990, 1996); F, France (1984, 1989); D, Germany (1989); I, Italy (1991); NE, Netherlands (1987, 1992); P, Portugal (1990); E, Spain (1980, 1990); SW, Sweden (1980, 1990); CH, Switzerland (1982, 1992); UK, United Kingdom (1993); US, United States (1987).

Sources: Wagstaff *et al.* (1999) and calculations by U. Häkkinen for Finland

Although the financing mixes and structures may change, the implications of the ECuity Project about the general effects of different structures should hold. Increases in co-payments since the early 1990s (as in Sweden or Germany), the introduction of not-for-profit institutions with fiscal incentives to insure these and other private payments (as in France) and the expansion of opportunities for private practice should increase the regressivity of the financing system, improve access for people with higher incomes and increase the expenditure on, and incomes earned in, the private sector and possibly overall.

The proportion of health spending financed by taxation is strongly and positively correlated with the progressivity of total health expenditure. Any statistically fitted relationship, however, would be dominated by the two outliers, the United States and Switzerland, in which private spending is both relatively high and very regressive. If these outliers are excluded, the correlation between tax financing and progressivity becomes less clear. Social insurance systems (low tax financing) may be either progressive or regressive, depending on their structure and policies. The key feature is comprehensiveness (Wagstaff *et al.* 1999). Germany has a ceiling on social insurance contributions and, in both Germany and the Netherlands, more affluent people are permitted or required to opt out and buy private coverage. In France, however, social insurance covers the whole population, without premium ceilings or floors. The result is actually more progressive than tax-financed Denmark, Finland and Sweden, despite the user charges and the privately funded mutual benefit associations. On balance, the ECuity Project data show most tax-financed systems to be more progressive, or less regressive, than most social insurance systems, but predominantly tax-financed systems show no clear pattern of system progressivity rising with the proportion financed by taxes.[4]

The contrast between the United Kingdom and Denmark, Finland and Sweden is striking. All rely heavily on tax financing, but the United Kingdom has the most progressive funding system of all those reported, and Denmark and Sweden are mildly regressive overall. Finland is especially interesting, having had one of the most progressive funding systems in 1990. The economic and fiscal crisis of the early 1990s led to a sharp reduction in the proportion of tax financing, a rise in the private share and a corresponding abrupt move from progressive to regressive.

General taxation was progressive in all countries studied but much more so in some than in others. This variation results partly from the tax mix. Tax revenue is raised through both direct and indirect taxation, with the former being consistently progressive and the latter regressive in all countries reported. The progressivity of direct taxation also differs across countries. Direct taxes in Sweden and Denmark have a very low degree of progressivity (reflecting the importance of proportional income taxes at the local level), in marked contrast to the United Kingdom. Direct taxes in Finland were formerly more progressive but have become much less so during the 1990s. When weakly progressive direct taxes are pooled with regressive indirect taxes, there is little overall progressivity left.

In general, the extent of reliance on tax financing among the countries studied in the ECuity Project appears to be inversely related to the progressivity of the tax system. Denmark and Sweden, which rely heavily on direct taxes, have relatively little progressivity in their direct tax structure. The United Kingdom, with more progressive direct taxes, increased the share of regressive indirect taxation in its tax mix from 43.2 per cent in 1985 to 53.9 per cent in 1993. These three countries, along with Italy and Spain, had the least progressive systems of general taxation of all countries studied.[5] By contrast, the countries with the most progressive systems of general taxation – the United States, Switzerland, the Netherlands and Germany – make least use of tax financing to support health care.

This pattern strongly suggests a political compromise in the conflict of economic interest between the healthy and wealthy and the unhealthy and unwealthy, in which what is lost on the roundabouts is made up on the swings. Every financing system has this conflict, but the terms of the compromise vary across countries not only in the extent of redistribution but also in the balance of financing sources through which it is achieved. A political coalition in support of tax financing can be assembled and maintained, so long as the redistribution is not too extreme.

The ECuity Project estimates suggest that the considerable egalitarian potential of tax financing is in practice much more limited.[6] But limited is not negligible. There is a sharp contrast between the tax-financed systems and the highly regressive distribution of the overall financing burden in the systems drawing heavily on private financing. Social insurance systems can go either way, depending on how they are structured.

Who gets – and when?

The experience of tax-financed systems since the early 1990s underlines the continuing tension between the economic interests of the healthy and wealthy and those of the unhealthy and unwealthy. Even proportional or mildly regressive tax-financed systems redistribute substantial sums, because the experience of illness and therefore the use of services (in the absence of financial barriers) is so much more regressive. Pressure for more private funding, for a shift of financing mix from tax financing to user charges, with or without private insurance, is therefore permanent in any tax-financed system. The arguments have changed little over the decades and the underlying economic interests have not changed at all.

Tax-financed systems seem to be especially vulnerable to this pressure, however, in times of general fiscal crisis. It is not difficult to understand why, when general incomes are falling, citizens should resist more taxation and governments should therefore respond by controlling public spending more strictly, including health spending. Nevertheless, why these cuts should be associated with a shift in the redistributional compromise is not so obvious. The answer may be found in exploring the next two distributional questions: Who gets? Who gets paid?

In principle, tax-financed and social insurance systems both answer the first question: people who need care get it – what they need when they need it. Ability to pay is the basis for determining individual contributions to financing health care but not the right to receive it. Need for care is, however, typically defined implicitly as whatever a qualified practitioner chooses to offer and a patient chooses to accept. Ability to pay, by contrast, is concretely expressed in specific revenue-raising measures. The stability of the political coalition supporting the financing compromise, especially in tax-financed systems, depends on the credibility of this public commitment to meet needs thus defined.

Wealthy people will always derive short-term economic benefit from a system with more private financing. They have the resources to meet their own needs, and the less they have to contribute to support that of others, the more they benefit economically. The unhealthy and unwealthy can be counted on to oppose private financing, which confronts them with either very heavy financial burdens or some exclusion from care. What is critical is the attitude of the broad middle group of the population, for whom the price of social solidarity – the discrepancy between what they pay and what they get – is on average much less than for the wealthy. For many people, it will turn out to be negative – the insurance motive is also very real for them.

But the tax-financed system must (be perceived to) meet their needs. If people in the middle band of the income distribution begin to feel that the public tax-financed system is no longer providing them with access to high-quality care, they will begin to look elsewhere. In two-tier tax-financed systems such as in Australia and the United Kingdom, coverage in the public system is universal, but patients who have the necessary resources can offer private payments for care that is more timely or convenient or perceived to be of higher quality.

Physicians who work both sides of the street practising both in the public system and privately can then manipulate waiting times and patient perceptions of quality to encourage these private payments. The opportunities for enhanced incomes through private charges can progressively undermine access in the public system, as appears to have happened for ophthalmological and orthopaedic surgery in the United Kingdom (Robinson and Dixon 1999: 67). The higher returns in private practice lead surgeons to limit both the time and the effort they commit to meeting their obligations in the public system, thus increasing the pressure on patients to offer private payment.

Private payments in the form of user charges within the tax-financed system may serve to reallocate access to care when supply is (perceived to be) inadequate. Since such charges primarily deter those with lower incomes, they improve access for those most able to pay (see Chapter 7). If user charges also draw in additional funds to support increased supply – to meet needs, as commonly claimed – they do so much more regressively than would an increase in either tax financing or social insurance funding.[7]

For people with the necessary resources, any form of partial out-of-pocket payment in a predominantly tax-financed system purchases preferred access to a service primarily paid from the taxes of others. As long as adequate access is perceived to be available for all, few are likely to be willing to pay for preference. But if a significant proportion of the population come to believe that the care provided through the tax-financed system is inadequate or inaccessible and that their health is being put at risk, the political support for private funding could build quite rapidly.

Who gets paid – and how much?

As noted above, the aggregate of income earned from the health care system is exactly equal to total health care expenditure. When health spending (P*Q) is cut, so are incomes (W*Z). Jobs are lost and/or rates of reimbursement (wages, profits and other forms of income) fall. This will be true regardless of whether such cuts have a massive or a negligible impact on either servicing levels or patients' health. Thus, everyone who draws income from the health system, whether as wages and salaries, as professional fees or as shareholder profits from corporate enterprises, has no economic interest in doing more with less.

The identity of expenditure and income explains why claims of underfunding – sectoral or system-wide – are a major part of the continuing political theatre of all health care systems. The claims may be more intense, and are certainly more focused, in tax-financed systems because they serve as the primary tool for extracting more funding from public payment agencies. Funds so extracted may be used either to enhance services or to increase rates of remuneration for those who produce the services, to raise Z and Q, or W and P, although the public claims will always focus on Q, on alleged needs for more and better services.

Identifying underfunding claims as political theatre does not imply that the level of resources available to the health care system does not matter. Clearly it does – health services contribute very importantly to health, and producing the services Q requires real inputs Z, whose owners must be paid for their use. But allegations of underfunding, coming from those who are paid for their services or hope to be, are not discernibly related to the adequacy or effectiveness of a health care system and certainly not to its level of funding. They are pressed as energetically in Canada, for example, as in the United Kingdom, and always have been, even though health spending per capita is more than 50 per cent higher in Canada (US$2175 compared with US$1391, converted to US$ using all-economy purchasing power parity (OECD 1999)). If the allegations were not income-driven, one might expect concerns about how effective or appropriate the care provided is or how efficiently it is produced to be pressed with equal vigour. They are not.

The relative parsimony of the National Health Service in the United Kingdom might lead one to expect that there, if anywhere, underfunding claims could be validated. However, attempts to determine whether the National Health Service is underfunded have led only to the conclusion that there is no satisfactory answer (Dixon *et al.* 1997). Conclusions may be reached and acted on at the political level – both the United Kingdom and Canada appear now to have a consensus that the health care system is seriously underfunded (albeit at very different funding levels!). Nevertheless, this has more to do, in both cases, with the success of the political theatre staged to manipulate public opinion (Maynard 1996).

In normal economic times, when rates of economic growth generate sufficient tax revenue to support a continuing increase in funding in the tax-financed health care sector, the underfunding claims emerge from a background of broad system support. But when funding is actually being cut, and people are losing jobs as well as suffering reduced wages and profits, the tone of the underfunding claims shifts dramatically. The continual, deafening chorus of complaint that Enoch Powell (1976), a former Minister for Health in the United Kingdom, described as rising day and night from every part of the National Health Service grows in volume and shifts to focus on lengthening waiting lists and increasing numbers of horror stories. The whole tax-financed system is alleged to be in danger of collapse.

Whatever the actual state of affairs, the experience of expenditure and income cuts in a major sector such as hospitals can lead to medical terrorism. There is an unfortunate asymmetry between the political theatre of tax financing and that of private care. Those whose work is paid by tax financing must negotiate for more funding primarily by emphasizing publicly the inadequacies of the health care system, whatever they may say in private. Those funded by private payments, by contrast, attract more funding by alleging the excellence of their work – essentially advertising. Private providers must puff their products; public providers must denigrate theirs. As long as funding is flowing steadily into the public system, this denigration is more likely to take the form of emphasizing how much better the system could be if it only had more money. When funding is shrinking, however, the public claims shift from marketing hope to marketing fear, a process that may undermine the tax-financed system itself.

Nor are provider responses limited to negative publicity. Unions and professional associations in both tax-financed and social insurance systems use various forms of job action, delays and limitations on access, up to and including full-blown strikes, to inconvenience and frighten patients and thus pressure governments to increase funding. In the process, such activities may also generate public support for private funding alternatives to tax financing. Freed from the constraints of public-sector bargaining, some providers would then be able to charge higher fees and expand servicing opportunities in the private sector, thus serving those able to pay.[8]

The distributional dynamics of both incomes and access to care, in times of fiscal crisis, are well illustrated by the recent Canadian experience. True funding cuts have led to increasing public unease as to system adequacy (who gets?), strongly encouraged by intense criticism from those who have lost jobs and incomes (who gets paid?). These reinforce the arguments of the economic interests permanently arrayed against tax financing (who pays?). The result has been a precipitous reduction in public satisfaction with the health care system and an almost universal sense of crisis among the general public. Those who have actually used the system continue to report relatively high satisfaction, and hospital use and outcome data show no deterioration (Roos 2000).

This process seems quite adequate to explain a general tendency for tax-financed systems to shift more towards private payment in times of fiscal crisis. What is less clear is whether they might later move back when the fiscal situation improves.

User charges introduced within a public system can later be removed if the ideological balance shifts and fiscal circumstances permit. The establishment of private markets for care outside the tax-financed system (and especially if supported by private insurance), however, may be a one-way street. Supplier interests thus established are much more difficult to displace. Where such markets exist, their participants – both those who pay and those who get paid – comprise concentrated, self-aware, well-organized and well-resourced interest groups. Moreover, the patients in private care tend in every country to be disproportionately members of the political and business elites, who after all have money as well as political influence.

This political reality points to the parallel between the economic interests of the healthy and wealthy and those of a subset of providers. Private markets not only place a heavier share of the financing burden on those on lower incomes, they also increase total expenditure on health care and thus the incomes generated from providing it. Social insurance systems show a more intermediate position, providing greater leverage for public regulation than private markets but less direct cost control than that available through public budgets. The role of different financing mechanisms in controlling expenditure is discussed in the following section.

Financing mechanisms and expenditure control

The two OECD (Organisation for Economic Co-operation and Development) countries relying most heavily on private financing, the United States and Switzerland, had in 1998 the most expensive and third most expensive health care systems, absorbing 14.0 per cent and 10.2 per cent of their country's gross domestic product (GDP), respectively (Anderson et al. 2000).[9] The percentage for the United States has been relatively stable since 1992; that for Switzerland has risen steadily since 1960 to reach its present level. Germany's and France's social insurance systems currently occupy the second and fourth rungs of this ladder, at 10.6 per cent and 9.6 per cent, respectively (Anderson et al. 2000). There is some overlap – Canada at 9.3 per cent outspends a cluster of social insurance and tax-financing countries at about 8.5 per cent.[10]

These expenditure rankings have changed over time and will surely do so again. Some tax-financed systems – the United Kingdom in particular – have always been relatively inexpensive, whereas others such as Canada and Sweden have been at or near the top of the rankings for extended periods. Each country has its own institutional history, and a formal statistical analysis is as likely to be misleading as helpful. What the experience in the OECD suggests, however, is that tax-financed systems provide more public control over health spending, both in short-term crisis and when long-term priorities change. How that control is exercised depends on political considerations specific to time and place.

Finland provides an especially dramatic example of response to acute economic and fiscal crisis, with a massive slash in spending in one year (1992–1993). In Canada, spending in the tax-financed sectors went down markedly between 1992 and 1997 during economic crisis while continuing to climb in the private sector. In both countries, the cuts brought the ratio of health spending to GDP back close to its pre-crisis level.

Public priorities throughout the OECD shifted towards increasing cost control in health care after the mid-1970s. Various administrative mechanisms were introduced to apply countervailing public authority (Abel-Smith 1992; Abel-Smith and Mossialos 1994), sufficiently similar as to be labelled (White 1995) the international standard. These mechanisms significantly and quite rapidly reduced the growth of health spending in most OECD countries.

Tax-financed systems seem to have had more success, as indicated by the current national rankings. Several countries have actually lowered the share of GDP spent on health care since 1990 (Anderson and Poullier 1999), all with tax financing. In addition to Finland and Canada, this ratio fell in Denmark, Ireland, Italy and Norway. Sweden's ratio peaked at 9.6 per cent in 1982; 4 years later it was 8.7 per cent and has remained there. Historically, Germany provides a leading example of cost control in a social insurance system. Very rapid cost escalation was brought sharply under control through regulatory legislation in the mid-1970s. But Germany in the 1990s is another story.

Tax-financed systems are clearly not consistently less costly than others; during the 1970s, several such systems were among the most costly in the OECD. They do appear to be more responsive to public priorities – at least as filtered through the national political system – when these require cost control or reduction. (After all, any health care system can cope with increasing resources!) Tax financing combines in one authority both the incentive and the capacity to contain costs to a greater extent than is possible with any of the other financing mechanisms.

However, as discussed above, this control comes at a political price in both public dissatisfaction and intensified provider criticism. Those who get paid always advocate continually expanding system costs; when these interest groups attract broad public support, they are difficult to resist. Severe fiscal crises both motivate governments to impose the tighter controls that tax financing makes possible and enable them to mobilize the necessary public acceptance, for a time at least. Severe constraints exact a further price in erosion of public support for tax financing itself, however, and the spread of more regressive private financing both within and alongside the tax-financed system. The redistributional compromise is never permanently settled and in times of strain it is reopened.

Cross-national surveys suggest that public satisfaction may be related to absolute levels of spending for health care, but the evidence is mixed.[11] Nevertheless, whatever the amount spent, any reduction or even cessation of growth leads to political difficulty and efforts to open up other sources of financing. It would appear that adequate funding for health care is defined, at least by providers, in terms not of any finite level of spending but of the rate of change.[12]

Tax financing thus provides those who are paid for health care a share of national income that is not only smaller than in other systems, but is potentially more vulnerable to changes in political priorities. Their responses include not only continuing pressures to maintain the flow of tax financing, but also efforts to modify the financing structure itself so as to make it less sensitive to shifting priorities.

One suggestion periodically brought forward is hypothecation – dedicating revenue from a particular tax or basket of taxes solely for the purpose of funding health care. The intent is to ensure the health care system a stable and growing revenue base outside political control. Nevertheless, the advantages of hypothecation seem to be more apparent than real.

Cosmetic hypothecation – describing a particular tax as a health tax – might have political advantages in reducing taxpayer resistance, in so far as spending on health care seems to be popular in all countries. If the designated taxes (or premiums) go into general revenue, however, then the label means nothing. Segregating the revenue in a special fund to pay for health care is equally meaningless if deficits (surpluses) are made up from (absorbed into) general revenue. Real hypothecation requires that revenue from the dedicated taxes actually determine health expenditure or, more accurately, that decisions on spending and tax rates are made so as to equate the two.

The tax source would thus have to be large, stable and growing in line with national income (preferably faster). Yet this is exactly the sort of revenue source that no government would want to give up. The arguments for hypothecation within the general revenue base seem to point more strongly towards social insurance financing outside government general revenue, a form of hypothecated tax, and indeed social insurance systems do seem, on balance, to offer providers the benefit of greater expenditure (see Chapter 3). Social insurance also offers the possibility of significantly enhancing the regressivity of financing, if that is part of the objective.

Covert tax financing

Tax-expenditure subsidies

Governments have several mechanisms, both fiscal and regulatory, by which to influence patterns of economic activity. Tax financing for health care involves raising revenue through various compulsory contributions to state revenue and then using that revenue either to provide or to pay for health care. Public authorities may also use the taxing power to exert influence more indirectly by offering relief from taxes that would otherwise be owed.

Private expenditure on favoured activities may be deducted from taxable income or credited in whole or part against other tax liabilities. Students of public finance refer to these as tax-expenditure subsidies to reflect the fact that tax concessions are as real a transfer from government to private resources as are direct subsidies. They have the same impact on the overall government budget and presumably on private behaviour. These tax-expenditure subsidies are often provided for certain forms or levels of out-of-pocket medical expenses. They are also used, in some countries, to promote and sustain private insurance well beyond what would otherwise be possible in a purely commercial insurance market.

Governments may also extend the reach of social insurance systems by paying premiums to enrol those who have no contributory earnings, or covering shortfalls of aggregate premium revenue from general taxation (see Chapter 3). These payments are direct subsidies, recorded in the public accounts, and can (or should) be included as part of the tax-financed component. Tax-expenditure subsidies, by contrast, do not show up in public expenditure or as tax financing for health care but rather reallocate tax liabilities from people who have made expenditure in the favoured categories to people who have not.

One might refer to this form of tax financing as indirect, except that the terms 'direct' and 'indirect' already have well-established meanings with respect to taxation. The label 'covert' reflects the fact that, unlike direct financial subsidies, tax concessions do not show up in the public accounts and are rarely open to public scrutiny and debate. Indeed, their exact value may be difficult to determine and estimates are contestable. The amounts reported for the countries of the OECD, for example, are both incomplete and unreliable. Although specialists understand covert tax financing well, it is largely invisible to the general public and governments are not held accountable for the amounts thus transferred or their destinations. Presumably in consequence, covert tax financing is typically regressive, often extremely so, whereas overt tax financing tends to be proportional or progressive.[13]

Tax-expenditure subsidies for private health insurance can be offered by simply providing that premium payments to approved insurers are in whole or part either deductible from taxable income or eligible as a credit against tax liability. An even less transparent form links the tax-expenditure subsidies to the purchase of private insurance by employers on behalf of employee groups. The employer deducts these premiums from taxable income, as part of employee compensation. Unlike wages, the employer-paid premiums are not taxed as income in the hands of the employee. It is quite feasible to treat employer-paid premiums as a taxable benefit. Failure to do so is a deliberate public policy intended to encourage the purchase of private insurance.

Although the employer may write the cheque to the insurer, most economists take the view that employees actually pay the premiums in the form of reductions in wages or other forms of compensation. Nevertheless, they pay these premiums from their before-tax income. For employees, the tax-expenditure subsidy is equivalent to purchasing health insurance coverage from after-tax income, like any other commodity, but then receiving a rebate from government of some proportion of the amount paid. Unlike the tax-expenditure subsidies, however, the cost of the rebate and the distribution of the benefits would be highly visible.

The covert tax financing of private payments has two redistributive effects, both regressive. To the extent that it promotes user charges or private insurance as a substitute for either overt tax financing or social insurance, it shifts the overall mix of financing sources in a more regressive direction. But the subsidy itself is also typically highly regressive, in so far as the effective rebate received by the covered individual is equal to the cost of the coverage provided multiplied by that individual's marginal income tax rate. Both tend to rise with income.[14]

The tax-expenditure subsidies for employer-paid private insurance are most significant in North America, especially in the United States. But Europe also furnishes good examples of regressive tax-expenditure subsidies. Portugal permits deduction of health expenditure from taxable personal income, co-payments and payments to private physicians being fully deductible and health insurance premiums up to a ceiling of €350. Since Portugal has a very high proportion of out-of-pocket payment (nearly 40 per cent in 1990), this tax-expenditure subsidy represents a substantial amount of money, estimated at 4.8 per cent of direct tax revenue or between 0.2 per cent and 0.3 per cent of GDP (Dixon and Mossialos 2000). Since the direct tax system is also quite progressive, these deductions are much more valuable to people with higher incomes. In Ireland, Wagstaff *et al.* (1999) find that accounting for the tax-expenditure subsidies reverses the apparent progressivity of expenditure for private insurance. Although affluent people buy more private insurance, the availability of tax concessions in a relatively progressive income tax system lowers its net cost at the upper end of the income distribution sufficiently to make the overall cost distribution regressive.

The tax-expenditure subsidies for private payments both illustrates and provides a vehicle for advancing the joint agenda of the healthy and wealthy and of people who draw their incomes from health care. It uses the fiscal power of the state to offset the severe limitations that private competitive markets place on the scope of private insurance in health care, thereby both enhancing the regressivity of the overall financing system and undermining public efforts to contain its cost (and the incomes it generates). Accordingly, one should expect to find advocacy of some form of tax-expenditure subsidies associated with proposals for expansion of private funding. Overt tax financing is an alternative to private financing; but covert tax financing is complementary, making high user charges more politically acceptable and protecting private insurance against the processes of competitive cream-skimming and experience rating that would otherwise severely limit its market.[15]

Regulation and compulsion

Governments may, however, preserve significant scope for private insurance by using various forms of regulation that restrict the competitive strategies of private insurers, for example by requiring them to offer community-rated coverage – a similar premium for all who apply – rather than risk-rating individuals or groups, charging different premiums on the basis of past experience or other correlates of risk. Since community rating is fundamentally inconsistent with maximizing profits, however, further regulation and various forms of subsidy or inter-insurer transfers are required to sustain it.[16]

Governments may go further, requiring all or some of their citizens to purchase private insurance, with characteristics and on conditions dictated by the state. Compulsion may be either directly by law or indirectly by excluding certain groups from tax-financed or social insurance coverage. Both are forms of covert tax financing, using state authority to encourage or compel the transfer of funds from individuals to insurers without passing through the public budget. Governments can thus report both lower overt taxation and public spending.

Mandatory private insurance has recently been introduced in Switzerland (1996) and in the province of Quebec in Canada (1997, for pharmaceuticals only).[17] In both jurisdictions, residents are now required by law to purchase a basic insurance package of defined benefits from private insurers. In both jurisdictions, the effect has been to achieve universal coverage while preserving (Switzerland) or extending (Quebec) both the market for private insurance and the extreme regressivity of the financing system – together with a steady and thus far uncontrollable escalation of total expenditure (Morgan 1998; Minder et al. 2000).[18]

Mandatory private insurance has thus advanced, in both jurisdictions, the agenda of the dual alliance above. It yields higher expenditure – incomes for providers – and a much more regressive financing structure than tax financing, while avoiding the political embarrassment of low-income uninsured people. Cost escalation may be its Achilles heel. Regardless of how it is financed, if health expenditure continues to rise relative to national income, it will inevitably return as a political problem.

In promoting private coverage, however, the covert forms of tax financing remove governments from any direct relationship with providers of care. Although governments commit public authority and, through tax-expenditure subsidies, public resources, they have neither explicit responsibility for costs nor obvious mechanisms of control or even negotiation. Any bargaining leverage over the provision of health care and its costs through the monopsony and regulatory powers associated with overt tax financing vanishes from the covert forms. It may be hard to get back.

Although neither tax-expenditure subsidies nor mandatory private insurance are major features in Europe, being aware of the implications of these forms of covert tax financing for the scale and distribution of health care costs is important. Covert tax financing may become increasingly attractive to European governments, not only for reasons of ideology or fiscal exigency but because international agreements, such as the European Union Treaties, commit them to cutting spending and shrinking the apparent size of government. Covert tax financing permits governments to appear parsimonious with public funds while subsidizing or compelling the uncontrolled expenditure of other people's money. At the same time, governments can advance a redistributive agenda that might not be acceptable to the general public if the process were explicit. Given the strength of the interests involved, one should expect to see continuing, and perhaps growing, advocacy for such policies to reinforce the trend towards more private funding in both tax-financed and social insurance systems.

Conclusions

This chapter has identified characteristic patterns of performance in tax-financed systems, contrasting them with systems relying more heavily on other revenue sources. Most health care systems draw to some extent on all four sources. Policy debates focus on the effects of shifting the balance at the margin – more or less tax financing or user charges or private insurance within a particular type of system. Comparisons across systems serve primarily to inform debates about these within-system shifts, although they may also be relevant to countries whose health systems are undergoing significant transformation.

Ideally, one would look for systematic differences in performance on a comprehensive range of important dimensions. But no individual country, let alone a large and representative group, generates sufficient information to support such a detailed characterization. This chapter has focused on financial comparisons, not because they are all that matter but because it is for them we have the most information.

Unfortunately but inevitably, the inherent conflicts of interest over financing intrude into the discussion of every other dimension of system performance in every health care system. Financial concerns distort and contaminate the analysis of all other issues or crowd them out entirely. Again, Enoch Powell (1976) discovered that the only subject a minister for health is ever destined to discuss with the medical profession is money.

One might hypothesize, for example, that the broader range of responsibilities of governments would lead tax-financed systems to show more interest in the non-medical determinants of health, rather than focusing exclusively on the one pathway of the health care system. Indeed, the exploration of social determinants has been more advanced in the countries with tax financing, most notably the United Kingdom – the Black Report (Department of Health and Social Security 1980) and the Acheson Report (Committee of Inquiry 1988) and a long and very powerful research tradition – but also Canada, Finland and Sweden. But one would be hard put to show a corresponding impact on resource allocation, let alone health outcomes. A cynic might say that, in tax-financed systems, the social determinants of health get attention and the health care system gets money.

Similarly, in a tax-financed system, one might hope that governments, acting as representatives of the general population, might be much more active in promoting the identification and dissemination of cost-effectiveness in health care. Again, the United Kingdom has long been the home of leading work on randomized clinical trials and on cost-effectiveness analysis more generally. Nevertheless, international comparative data on the outcomes of care are very thin. The greater interest in cost-effectiveness in the United Kingdom may be motivated more by the need for a relatively tight budget than by any predisposition in tax financing *per se*.

Any attempt to redirect funding, whether from less to more effective forms of health care or from health care to other determinants of health, must threaten some provider incomes. The same is true of efforts to improve the efficiency of provision by doing more with less rather than more with more. Accordingly, any broad public concern that might predispose tax-financed systems to address these issues tends to be offset by the political costs of provoking conflicts with concentrated provider interests. Public-spirited philosopher-kings are scarce, perhaps because they have such short tenure.

Providers in tax-financed systems are often said to be less responsive and accountable to their patients, paying insufficient attention to their concerns, let alone their convenience. Yet similar complaints arise in all systems, with their focus related more to how providers are funded than to how the system is financed. Tax-financed or social insurance systems in which provider budgets and remuneration of personnel are insensitive to patient choices and concerns generate little incentive for responsiveness. The redesign of funding systems to extend the range and influence of patient preferences is of world-wide concern.

The financing mix can, however, affect provider responsiveness at both the practice and the system level. A mixed public–private system may permit providers in a tax-financed system to collect additional payments directly from patients either formally as extra billing or informally, under the table and untaxed. In addition, providers may be able to operate private practices on the side for their better-off patients. In either case, those unwilling or unable to pay more receive less time and attention. At the system level, responsiveness to patients can deteriorate quite sharply in tax-financed or social insurance systems if dissatisfied providers adopt various pressure tactics to extract more money. In the universal struggle over income shares, patients are hostage to both sides.

We therefore return to the dimensions of performance for which comparative conclusions do seem to be justified. It is quite unambiguous that (overt) tax-financed systems are relatively progressive and privately financed systems are highly regressive. Any shift in the mix of funding sources towards more tax financing (private payment) increases the share of the financing burden borne by those on higher (lower) incomes. Nevertheless, this redistributive effect turns out to be greatly tempered in practice; countries making most use of tax financing tend to have relatively less progressive tax systems.[19] Countries with the most progressive tax systems, by contrast, seem most reluctant to use them to finance health care.

More generally, within each country the mix of financing sources reflects a compromise among conflicting economic interests that is always in debate and shifts according to their varying strengths. The time path of this compromise is complex, because interests that are in opposition along one of the three axes of conflict detailed above may be congruent along another. The outcome depends on their shifting coalitions.

The terms of this compromise over financing are especially sensitive to another compromise – that over access to high-quality care. In principle, a tax-financed system provides all citizens with the same access to equivalent care, regardless of how much they contribute. This may be broadly acceptable, and the tax-financed system retains solid support so long as most of the population believe that they are receiving all necessary care, of high quality and in a timely manner.[20]

Those at the top of the income distribution can always get preferred treatment at lower cost by opting out of a collective, income-based financing system, as in Germany and the Netherlands. Tax financing does not permit this explicitly, but an indirect form of opting out may be achieved, as in the United Kingdom, through a relatively spartan universal tax-financed system combined with an upper tier in which better-off patients can jump the queue or receive enhanced quality care. For them, the extra payments are more than compensated by lower taxes, at least relative to what it might cost to provide care of private standard to everyone through tax financing.[21] Countries with tax financing such as Canada or Sweden that have maintained a universal standard high enough to discourage private care have found this expensive.

If a significant proportion of the population come to believe that they are not getting adequate care, then the coalition supporting tax financing may begin to weaken. A sudden shock to the fiscal capacity of the state, as in Canada or Finland, followed by sharp cuts in health care funding, encourages the belief that governments are no longer capable of paying for high-quality care for all. (The people at the top of the income distribution have an interest in encouraging this belief, as in Canada.) *Sauve qui peut* – those who can afford to had better look after themselves or at least supplement what the tax-financed system can pay. If not all needs can be met, more of those in the middle of the income distribution may begin to see their interests as lying with those at the top, not those at the bottom. Support may grow for private payment and lower taxes – the agenda of the wealthy.

The compromise between providers and payers becomes a critical element in generating public perceptions. As noted above, providers' operational definition of adequate financing seems to be more. Health care is always underfunded, no matter at what level, and only continuing relatively rapid growth in expenditure is satisfactory. Failure to grow is a funding crisis and actual cuts are a catastrophe – imminent system collapse. This, at least, is the message from the political theatre. In a tax-financed system, the complaints of providers are translated directly into political pressure on governments, as provider representatives have become increasingly sophisticated at finding the pressure points of vulnerable governments.

Growing concern, therefore, is being expressed in many countries about the sustainability of tax financing for health care. The common argument that countries cannot afford to meet growing needs for health care through tax financing and must therefore draw in other sources of financing makes no economic sense. A country's ability to sustain a given level of expenditure is not increased by moving money through one financing source rather than another. A given level of care actually costs more, not less, if financed through private insurance, because the administrative costs are greater. The real argument runs deeper.

Tax-financed systems, faced with providers' ambitions for an ever greater share of national income, find themselves on the horns of a dilemma – concede growing expenditure or confront growing provider dissatisfaction. Both responses threaten the coalitions that support the relatively progressive pattern of transfers found in tax-financed systems. Increasing total expenditure requires an increasing amount of income transferred from the healthy and wealthy to cover the increasing costs of care for the unhealthy and unwealthy. Since health expenditure comprises a large share of public budgets in tax-financed systems, these increasing transfers may generate increasing taxpayer resistance, especially from strategically placed elites. Public surveys routinely find that increases in health care spending draw wide public support – adding to the difficulties of cost control – but that support does not necessarily translate into electoral support for increased taxation and public spending (Glennerster 1997).

In contrast, effective cost containment leads, through the identity of income and expenditure, to increasing provider efforts to convince the general public that the health care system is deteriorating and placing their health at risk. Discontented providers also have a variety of ways to impede access to tax-financed care, reinforcing their message of underfunding. To the extent that these are successful, the result is not only greater political pressure on governments to relax the cost controls, but increased efforts by individuals to find more timely access or perceived better quality care through private purchase.[22] The tax-financed system can suffer slow erosion even while it enjoys, in principle, broad popular support and willingness to contribute further, if an increasing proportion of the population become unwilling to accept a universal standard of care that they believe to be inadequate.

There seem to be two possible ways to resolve this dilemma. If general economic growth is sufficiently rapid, the health care system can continue to expand without requiring an increasing share of income to be transferred across income classes. Tax-financed systems have functioned very successfully under these conditions in the past but are then hostage to both the performance of the general economy and the relative forbearance of providers. The threat from economic downturns has already been demonstrated; over the longer run, the increasing role of for-profit organizations in health care (especially pharmaceuticals) could significantly increase the pressure from providers.

Alternatively, shifting the public debates away from the political theatre of income claims to focus more on actual measures of system performance may be possible. Governments in tax-financed systems have played a relatively limited role in system management, delegating most operational control to providers of care. They have made minimal efforts to collect and disseminate reliable information on system performance at a level of detail that could substantiate or refute claims of unmet needs or system failure.[23] (When they are substantiated, an appropriate response must be, and be seen to be, forthcoming.) Broadly based public support, combined with prosperity sufficient to maintain the compromises with providers, has permitted this relatively disengaged approach. But it has left tax-financed systems hostage to the good will, or at least grudging acceptance, of providers, and poorly placed to deal with the strong economic interests pushing for both system expansion and creeping privatization.

Students of health care systems seem to broadly agree that all industrialized countries have substantial scope for increasing efficiency and effectiveness without sacrificing the quality of care. Claims that external trends – ageing populations, changing technologies and public tastes – will force wealthy industrialized societies to choose between spending an ever-increasing share of their incomes on health care, letting the standard of care for the whole population fall steadily behind the technically possible, or accepting multi-tiered care, regressively financed and graded by ability to pay, are simply false.[24] The evidence, however, has made little headway against the entrenched interests of providers. The gap between research evidence and public perceptions appears to be widening (Roos 2000), and the economic motivations drawing it apart are not at all obscure. The long-run sustainability of tax-financed systems, despite or perhaps because of their successes, may well depend on finding ways to bridge this gap.

Notes

1 This is an edited version of a longer paper: Evans, R.G. (2000) Financing health care: taxation and the alternatives. HPRU 2000: 15D Working Paper. Centre for Health Services and Policy Research, University of British Columbia, Vancouver.

2 Financing systems have several different distributional effects, although that between income classes (vertical equity) turns out to be the most significant (van Doorslaer et al. 1999). The burden distribution within classes (horizontal equity) also varies; user-charge financing distributes that burden according to illness, or at least use of care, and (competitive) private insurance distributes it according to probability of use – generally estimated from past use. Social insurance systems treat equals more or less equally depending on the range of different premium and benefit structures. Individuals may also be re-ranked within the income distribution, apart from any changes in the distribution itself.

3 Italy is classified in the ECuity Project as having roughly equal parts of tax financing and social insurance financing. Elsewhere in this study, however, the Italian social insurance share is classified as tax financing because it is raised through a payroll tax (D'Ambrosio and Donatini 2000). Compulsory contributions to public agencies look very much like taxes, whether or not they are pooled with state general revenues. A similar ambiguity arises with respect to Switzerland, where basic private coverage is now compulsory, leading the OECD to classify that system as predominantly public. The ECuity Project data pre-date this change but are unlikely to be greatly affected by it.

4 The picture appears clearer in Wagstaff *et al.* (1993: 44) and Klavus and Häkkinen (1998, figure 2). But the earlier data (Wagstaff and van Doorslaer 1992) have been revised in Wagstaff *et al.* (1999), moving France onto the progressive side. Also, between 1980 and 1990, Portugal shifted about 10 per cent of its total health costs from tax financing to user charges, becoming the ECuity Project country with the highest share of user charges. Although still predominantly tax-financed, Portugal's overall system is now about as regressive as that of Germany.

5 Spain, in increasing its share financed by taxes, also increased the role of highly regressive indirect taxes, such that the progressivity of its overall tax system fell somewhat further. Italy, in contrast, has a moderately progressive tax system if the payroll tax classified as social insurance is included in taxation.

6 Canada might appear to be an exception, combining both tax financing and relatively progressive general taxation. But the universal public insurance plans cover only hospital and physicians' services. Other forms of health care – drugs, dentistry, much of non-hospital long-term care – are covered through a patchwork of provincial and private insurance plans, partial in their coverage of both the population and their costs. The proportion of total health care costs paid out-of-pocket, 16 per cent in 1997, was almost the same as in the United State at 17 per cent. The proportion of private funding in Canada, now over 30 per cent, is one of the highest in the OECD before it was expanded in the 1990s. This observation is again consistent with a political trade-off – quite progressive tax financing, but covering a smaller share of total health expenditure.

7 In countries with no capacity to mobilize tax revenues, informal payments occur regardless of policy. In such circumstances, there might be a rationale for explicit private payments (see Chapters 8 and 9); where tax financing is impossible, some forms of user charges might be preferable to others.

8 Private markets also withhold services from those unwilling or unable to pay what providers demand, as in the United States health care system. The withholding is limited to a small, although growing, proportion of the population who do not have insurance or personal resources – or significant political influence. Currently, about 45 million people are estimated to be uninsured in the United States. This may increase to 60 million – more than 20 per cent of the population – by 2008 (Iglehart 2000). In tax-financing or social insurance systems, provider job actions affect all or most of the population and thus have greater political effect.

9 This refers to a subset of the current OECD membership before its expansion in the 1990s; some of the more recent entrants have lower expenditure and higher private shares.

10 Canada's continuing relatively high ranking is related to the fact that it has a relatively high proportion of private spending, even though public coverage for acute care hospitals and physicians' services is nearly 100 per cent. If private-sector expenditures in Canada had risen only at the same rate as those in the public sector between 1992 and 1999 (15.1 per cent), rather than the actual 44.8 per cent (Canadian Institute for Health Information 1999), Canada would now also be spending about 8.6 per cent of its GDP on health care.

11 The ten-country survey reported by Blendon *et al.* (1990) showed an almost linear relationship between reported satisfaction and spending per capita, with the exception of the United States where spending was highest and satisfaction was lowest. But subsequent results for five countries (Donelan *et al.* 1999) show a very clear relationship between plummeting satisfaction and funding cuts, with relatively high satisfaction in the United Kingdom where funding was by far the lowest but seemed poised to increase.

12 Even in the United States, where health spending reached 14 per cent of national income in 1992, the subsequent stabilization at that level has been associated with

widespread dissatisfaction. Because the limitations on access have been imposed only on a portion of the population – those in managed care programmes and the increasing numbers with no insurance at all – the political impact has been limited. Private systems fragment and diffuse public unhappiness, providing it with no focus or point of leverage.

13 Highly regressive but invisible subsidies to private insurance can be very resistant to change. Thirty years of criticism of the tax-expenditure subsidies in the United States from economists of every political stripe has had no impact. Proposed Canadian legislation, in the late 1970s, to remove the tax-expenditure subsidies for private insurance was withdrawn in the face of pressure from private insurers and providers (in particular dentists). In contrast, tax-expenditure subsidies for private payments were eliminated in Finland in 1992, and limited tax-expenditure subsidies for private insurance were eliminated in the United Kingdom in 1997. The key factors may be the scale and concentration of the affected private interests.

14 In the United States, with a relatively progressive income tax system and private insurance coverage, which, although extensive, varies considerably by income level (Kronick and Gilmer 1999), the total value of the tax-expenditure subsidy rebate is very large – an estimated US$124.8 billion in 1998, 10 per cent of total health expenditures and about one-third of outlays by private insurers. It is also very steeply regressive, being worth an estimated US$2357 per year to families with incomes over US$100,000, but only US$71 to families with incomes under US$15,000 (Sheils and Hogan 1999). It is difficult to believe that an overt tax financing programme of this magnitude and benefit pattern could survive public scrutiny.

15 Even with the tax-expenditure subsidies, rates of private coverage in the United States have been showing a downward trend; the ever-rising costs may be pricing people out of this market (Kronick and Gilmer 1999). Public subsidies – overt tax financing – for private insurance purchase are now being suggested to shore up the private insurance system, but it is estimated that they would have to be extremely expensive to have even a modest effect (Gruber and Levitt 2000). Emmerson *et al.* (2000) make a related point, that attempting to promote the spread of private insurance through tax-expenditure subsidies so as to reduce the demand on the NHS in the United Kingdom would be extremely unlikely to save more than its revenue cost.

16 The Australian Government, for example, has wanted to preserve voluntary private insurance alongside the public system for ideological and budgetary reasons. But it also wants to promote competitive markets, which force insurers to adjust their premium structures to attract only the better risks. The government responded to shrinking coverage by requiring private insurers to offer community-rated coverage, setting off a classic vicious circle of disenrolment by the better risks, insurer losses, premium increases and further selective disenrolment. Government then introduced public subsidies for private coverage – to preserve the private market! The only other alternative is to make private insurance *de facto* compulsory for some or all of the population.

17 Pharmaceuticals outside hospitals are not covered by the federal–provincial health programme in Canada; provinces may provide whatever coverage, if any, they choose.

18 The details matter, of course. Switzerland requires all residents to purchase a basic package of hospital and medical benefits from private insurers that must set premiums on a community-rated basis, at levels yielding no profit on this portion of their business. Lower-income individuals receive a subsidy to support this private purchase. Quebec mandates private coverage only for employee groups; many but not all previously had this coverage. The public plan that previously covered people older than 65 years or on social assistance was expanded to include everyone else.

But there is a major difference. The public plan, previously entirely tax financing, now includes a structure of co-payments, differentiated by class of enrollee. There has been a substantial increase in the user-charge component of the pharmaceutical financing mix, a lesser but significant increase in private insurance outlays and a large reduction in tax financing. Total expenditure increased.

19 Not in the United Kingdom and Finland – but the progressivity of the tax system has declined significantly in both countries.

20 No real-world system can provide either access to, or quality of, care that is equivalent for all, nor are all needs ever met. Health is a state of inadequate diagnosis. Public acceptance depends rather on perceptions and on scale.

21 This presumes that the private standard really is more expensive. The easiest way to encourage patients to go private and pay extra is simply to manipulate access to the public system. A single-tier system might in fact be able to offer the same standard of care, on average, and at lower cost – but with lower incomes for some physicians.

22 The point is not that provider concerns and claims are necessarily false but rather that, in so far as they arise out of the income–expenditure identity, their truth value is irrelevant to the process of extracting more funding.

23 Shroud-waving (United Kingdom) and medical terrorism (Canada) thrive in an information vacuum.

24 In less wealthy societies, however, with a very wide dispersion of incomes, the economic constraints may well be binding. If the costs of health care for the whole population at the standards now prevailing in the industrialized countries are simply beyond the means of the country as a whole but well within the means of its upper-income groups, then there is probably no politically feasible option but multi-tiered care. The wealthy will not accept the best standard of universal care that a tax-financed system could afford. The only question is whether, with increasing prosperity, a country can move towards tax financing (or universal social insurance) or whether private financing becomes so deeply entrenched, as in the United States, that it is impervious to change. The answer may well depend on whether incomes become more or less dispersed as economic growth proceeds.

References

Abel-Smith, B. (1992) Cost containment and new priorities in the European Community, *Milbank Quarterly*, 70: 393–416.

Abel-Smith, B. and Mossialos, E. (1994) Cost containment and health care reform: a study of the European Union, *Health Policy*, 28: 89–132.

Anderson, G.F. and Poullier, J-P. (1999) Health spending, access, and outcomes: trends in industrialized countries, *Health Affairs*, 18(3): 178–92.

Anderson, G.F., Hurst, J., Sotir Hussey, P. and Jee-Hughes, M. (2000) Health spending and outcomes: trends in OECD countries, 1960–98, *Health Affairs*, 19(3): 150–7.

Blendon, R.J., Leitman, R., Morrison, I. and Donelan, K. (1990) Satisfaction with health systems in ten nations, *Health Affairs*, 9(2): 185–92.

Canadian Institute for Health Information (1999) *National Health Expenditure Trends, 1975–1999*. Ottawa: Canadian Institute for Health Information.

Committee of Inquiry (1988) *Public Health in England*. The report of the Committee of Inquiry into the Future Development of the Public Health Function (Acheson Report). London: HMSO.

D'Ambrosio, M.G. and Donatini, A. (2000) *Health Care Systems in Transition: Italy*. Copenhagen: European Observatory on Health Care Systems.

Department of Health and Social Security (1980) *Inequalities in Health: Report of a Working Group* (the Black Report). London: Department of Health and Social Security.

Dixon, A. and Mossialos, E. (2000) Has the Portuguese NHS achieved its objectives of equity and efficiency?, *International Social Security Review*, 53(4): 49–78.

Dixon, J., Harrison, A. and New, B. (1997) Is the NHS underfunded?, *British Medical Journal*, 314: 58–61.

Donelan, K., Blendon, R., Schoen, C., Davis, K. and Binns, K. (1999) The cost of health system change: public discontent in five nations, *Health Affairs*, 18(1): 206–16.

Emmerson, C., Frayne, C. and Goodman, A. (2000) *Pressures in UK Healthcare: Challenges for the NHS*. London: Institute for Fiscal Studies.

Glennerster, H. (1997) *Paying for Welfare: Toward 2000*, 3rd edn. London: Prentice-Hall.

Gruber, J. and Levitt, L. (2000) Tax subsidies for health insurance: costs and benefits, *Health Affairs*, 19(1): 72–85.

Iglehart, J.K. (2000) The painful pursuit of a competitive marketplace, *Health Affairs (Millwood)*, 19(5): 6–7.

Kakwani, N.C. (1977) Measurement of tax progressivity: an international comparison, *Economic Journal*, 87(March): 71–80.

Klavus, J. and Häkkinen, U. (1998) Micro-level analysis of distributional changes in health care and financing in Finland, in M.L. Barer, T.E. Getzen and G.L. Stoddart (eds) *Health, Health Care and Health Economics: Perspectives on Distribution*. Chichester: John Wiley.

Kronick, R. and Gilmer, T. (1999) Explaining the decline in health insurance coverage, 1979–1995, *Health Affairs*, 18(2): 30–47.

Maynard, A. (1996) *Table Manners at the Health Care Feast: The Case for Spending Less and Getting More from the NHS*, LSE Health Discussion Paper No. 4. London: London School of Economics and Political Science.

Minder, A., Schoenholzer, H. and Amiet, M. (2000) *Health Care Systems in Transition: Switzerland*. Copenhagen: European Observatory on Health Care Systems.

Morgan, S. (1998) *Quebec's Drug Insurance Plan: A Model for Canada?*, Discussion Paper HPRU 98:2D (February). Vancouver: Centre for Health Services and Policy Research, University of British Columbia.

Mustard, C.A., Shanahan, M., Derksen, S. *et al.* (1998a) Use of insured health care services in relation to income in a Canadian province, in M.L. Barer, T.E. Getzen and G.L. Stoddart (eds) *Health, Health Care and Health Economics: Perspectives on Distribution*. Chichester: John Wiley.

Mustard, C.A., Barer, M., Evans, R.G. *et al.* (1998b) Paying taxes and using health care services: the distributional consequences of tax financed universal health insurance in a Canadian province. Paper presented to the Centre for the Study of Living Standards conference on the State of Living Standards and the Quality of Life in Canada, 30–31 October, Ottawa. http://www.csls.ca/oct/must1.pdf (accessed 25 February 2001).

OECD (1999) *OECD Health Data 99: A Comparative Analysis of 29 Countries*. Paris: Organisation for Economic Co-operation and Development.

Powell, J.E. (1976) *Medicine and Politics: 1975 and After*, revised edn. Tunbridge Wells: Pitman Medical.

Rasell, E., Bernstein, J. and Tang, K. (1993) *The Impact of Health Care Financing on Family Budgets*. Washington, DC: Economic Policy Institute.

Rasell, E., Bernstein, J. and Tang, K. (1994) The impact of health care financing on family budgets, *International Journal of Health Services*, 24(4): 691–714.

Robinson, R. and Dixon, A. (1999) *Health Care Systems in Transition: United Kingdom*. Copenhagen: European Observatory on Health Care Systems.

Roos, N.P. (2000) The disconnect between the data and the headlines, *Canadian Medical Association Journal*, 163(4): 411–12.

Sheils, J. and Hogan, P. (1999) Cost of tax-exempt health benefits in 1998, *Health Affairs*, 18(2): 176–81.

van Doorslaer, E., Wagstaff, A., van der Burg, H. *et al.* (1999) The redistributive effect of health care finance in twelve OECD countries, *Journal of Health Economics*, 18(3): 291–313.

Wagstaff, A. and van Doorslaer, E. (1992) Equity in the finance of health care: some international comparisons, *Journal of Health Economics*, 11(4): 361–87.

Wagstaff, A., Rutten, F. and van Doorslaer, E.K.A. (eds) (1993) *Equity in the Finance and Delivery of Health Care: An International Perspective*. Oxford: Oxford University Press.

Wagstaff, A., van Doorslaer, E., van der Burg, H. *et al.* (1999) Equity in the finance of health care: some further international comparisons, *Journal of Health Economics*, 18(3): 263–90.

White, J. (1995) *Competing Solutions: American Health Care Proposals and International Experience*. Washington, DC: Brookings Institution.

chapter three

Social health insurance financing

Charles Normand and Reinhard Busse[1]

The social health insurance model

Funding access to health care through social health insurance has its origins in Germany in the nineteenth century. The earliest versions of health insurance developed without any significant government intervention. Industrialization brought with it the emergence of large firms, and the workers in these firms started to organize themselves into trade unions. Sickness funds organized by the workers for mutual support often attracted support from employers, who saw benefits in their workers having access to better health care. Thus, a model arose in which health insurance was provided for some or all the workers in a firm, with much of the control remaining with the workers but with some management and financial input from employers.

The early sickness funds varied in their structures and governance but were mainly based on mutual support (in which contributions were based on income) and provided access to care based on need. In Germany, under Chancellor Bismarck, the sickness funds were formalized into a broader and more consistent system of health insurance. This led to the eventual development of territorial funds, which provided health insurance for those who were unable to obtain benefits through large formal employers (Altenstetter 1999; Busse 2000). The current arrangements in Germany have evolved slowly and in response to problems that emerged. In addition, traditions and unwritten rules have a strong role in the German system. These are just as important as the formal rules. It has continued to use the language and traditions of insurance, despite formal similarities to systems of government financing of care. It has also given priority to allowing choice of provider.

This chapter is organized into five sections. The first outlines the key features of social health insurance and how it operates. The second considers the variation in social health insurance in western Europe, in particular in France,

Germany and the Netherlands. The third section analyses recent reforms in western Europe and considers to what extent they have met their objectives. The fourth section evaluates social health insurance and presents its strengths and weaknesses, and the final part draws conclusions about the lessons from western European experience for the development of social health insurance in other countries.

There is substantial literature on the structures, operation and various technical aspects of social health insurance (Roemer 1969; Ron *et al.* 1990; Normand and Weber 1994). In this section, we outline the key features of social health insurance and how it operates.

Social health insurance has no uniformly valid definition, but two characteristics are crucial. Insured people pay a regular, usually wage-based contribution. Independent quasi-public bodies (usually called sickness funds) act as the major managing bodies of the system and as payers for health care. These two basic characteristics have certain limitations. In France's mutual benefit associations, contributions are based on income and usually split between employers and employees – but insurance is entirely voluntary (also called private social health insurance). A part of Switzerland's compulsory health insurance is not run by sickness funds but by privately owned insurance companies. We therefore use a pragmatic definition that also leaves room for innovative approaches: social health insurance funding occurs when it is legally mandatory to obtain health insurance with a designated (statutory) third-party payer through contributions or premiums not related to risk that are kept separate from other legally mandated taxes or contributions. In Figure 3.1, these two characteristics relate to the arrow C and the box 'payer/purchaser'.[2]

Several other characteristics are frequently found in social health insurance funding and fund management, although they are not essential features of the model.

1 *Social health insurance is compulsory for the majority or for the whole population.*
   Early forms of social health insurance normally focused on employees of large firms in urban areas. Over time, coverage has expanded to include small firms and, recently, self-employed people and farmers. It is today typically compulsory for most or all people, although some countries exclude people on high incomes from social health insurance (such as the Netherlands) or allow them to opt instead for private insurance (such as Germany).
2 *There are several funds, with or without choice and with or without risk-pooling.*
   Some countries have more than one sickness fund but little choice, since people are assigned to funds based on their geographical location, occupation or both. In others, there is a choice among funds, which stimulates competition but may also bring potential difficulties in ensuring equal access to care for all. Four broad types of organization of sickness funds can therefore be differentiated: a single fund for the entire population of a country; single funds serving geographically distinct populations within a country; multiple funds serving the population in the same geographical area but that do not compete for insurees; and multiple competing funds. Where there is more than one (competing or non-competing) fund, risk-pooling should ensure that funds with low-cost and/or high-income members subsidize those with high-cost and/or low-income members. However, this is politically and technically difficult.

Figure 3.1 Simplified model of the financing functions and monetary flows in countries with social health insurance

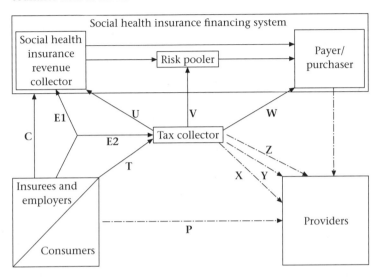

Key:
C = contributions (both income-related and non-income-related);
E = earmarked health taxes;
P = private expenditure (cost-sharing for social health insurance services; voluntary health insurance; and out-of-pocket payments for non–social health insurance services);
T = (general) taxes;
U = tax-financed contributions, such as for non-employed people;
V = general subsidies for pooled social health insurance financing;
W = subsidies for individual sickness funds;
X = reimbursement of services for people not covered by social health insurance;
Y = reimbursement for non–social health insurance services (such as public health);
Z = non-service-related payments (such as for investment) or subsidies.

Note: The dotted lines are outside the scope of this chapter

3 *Contributions made by government (or special funds) on behalf of people not in employment are usually channelled through the sickness fund(s).* In any social health insurance system, some people cannot contribute directly and some people are likely to need government support. If funding for these people is channelled through the social health insurance system, this can increase the size of the risk pool. It can also ensure that all people get the same service (if there is a single sickness fund or multiple funds with a common benefit package), and there is less danger of the service for poor people becoming a poor service.

4 *Both employers and employees pay contributions and share responsibility for managing fund(s).* As employers make significant financial contributions to social health insurance, it may be important that they feel some control over it.

In summary, the key features of social health insurance funding of health services are that contributions are paid based on ability to pay and the system provides a separate, transparent system for the flow of funds from the contributors to the sickness fund (and on to providers of services).

Variation in systems of financing social health insurance in western Europe

This section uses the countries with social health insurance systems in western Europe (Austria, Belgium, France, Germany, Luxembourg, the Netherlands and Switzerland) to illustrate the variability in arrangements outlined in the first section. These include the definition of 'insured', the organization of the sickness funds and the determination, collection, pooling and redistribution of contributions. The major findings are summarized in Table 3.1.

Who is insured (and are the conditions equal)?

As social health insurance has its roots in work-related insurance, population-wide coverage was not the original intention. Although coverage has been gradually expanded to non-working parts of the population in all countries, population-wide coverage was only very recently achieved in Switzerland (1996), Belgium (1998) and France (2000). An exception to this is the universal AWBZ insurance under the Exceptional Medical Expenses Act in the Netherlands, which was introduced in 1968; as the so-called first compartment, it covers long-term care and population-wide disease prevention programmes.

Austria and Luxembourg have *de facto* universal coverage, although a few people (1–3 per cent of the population) remain uninsured, mostly wealthy people in Luxembourg (Kerr 1999). Germany has a large proportion of the population (74 per cent) mandatorily insured and a small portion legally excluded,[3] leaving a third group (mainly employed people with income above a threshold) with a choice between statutory and private health insurance (Busse 2000). For acute care, the Netherlands strictly separate along an income limit between the mandatory scheme governed by the Sickness Funds Act (ZFW) and private health insurance, with no choice between the two systems. The ZFW income limits in 2000 were €29,300 for people younger than 65 years and €18,700 for people older than 65 years.

Coverage does not necessarily mean insuring everybody for the same benefits. Although this is usually the case, Belgium has a two-tier system for the 88 per cent of people in the 'general regime' (with a comprehensive benefits package) and the 12 per cent in the 'regime for self-employed' (for whom the benefits package covers 'major' risks only) (Nonneman and van Doorslaer 1994).

How are the sickness funds organized (and is there any choice among them)?

The number of funds and their size and structure vary widely, as does the extent to which they compete for members. Austria, France and Luxembourg have comparatively small and stable numbers of non-competing funds, as these are defined based on occupational status and, for Austria, place of residence. Luxembourg, for example, has nine sickness funds: one each for manual

Table 3.1 Important characteristics of social health insurance systems in western Europe relating to financing, 1999 or 2000 (unless stated otherwise)

	Austria	Belgium	France	Germany	Luxembourg	Netherlands	Switzerland
Social health insurance coverage (percentage of population)	99%	99–100%	100%	88%	97–99%	AWBZ 100%, ZFW 64%	100%
Number of sickness funds	24	About 100 (all but 2 organized in 5 mutual benefit associations)	19	420 (in 7 associations)	9	30	109
Percentage of insured people with choice of fund	0%	About 99%	0%	96%	0%	100%	100%
Contribution rate: uniform or varying, percentage of wage (distribution employer : employee)	Varying by profession: 6.4–9.1%[a]	Uniform: 7.4% (52 : 48)	Uniform: 13.6% (94 : 6)	Varying by fund: mean 13.6% (50 : 50)	Uniform: 5.1% (50% : 50%) + 0.3–5.0% sick pay (50 : 50)	Uniform: AWBZ 10.3% (0% : 100%), ZFW 8.1% (78 : 22)	No
Ceiling on contributory income	Yes (€44,000)	No	No	Yes (west: €40,000; east: €32,000)	Yes (€70,000)	Yes (AWBZ €22,000, ZFW €29,000, €19,000 for pensioners)	Not applicable
Other personal contributions to funds (excluding co-payments to providers)	No	Plus a nominal premium per capita (varying by fund)	General social contribution 7.5% + social debt repayment contribution 0.5%	No	No	Plus premium per capita (varying by fund), mean €180 annually	Only premium per capita
Determines contributions	Government	Government[b]	Government	Individual funds	Union of Sickness Funds	Government[b]	Individual funds or insurers

Table 3.1 (cont'd)

	Austria	Belgium	France	Germany	Luxembourg	Netherlands	Switzerland
Collects contributions	Individual funds	National Social Security Office[b]	Local government agencies, transferred to Central Agency for Social Security Institutions	Individual funds	Union of Sickness Funds	AWBZ/ZFW Fund managed by Board for Health Care Insurance[b]	Individual funds or insurers
Mechanism for pooling or financial risk-sharing among funds	No, but funds in deficit may apply for transfers from other funds	Mainly joint expenditure; limited prospective allocation to funds (1999: 4%; 2000: 7.5%)	Subsidies from major funds (up to 42%) and government to smaller funds	Risk-structure compensation mechanism at the federal level (for > 90% of income)	Joint expenditure	Mainly joint expenditure; limited prospective allocation to funds (ZFW 35% in 1999)	Risk-structure compensation at the cantonal level
Tax financing of social health insurance (if available: percentage of fund income)	Generally no, except 23% for farmers fund: 0.5% of the total	Yes, 35–40%	Yes (up to 8%); plus special taxes (up to 34%)[c]	Generally no, except 52% for farmers' funds: < 1% of the total	Yes, maximum 40%[d]	Yes, AWBZ < 1%, ZFW 25%	Only indirect subsidies (to insurees rather than to funds)
Social health insurance expenditure as a percentage of total health expenditure	48% (1996)	62% (1994)	74% (1996)	61% (1994)[e]	75% (1997)	73% (1999): AWBZ 37%, ZFW 36%	28% (1997)[e]

[a] Manual workers 7.9% (50% : 50%) + 2.1% sick pay (100% : 0%), white-collar workers 6.9% (51% : 49%), civil servants 7.1% (44% : 56%), self-employed 9.1%, farmers 6.4%.

[b] Individual funds for per-capita premiums.

[c] On car insurance, alcoholic drinks and pharmaceutical marketing.

[d] 250% supplement on pensioners' contributions, 10% on other contributions.

[e] Plus health expenditure from other social insurance schemes (4% and 7%, respectively for Germany and Switzerland).

workers, white-collar workers in the private sector, self-employed people, the agricultural sector, civil servants of the state, civil servants of local authorities, manual workers at ARBED (a private company), white-collar workers at ARBED and the Luxembourg railways.

Western European countries with competing funds have more funds, but the numbers are decreasing. In 1993, Germany had 1221 funds, but these were merged into 420 funds in 2000 and are classified into seven groups: 17 general regional funds, 12 substitute funds, 337 company-based funds, 32 guild funds, 20 farmers' funds, one miners' fund and one sailors' fund. Belgium has about 100 funds organized according to religion and political affiliation. All but two funds are members of five associations (Christian, Free and Professional, Liberal, Neutral and Socialist), the remaining ones being the Auxiliary Fund and the Fund of the Belgium Railway Company. In the Netherlands, mergers between 1985 and 1993 halved the number of sickness funds from 53 to 26. The number has since increased slightly to 30, as competition among funds was introduced in 1995. In Switzerland, sickness funds and private insurance companies offer compulsory health insurance (the companies may only profit from supplementary insurance), and the number of insurers declined from 207 in 1993 to 109 in 1999 (Minder *et al.* 2000).

The presence of more funds in a country does not necessarily mean more choice, as demonstrated by Germany, where membership of most funds was legally assigned until 1995. Since 1996, most insured people may choose which fund to join; only farmers, miners and sailors are assigned membership to the corresponding funds. Insured people in Belgium have traditionally had a choice among funds (except for railway employees) but not insured people in Austria, France and Luxembourg. If insured people are allowed to choose and switch between funds, countries need to decide how often this should be allowed. When the Netherlands opened their funds to competition in 1995, they opted for a 2 year interval but changed to an annual option from 1997. People may switch every 3 months in Belgium, every 6 months in Switzerland and every 12 months in Germany (generally). However, voluntary members earning above the threshold in Germany could always – and still can – move from one fund to another at any time with 2 months' notice. However, a decision to leave the social health insurance system and obtain private insurance cannot be revoked.

Paying contributions: rates, ceilings and supplementary contributions

Contributions are mainly based on wages and are shared between employers and employees in all countries (except Switzerland[4]). Nevertheless, there are important differences relating to:

- the uniformity of the rate;
- the distribution of contributions between employer and employee;
- the existence of an upper contribution ceiling;
- the existence of additional non-wage-related contributions.

Insured people have the same contribution rate regardless of sickness fund and membership status in Belgium, France, Luxembourg and the Netherlands. In Austria, rates vary between 6.4 and 9.1 per cent according to employment status but not between funds for a given employment status. In Germany, the contribution rates differ among funds but not by employment status.[5]

The employer and employee each pay about half in Austria, Belgium, Germany and Luxembourg. In France, the employers paid 70 per cent for a long time, but the employees' contribution has been reduced to 6 per cent in favour of a health tax. In the Netherlands, employers cover most of the ZFW but nothing of the AWBZ; in total, employers pay 35 per cent for those insured under both schemes.

Austria, Germany,[6] Luxembourg and the Netherlands have ceilings on contributions (differing between the insurance schemes in the Netherlands) but not Belgium and France.

Belgium, France and the Netherlands impose additional contributions to the wage-based contributions. In Belgium and the Netherlands, insured people pay a non-income-related per-capita premium on top of their contributions. These premiums, which vary among funds, are currently small in Belgium but are about €180 a year in the Netherlands (about one-tenth of the income of sickness funds) and are levied not only on sickness fund members but also on their covered dependants.

France has replaced the employee's part of the contributions with a general social contribution that is also based on non-wage income; in addition, a social debt repayment contribution is charged. The reasons for these complementary premiums differ: in France, containing costs and increasing the financial base of the funds was the driving force; in the Netherlands, the charges aimed to introduce an element of price competition among funds.

Negative supplementary contributions are also theoretically possible. For example, Germany experimented with no-claim bonuses – a refund of contributions if no services were used – after 1989 and opened up this option as a market instrument for all funds in 1997, despite evaluations demonstrating that only insurees with low utilization benefit (Malin and Schmidt 1996). As a typical instrument used by private health insurance schemes, the bonuses are no longer considered compatible with the basic philosophy of social health insurance and were abolished by a new parliamentary majority in 1998.

As contributions are based on wages, contributions for non-waged people must be determined. For the largest group, pensioners, contributions vary between countries, both regarding how much they pay and who actually pays. In most cases, pensioners pay the same rate on their pension as employees pay on their income (or, in Switzerland, the same per-capita premium). This amount is split between the pensioner and the statutory pension fund (substituting for the employer) in Germany and Luxembourg and placed entirely on the pensioner in the Netherlands. In Belgium, pensioners pay only the employees' part of 3.55 per cent; the contribution rate is more than 11 per cent for pensioners in Austria. As pensioners in Austria pay only as much as working members on average (3.75 per cent), pension funds pay two-thirds of the contribution (European Commission 2000).

Decision-making powers

Although sickness funds are self-governing in most countries, the government or parliament decisively influence the setting of contributions. In France, for example, the government, representatives of employees and employers and the social security organizations negotiate contribution rates, but the government ultimately decides. In the Netherlands, the Health Care Insurance Board (College voor zorgverzekeringen, CvZ), which runs the Central Funds of ZFW and AWBZ, recommends contribution rates for the following year to the Ministry of Health, Welfare and Sport, which sets the rates. Only Germany and Luxembourg have delegated the power to determine contribution rates to self-governing bodies subject to government approval – in Germany to the individual funds and in Luxembourg to the Union of Sickness Funds. Similarly, insurers in Switzerland set their own community-based premiums under the supervision of the Federal Office for Social Insurance. The government amends the contribution ceilings annually in all countries, taking into account changes in wages. The sickness funds in Belgium and the Netherlands set their own per-capita premiums. These differ in the Netherlands because of competition (see previously) but have mostly remained uniform in Belgium: only one fund lowered its rate from the usual €2.20 per month to €1.20 in 1998 but reverted in 1999 (Schut and van Doorslaer 1999).

Collection of contributions and other social health insurance revenue

The sickness funds collect the contributions in Austria, Germany and Switzerland. Associations of funds (Luxembourg) or government agencies may also collect contributions. In Belgium, contributions are paid directly to the National Social Security Office (RSZ/ONSS), which, in turn, redistributes the money to the respective government agencies responsible for administering different sectors of social security, such as unemployment and pensions. The agency responsible for health benefits is the National Institute for Sickness and Invalidity Insurance (RIZIV/INAMI). Similarly, in France, revenue is collected by local government agencies that collect social security and family allowance contributions. The money is passed to a national agency, the Agence Centrale des Organismes de Sécurité Sociale (Central Agency for Social Security Institutions), which manages and allocates the money to the different social security organizations and their branches.

Risk-pooling and allocation among funds

The next issue in social health insurance financing is risk-pooling among funds and (re)allocation of financial resources to the individual funds. In Belgium and the Netherlands, before the mid-1990s, complete national pooling of contributions went hand-in-hand with *de facto* joint expenditure: retrospective allocation of contributions to funds according to actual expenditure.

The reforms have led to the gradual introduction of per-capita risk-adjusted allocations to the sickness funds. In Belgium, the prospective allocation amounted to 10 per cent of the total health care budget for 1995–96 and 1996–97 and was raised to 20 per cent for 1998–99 and 30 per cent for 2000–2001. Since the funds were only financially responsible for 15, 20 and 25 per cent of that allocation in the respective years, the actual percentages 'at risk' amounted to only 1.5, 4.0 and 7.5 per cent. The Netherlands went ahead more rapidly, from 3 per cent in 1993–95 to 15 per cent in 1996, 27 per cent in 1997, 29 per cent in 1998 and 35 per cent in 2000 – but a special provision that expenses for extremely expensive patients are shared provides a 'safety net' for the funds (Schut and van Doorslaer 1999). Since the Union of Sickness Funds in Luxembourg covers directly the expenses for services delivered on a contract basis (such as hospital care), the retrospective approach is only used for services with patient reimbursement such as physicians' services. France has both a compensation scheme among the local sickness insurance funds as well as support for some of the smaller funds (those with insured people with lower earnings) from the National Sickness Fund as well as through taxes.

Ensuring an equitable financial basis in countries where individual funds collect the contributions is much more difficult. There are two reasons for this. First, money not only has to be allocated according to some criteria but actually needs to be reallocated; the money necessary for compensating one sickness fund has to be taken from another fund. However, the better-off funds tend to regard the contributions they collect as 'theirs', so that the issue becomes politically contentious. The second reason is more technical: the reallocation not only has to consider 'need' factors (or other factors determining utilization and expenditure) but also the differing contribution bases of the funds. Thus, although revenue collection and risk-pooling are two distinct functions, the organizational forms used appear to be related.

Not surprisingly, risk-structure compensation is discussed fiercely in Germany and Switzerland. In both countries, all of the expenditure required to cover the uniform benefits basket – more than 90 per cent of all income – is liable to pooling and redistribution. The Federal Insurance Office carries out the risk-structure compensation in Germany[7] and the joint organization of insurers offers compulsory health insurance (known as Foundation 18 based on the relevant paragraph in the health insurance law) in Switzerland. Austria has no formal mechanism for financial redistribution, but funds in financial difficulty may apply to the association of social insurance funds for financial aid from other funds.

The role of taxes in funding social health insurance

The common assumption that social health insurance countries rely mainly on contributions to finance their health systems has to be questioned. International statistics on sources of health care funding often do not specify whether expenditure through taxation includes tax-financed payments to the social health insurance financing system (U + V + W in Figure 3.1) or whether these are included as social health insurance expenditure. Austria and Switzerland, for example, finance a substantial part of hospital care directly through taxation, and social health insurance therefore covers a relatively low proportion of expenditure. In other countries, such as the Netherlands, the sickness funds exclusively finance hospital care and, in turn, receive substantial subsidies from general taxation. Besides the Netherlands, subsidies from taxes – which are paid to a joint fund administered by the sickness funds (V in Figure 3.1) – are quite substantial in Belgium and Luxembourg. In Austria, on the other hand, as in Germany, funds receive no subsidies from taxes (except for the farmers' funds in both countries, indicated by W in Figure 3.1). France has a mixed approach. Its direct tax subsidies are rather low and limited to funds with members with a low income or high need such as the farmers' fund, but it allows the funds to accumulate sizeable deficits that were covered by the state and are now being paid off through a special social debt repayment contribution (E2 in Figure 3.1) – a mechanism by which social health insurance financing is retrospectively changed into tax financing.

Two factors have to be combined to estimate the extent to which countries rely on social health insurance contributions based on wages: the percentage of social health insurance income through contributions ($C/(C + E1 + U + V + W)$ in Figure 3.1) and the percentage of overall health expenditure covered by social health insurance ($(C + E1 + U + V + W)/(C + E + P + T)$). Based on such a calculation, Germany and the Netherlands are the only countries in western Europe that cover more than 60 per cent of total health care expenditure through wage-related contributions. Until 1997, France was the country that relied most heavily on such contributions, but since it shifted to a wider base for contributions, the share is currently below 60 per cent. Austria and Luxembourg finance a little less than 50 per cent and Belgium even less than 40 per cent of total health care expenditure through wage-related contributions (Table 3.1). In some respects, the Belgian system is more properly classified as mixed in terms of funding sources, as taxes accounted for 38 per cent of expenditure versus 36 per cent from social security contributions in 1994 (Crainich and Closon 1999).

Reforming social health insurance systems in western Europe

Since the 1980s, reforms in financing in the social health insurance countries have had several, partly conflicting objectives: to increase equity, efficiency or choice for insurees and to stabilize contributions without adversely affecting the labour market. This section discusses the reforms aiming at different objectives in the Netherlands, Germany and France.

Reforms to ensure equitable financing in the Netherlands

In the 1980s, the system of voluntary insurance for elderly and self-employed people collapsed because private insurers were offering low premiums to young and healthy people. High-risk groups were left with a choice between a policy with high deductibles or leaving the voluntary scheme. The government was forced to take action and introduced two acts in 1986: the Access to Health Insurance Act (WTZ) and the Act on Co-financing the Overrepresentation of Elderly People in the Sickness Fund Scheme (MOOZ).

The WTZ guarantees access to insurance, as private insurers are obliged to accept applicants from certain defined groups, and authorizes the Minister for Health, Welfare and Sport to determine a guaranteed benefits package and its associated premiums. However, premiums for this scheme were insufficient to cover expenditure. In accordance with the legislation, an equalization fund was set up, administered by representatives of the private insurers, to redistribute funds to compensate for insurees in these specific categories (corresponding to about 40 per cent of the total costs of the private schemes). The law also enforces income solidarity among privately insured people, since they have to pay a fixed amount per month to the equalization fund to compensate for the costs of the insurees covered by the standard package policy. The MOOZ requires solidarity payments to be transferred from privately insured people to the Central Fund of the ZFW scheme. This compensates for the numbers and costs of elderly people, who are over-represented in the statutory scheme.

The Council for Public Health and Healthcare (Raad voor de Volksgezondheid en Zorg 2000) has said that both the WTZ standard package and the MOOZ regulations could violate European Union (EU) law on fair competition and recommends that the role of the EU and that of EU countries in health care be redefined (Sheldon 2000).

Introducing choice of sickness fund and risk-pooling in Germany

Traditionally, most insured people in Germany were assigned to a sickness fund based on place of residence and/or occupation. This led to greatly varying contribution rates because the income and risk profiles of different occupations vary. White-collar workers had a choice of fund on joining or when changing jobs. Only voluntary members, those with an income above a certain threshold, had the right to choose among several funds and to change funds.

The Health Care Structure Act of 1993 extended the right to choose a sickness fund freely and to change funds each year (from 1996). All general regional funds and all substitute funds were legally obligated to accept all applicants for membership. The company-based funds and the guild funds may choose whether to restrict access. However, if they opt to allow unrestricted access to members, they are also obligated to accept all applicants. Only the farmers', the miners' and the sailors' funds still retain the system of assigned membership.

To ensure that all sickness funds started from an equal position when competition was introduced, a scheme for risk-structure compensation was introduced in two steps (1994 and 1995). In the second stage, retired insurees were included. Previously, funds had shared the actual expenses of retired people.

The aim of the scheme for risk-structure compensation was to reduce differences in contribution rates resulting from different income levels and expenditure because of the age and sex composition of members. The compensatory mechanism requires all sickness funds to provide or receive compensation for the differences both in their contributory incomes and in their average (standardized) expenditure (Busse 2001).

Free choice and the compensation scheme affected the social health insurance system as follows.

- Movement between funds increased. Changes in membership are correlated with contribution rates: funds with higher than average contribution rates lose members, whereas those with lower than average rates gain members (Müller and Schneider 1999).
- For people who have moved from one fund to another, 58 per cent cited lower contributions as the main motive, whereas for people considering a move, both the contribution rate and better benefits are equally important. People not considering a move regard 'better benefits' – despite almost identical benefit packages – to be more important (Andersen and Schwarze 1998).
- The risk-compensation scheme has narrowed differences in contribution rates between funds. This trend is especially observable in western Germany but recently also in the east. In 1994, 27 per cent of all members paid a contribution rate differing by more than one percentage point from the average, and this figure declined to 7 per cent in 1999.
- The movement of members between funds has not equalized the different risk structures but has segregated membership further: the healthier, younger, higher-earning people move more often and towards cheaper funds.

Replacing payroll contributions by an earmarked health tax in France

France's social security system was in constant deficit in the 1990s, with health care being the main reason. Social contributions were blamed for increasing labour costs and for adversely affecting employment. They were also considered as an insecure source of revenue, as they depend heavily on employment levels and economic activity. In an effort to address structural and financial difficulties, Prime Minister Alain Juppé presented a plan to reform the social security system in December 1995. There were three main aims: to avoid negative effects on the labour market, to reduce the public deficit and to achieve consistency between the founding principles of social security and funding mechanisms (Bouget 1998).

One of the main proposals was to widen the base of the general social tax. This tax, levied on all types of income, including savings, subsidies, pensions and capital income, was set at 1.1 per cent in 1991 and was initially allocated to family benefits. In 1996, it was earmarked for health. The employees' payroll contributions for health were largely replaced by an increase in the earmarked health tax from 1998: while the payroll contribution rate decreased from 5.5 to 0.75 per cent, the earmarked health tax increased from 3.4 to 7.5 per cent – thereby reducing the overall percentage but widening the base on which it has to be paid. The employer's contribution was maintained. Another measure was to create a new tax, the social debt repayment tax to clear the debt of the social security system (Lancry and Sandier 1999). Starting from 1996 and due to last for 13 years, this new tax is set at 0.5 per cent of total income and is levied on the whole population, except those receiving state benefits and disability pensions. France has three different income bases for financing the social security system: one for social contributions, a second for the earmarked health tax (E1 in Figure 3.1) and a third for the social debt repayment tax (E2 in Figure 3.1). Future debates will focus on the collective choice between proportional taxes, notably the earmarked health tax, and progressive taxes such as income tax (Bouget 1998).

Conclusion

In effect, reforms in these countries were often aimed at achieving more than one of the objectives. By introducing monetary transfers from private health insurance to statutory health insurance, the reform in the Netherlands not only improved the equity of the system but also addressed the revenue crisis within the statutory scheme. Germany's main aim was increasing choice, but the desire to increase efficiency was also important (mainly through better contracting with providers, which is not the topic of this book). Eliminating the previous inequality between white- and blue-collar workers was a third aim – and secured the support of the Social Democratic Party of Germany, which was in opposition at the time. A mix of objectives is also visible in France: widening the contributory base and increasing equity.

Nevertheless, reforms in different countries with the same objectives may lead to different outcomes; for example, the pro-competition reforms in Germany and the modified Dekker Plan in the Netherlands. In Germany, the risk-structure compensation narrowed the traditionally large differences in contributions (ensuring increased equity). In the Netherlands, however, the non-income-related per-capita premium had the effect of widening differences in contribution (decreasing equity).

Reforms within one country may have both conflicting aims and/or outcomes. For example, the WTZ and MOOZ reforms in the Netherlands increased equity in financing, but the subsequent Dekker/Simonis reform decreased equity in financing by introducing a non-income-related per-capita premium.

Strengths and weaknesses of social health insurance financing in western Europe

Properly discussing the strengths and weaknesses of social health insurance financing requires clarity on the objectives of health policy. The policy objectives considered here are financial sustainability, equity, efficiency, responsiveness and satisfaction.

Although the models of social health insurance and general taxation are similar, they differ systematically in practice. First, the separate structures for collecting and managing funds tend to result in greater transparency. However, the organizational autonomy of social health insurance funds also requires adequate systems of accountability. Second, that access to care depends on contributions to the fund gives the patient the status of a customer. The relationship between insurer and member is therefore more contractual, and thus the benefits to which the contributors are entitled have tended to be more explicitly defined. Third, revenue is determined by contributions and not by political preferences; social health insurance is thus less politicized.

Since there is no simple answer to the question of how much should be spent on health care, adequacy is best judged in the context of a country's total resources and other development priorities (Cichon *et al.* 1999). There are several reasons and some evidence to suggest that separating health care spending from other government-mandated spending can increase funding for health services. Most importantly, perhaps, greater social willingness to pay for health care seems to be associated with the hypothecation of funds inherent in a transparent arrangement for funding social health insurance. This also appears to translate into greater population satisfaction with social health insurance systems than with systems funded by general revenue or voluntary insurance (Ferrera 1993; Mossialos 1998). Separating health care financing from government financing allows people to consider separately the desirability of higher contributions for better services, secure in the knowledge that any additional contributions will not be diverted to other government programmes they may consider to be of lower priority.

Most systems of social health insurance use current employment income as the contribution base, in part because they originated as employer-sponsored systems. Since income from employment has historically been a good proxy for ability to pay, this has generally been fair. However, this narrow base is becoming less satisfactory for several reasons. First, the trend towards self-employment is increasing at the expense of employment. Second, more people have more than one job. Third, wealth affects ability to pay but is not taken into account. Fourth, capital income is an increasing proportion of income. The introduction of social health insurance in the countries of central and eastern Europe has shown that there are problems with this narrow contribution base, and ways may be needed to take into account wealth and non-employment income in assessing contributions to increase revenue and improve equity.

The issue of who actually pays for social health insurance systems is not straightforward, despite the visible division between insurees and employers. Much depends on the amount of competition in product and labour markets. If markets are very competitive, then firms will only survive if they contain the total cost of employment, so that the total amount spent on wages and insurance contributions is likely to be constant. If insurance contributions rise, then wages over time are likely to fall. Thus, in economic terms, the employers may shift their share of the payroll contribution to employees in the form of reduced wage growth. The tax treatment of insurance contributions is also important. If contributions are exempt from tax, then contributions cost the same for employers to pay as increasing wages and for employees to pay and in principle it makes no difference who pays.

A tax is progressive if the proportion of income paid in tax rises as income rises. In a regressive system, the proportion falls as income rises. Health care financing can be analysed similarly – funding is progressive if the proportion of income paid for health care rises as income rises. The findings of the ECuity Project (van Doorslaer *et al.* 1993; Wagstaff *et al.* 1999) suggest that social health insurance is, on average, slightly less progressive than tax financing but much more progressive than private financing arrangements. Although *The World Health Report 2000* (WHO 2000) confirms the results regarding private financing, social health insurance and tax financing do not differ systematically in financial equity according to that calculation.[8]

While differences within tax-financed systems depend on the mix between (progressive) income taxes and (regressive) indirect taxes as well as how completely they are collected, equity differences among social health insurance countries depend on several factors:

- the extent to which contributions are based on income (rather than per-capita premiums);
- whether richer and/or healthier people are paying relatively less (through income ceilings or no-claim bonuses) or are allowed to stay out of the system altogether;
- the extent to which the contributions to different funds are pooled, i.e. adjusted for differing risks; and
- the extent to which benefits are fully covered or require cost-sharing.

All these points have to be considered with special attention to including or excluding dependants: equity decreases further if per-capita premiums are charged for members and dependants. Including dependants might lead to greater inequity if a ceiling exists: an affluent couple with one non-employed spouse pays once, whereas a middle-class double-income couple pays twice.

Historically, many countries, most notably Germany, have had multiple funds but not competing funds. This is changing as the right to choose insurer has been introduced. Equity is not related to the existence or lack of competition, but rather to the existence or lack of functioning pooling mechanisms; in other words, regional monopoly funds can be inequitable if resources are not pooled and competing sickness funds can be equitable if resources are effectively pooled.

If a perfect system of risk adjustment is introduced and full allowance is made for differences in incomes, then full choice and competition between funds and full solidarity are theoretically possible. However, such mechanisms are complex and expensive, and increased diversity and choice can also increase inequality in access to care. For a more detailed discussion of risk-adjustment mechanisms between competing insurance funds, see Chapter 11 and Busse (2001) for Germany, Chinitz and Shmueli (2001) for Israel and Okma and Poelert (2001) for the Netherlands.

International comparisons show that social health insurance systems have higher expenditure than tax-funded systems. The important question is whether this higher spending reflects a higher volume of services or simply higher costs of producing care, because of higher transaction costs and/or higher provider income. The available evidence is limited and allows no clear conclusions. Again a combination of *a priori* reasoning and evidence is helpful.

Efficiency in the production of care requires structures, skills, motivation and incentives. Structures affect efficiency both through the market power of buyers and sellers and by affecting transaction costs. A serious issue in assessing the efficiency of different financing systems is how to minimize management and transaction costs. Evidence on the relationship between management costs and performance is still poor (Street *et al.* 1999). Although much of the transaction costs in social health insurance systems are related to contracting and purchasing services (and whether funds do this individually or collectively is a major determining factor), only the transaction costs of collecting, pooling and allocating contributions are relevant here. Unfortunately, the management costs of sickness funds are not broken down into collecting and pooling versus contracting and purchasing, and we do not have comparative data from tax-based systems on the transaction costs of collecting taxes and allocating them to, for example, health authorities. If, however, sickness funds are small and have differing contribution rates and different ways of collecting contributions, the danger of inefficiency is great – but there is no reason why social health insurance should necessarily involve higher transaction costs than tax financing.

However, as the desire for diversity and choice increases, the tendency to incur high costs and to reduce the downward pressure on costs is a major risk (Normand and Weber 1994). The choice of simple contracting arrangements in Germany is in part a response to the need to contain costs, although it will be interesting to see the effects of the current trend towards increasing competition between funds. Between 1995 and 1999 (since the introduction of competition), the visible administration costs of the funds as a percentage of all expenditure have increased from 5.24 to 5.76 per cent (Bundesministerium für Gesundheit 2000). To a certain extent, this results from employers shifting costs to the funds in company-based funds.

Because resources are never sufficient to satisfy all demands, some form of rationing or priority-setting is inevitable. A shift from tax financing to social health insurance does not change this. However, it may change who is responsible for choosing which services are provided and may shift blame for constraints (at least in part) away from governments.

Social health insurance systems tend to be associated with high levels of satisfaction in the population. The sources of this satisfaction are interesting, including a combination of solidarity (although less than with general revenue funding) and transparency (a clear advantage of social health insurance systems). To some extent, social health insurance may make every patient a private patient. Social health insurance systems have certainly been associated with attitudes to patients that treat them as valued customers and not simply a nuisance, as suggested by the high responsiveness ratings in *The World Health Report 2000* (WHO 2000).[9]

Conclusions

Learning from the experiences of others is positive but should not lead to copying systems originating in different settings. Social health insurance in western Europe has been very successful at meeting particular goals, especially in providing near-universal access to care. It provides services that are acceptable to the public and that have some solidarity. The details of the organization of funds and provision of care have often arisen as a result of slow evolution and adaptation of institutions to meet new challenges. There are many clear advantages. The problems are mainly in the risk of cost escalation, excessive reliance on too narrow a contributions base, and the potentially high costs of management and transactions in contracting and purchasing.

Countries that are considering developing social health insurance need to be aware of the trade-offs between costs and the range of services available, between costs and the extent of diversity and choice, and between competition and the objectives of equity and containing management costs. History and tradition have played very important roles in determining exactly how social health insurance operates. Germany's system appears to be very diverse and pluralistic but is also a uniform system, since contracting between all funds and all providers is collective. It has developed into a system of cooperation with important elements of diversity. As reforms are increasing competition, it will be interesting to see whether the (often very important) traditions and unwritten rules can withstand the changes. The recent reforms in France and the Netherlands have been grappling with the different objectives of universality, containing the costs of services and of administration (and increasing the income of the funds), while retaining the features of the systems that users value.

Social health insurance has many variants, and the performance of social health insurance systems may depend significantly on how contributions are collected, pooled and allocated to sickness funds as purchasers of care. However, the main argument in favour of social health insurance systems is that they are proportional and thus a way of collecting revenue that is relatively more equitable than private health insurance. Income ceilings limit the extent of progressivity, especially compared with general tax funding. The financial flows are more transparent, thus making (high) contributions by the public acceptable. The combination of employer and employee contributions mobilizes additional revenue but may adversely affect job mobility and economic competitiveness. Pooling funds under the control of independent bodies increases the autonomy of decision-making from the political process. The insurance relationship persists in the explicitness and transparency of benefits and the handling of patients as customers.

However, social health insurance risks becoming too dependent on the payroll for contributions at a time when the proportion of people with permanent jobs in large organizations is declining. Developing social health insurance is easier when the pattern of employment includes large firms and formal employment as the norm. Social health insurance can be emphasized as the organizational form for pooling funds and purchasing services, while general taxation (or a mix of general and payroll taxation) can be the main source of funds.

The fact that social health insurance systems have evolved and survived suggests that this model of quasi-independent funds can offer a sustainable model that can adapt to different conditions. Most systems are significantly regulated by government, and systems vary from being close to hypothecated taxes to those where government loosely supervises the independent funds. Many systems have some tax-financed components (not all of which are visible and fully acknowledged), while others have government guarantees for debt. Social health insurance countries typically spend more on health than those that use tax financing. One reason is that the financial flows are more transparent and funding for health care is more acceptable. Serious consideration has been given recently to developing competition in collecting and managing the funds. It remains to be seen whether market forces can play a useful role in forcing costs down while avoiding the potential problems of inequity and high transaction costs.

Notes

1 We thank Jan Bultman and Fons Berten for providing background material on social health insurance in the Netherlands and Anne-Pierre Pickaert for information on France.
2 The usual attribution of other characteristics to social health insurance systems, such as contracts between funds and providers or the relatively unrestricted access of patients to providers, are outside the scope of this chapter. These relationships and financing flows are therefore shown as dotted lines in Figure 3.1.
3 Self-employed people are excluded from social health insurance unless they have been a member previously (except those who fall under mandatory social health insurance coverage like farmers), and active and retired permanent public employees such as teachers, university professors, employees in ministries, and so on, are excluded *de facto* as they are reimbursed by the government for most of their private health care bills (most of them receive private insurance to cover the remainder).
4 Since compulsory health insurance was introduced in 1996, Switzerland has had a system of community-rated health insurance premiums. These differ between insurers but are community rated for all people insured by each insurer in a certain region (usually the canton).
5 This rule has exceptions. The largest group treated differently were pensioners (until 30 June 1997), since their contributions were based uniformly on the average contribution rate of all funds. For that purpose, the average rate on 1 January each year was applied 6 months retrospectively and 6 months prospectively (from 1 July of the previous year until 30 June of the same year). Since 1999, workers who earn less than €322 per month have been required to pay a uniform rate of 10 per cent, and this group was not mandatorily insured before. Students pay a uniform premium per person.
6 The only exemption being the ceiling for miners (mandatorily insured in the miners' fund), which is one-third higher than normal.
7 The Federal Insurance Office is charged with supervising sickness funds operating country-wide and with the risk-structure compensation mechanism between all sickness funds. Before 1994–95, Germany had a mixed system: expenditure for pensioners was covered jointly by all funds (as in Luxembourg), whereas contributions and expenditure for all other insurees were not reallocated at all (as in Austria).

8 The top 12 countries in the world in fairness in financing include Austria, Belgium, Germany and Luxembourg, as well as Denmark, Finland, Ireland, Norway and the United Kingdom (whereas France, the Netherlands and especially Switzerland rank lower).

9 Switzerland, Luxembourg, Germany and the Netherlands rank second, third, fifth and ninth in the world in terms of responsiveness, whereas of the tax-financed systems in western Europe, only Denmark achieves a comparable position (fourth).

References

Altenstetter, C. (1999) From solidarity to market competition? Values, structure and strategy in German health policy 1883–1997, in F.D. Powell and A.F. Wessem (eds) *Health Care Systems in Transition*. Thousand Oaks, CA: Sage Publications.

Andersen, H.A. and Schwarze, J. (1998) GKV '97: Kommt Bewegung in die Landschaft? Eine empirische Analyse der Kassenwahlentscheidungen [Statutory health insurance 1997: is there movement in the landscape? An empirical analysis of decisions to change sickness funds], *Arbeit und Sozialpolitik*, 52(9/10): 11–23.

Bouget, D. (1998) The Juppé plan and the future of the French social welfare system, *Journal of European Social Policy*, 8(2): 155–72.

Bundesministerium für Gesundheit (Federal Ministry of Health) (2000) *Statistisches Taschenbuch Gesundheit 2000* [*Statistical Report Health 2000*]. Bonn: Bundesministerium für Gesundheit.

Busse, R. (2000) *Health Care Systems in Transition: Germany*. Copenhagen: European Observatory on Health Care Systems.

Busse, R. (2001) Risk structure compensation in Germany's statutory health insurance, *European Journal of Public Health*, 11(2): 174–7.

Cichon, M., Newbrander, W., Yamabana, H. *et al.* (1999) *Modelling in Health Care Finance: A Compendium of Quantitative Techniques for Health Care Financing*. Geneva: International Labour Organization.

Crainich, D. and Closon, M-C. (1999) Cost containment and health care reform in Belgium, in E. Mossialos and J. Le Grand (eds) *Health Care and Cost Containment in the European Union*. Aldershot: Ashgate.

European Commission (2000) *MISSOC* (*Mutual Information System on Social Protection in the European Union*): *Comparative Tables*. Brussels: Directorate-General for Employment and Social Affairs, European Commission. http://europa.eu.int/comm/employment_social/soc-prot/missoc99/english/f_tab.htm (accessed 25 February 2001).

Ferrera, M. (1993) *EC Citizens and Social Protection: Main Results of a Collaborative Survey*. Brussels: European Commission.

Kerr, E. (1999) *Health Care Systems in Transition: Luxembourg*. Copenhagen: European Observatory on Health Care Systems.

Lancry, P-J. and Sandier, S. (1999) Twenty years of cures for the French health care system, in E. Mossialos and J. Le Grand (eds) *Health Care and Cost Containment in the European Union*. Aldershot: Ashgate.

Malin, E-M. and Schmidt, E.M. (1996) Beitragsrückzahlung: keine Auswirkungen auf die Leistungsinanspruchnahme [Contribution repayment: no effect on service demand], *Die Betriebskrankenkasse*, 84(8): 379–83.

Minder, A., Schoenholzer, H. and Amiet, M. (2000) *Health Care Systems in Transition: Switzerland*. Copenhagen: European Observatory on Health Care Systems.

Mossialos, E. (1998) *Citizens and Health Systems: Main Results from a Eurobarometer Survey*. Brussels: Directorate-General for Employment, Industrial Relations and Social Affairs, European Commission.

Müller, J. and Schneider, W. (1999) Entwicklung der Mitgliederzahlen, Beitragssätze, Versichertenstrukturen und RSA-Transfers in Zeiten des Kassenwettbewerbs – empirische Befunde im dritten Jahr der Kassenwahlrechte [Trends in membership levels, contribution rates, types of insurees and risk adjustment transfers during the period of insurer competition – empirical findings in the third year of fund choice], *Arbeit und Sozialpolitik*, 53(3/4): 20–39.

Nonneman, W. and van Doorslaer, E. (1994) The role of the sickness funds in the Belgian health care market, *Social Science and Medicine*, 39(19): 1483–95.

Normand, C. and Weber, A. (1994) *Social Health Insurance: A Guidebook for Planning*, Document WHO/SHS/NHP/94.3. Geneva: World Health Organization.

Okma, K. and Poelert, J. (2001) Implementing prospective budgeting for Dutch sickness funds, *European Journal of Public Health*, 11(2): 178–81.

Raad voor de Volksgezondheid en Zorg (Council for Public Health and Healthcare) (2000) *Europe and Healthcare*. Zoetermeer: Raad voor de Volksgezondheid en Zorg. http://www.rvz.net/Samenvat/Werk99/europe.htm (accessed 25 February 2001).

Roemer, M. (1969) *The Organization of Medical Care under Social Security*. Geneva: International Labour Office.

Ron, A., Abel-Smith, B. and Tamburi, G. (1990) *Health Insurance in Developing Countries: The Social Security Approach*. Geneva: International Labour Organization.

Schut, F.T. and van Doorslaer, E.K.A. (1999) Towards a reinforced agency role of health insurers in Belgium and the Netherlands, *Health Policy*, 48(1): 47–67.

Sheldon, T. (2000) EU law makes Netherlands reconsider its health system, *British Medical Journal*, 320(7229): 206.

Shiveli, A. and Chinitz, D. (2001) Risk-adjusted capitation: the Israeli experience, *European Journal of Public Health*, 11(2): 182–4.

Street, A., Carr-Hill, R. and Posnett, J. (1999) Is hospital performance related to expenditure on management?, *Journal of Health Services Research and Policy*, 4(1): 16–23.

van Doorslaer, E., Wagstaff, A. and Rutten F. (1993) *Equity in the Finance and Delivery of Health Care: An International Perspective*. Oxford: Oxford University Press.

Wagstaff, A., van Doorslaer, E., van der Burg, H. *et al.* (1999) Equity in the finance of health care: some further international comparisons, *Journal of Health Economics*, 18(3): 263–90.

WHO (2000) *The World Health Report 2000. Health Systems: Improving Performance*. Geneva: World Health Organization.

chapter four

Health financing reforms in central and eastern Europe and the former Soviet Union

Alexander S. Preker, Melitta Jakab and Markus Schneider[1]

Introduction

The transition economies of central and eastern Europe (CEE) and the former Soviet Union (FSU) confront the same challenge as established market economies in health financing: how to mobilize and allocate resources equitably and efficiently to satisfy a growing need and demand for health services. In transition economies, solutions have been attempted amid profound social, political and economic transformation. Health-sector reform has been characterized by the same themes that have characterized the social and economic transition from central planning to markets. This has included reducing direct state involvement (including decentralization, privatization and organizational reform), increasingly subjecting various actors to market forces and competition, and relying on market signals to guide resource allocation decisions.

In this chapter, we review the experience of transition economies with health financing reform since the early 1990s, based on a sample of 16 countries representing both CEE and FSU countries: Albania, Azerbaijan, Croatia, Czech Republic, Estonia, Georgia, Hungary, Kazakhstan, Kyrgyzstan, Latvia, Poland, Republic of Moldova, Romania, Russian Federation, Slovakia and Slovenia. Most countries entered the transition phase with a similar inheritance in terms of health financing systems characterized by high levels of financial and risk protection and equity. A decade into transition, however, these systems have diverged significantly. Three patterns seem to have emerged:

1 The first group includes countries that, despite the decline in economic output and public resources, have managed to maintain high levels of financial protection. These countries, which include Croatia, the Czech Republic and Hungary, are characterized by higher per-capita incomes, less severe economic decline and early health reforms implemented consistently throughout the country.

2 The second group comprises countries that have experienced deterioration in financial protection and equity. This group has had lower per-capita incomes and more severe economic decline with prolonged and inconsistent economic and political transition. Health system reform was also initiated more recently and is typically more fragmented. Representative countries include Albania and the Russian Federation.

3 Finally, the third group comprises countries that experienced serious deterioration in their health systems resulting from a drastic decline in economic performance in addition to their low initial income per capita. In these countries, which include Azerbaijan, Georgia and the Republic of Moldova, public financing has collapsed with a massive loss of resources for social services such as health care.

The same three clusters emerge in health financing reforms. The first group has moved to a Bismarck model predominantly financed by payroll taxes. This transition has been complex. In particular, introducing a social insurance model for health financing, with semi-autonomous quasi-state organizations, has been institutionally challenging. The main dilemmas included: whether to establish social insurance on a competitive or single-payer basis; adopting national versus decentralized revenue collection and pooling and/or purchasing systems; building management capacity in the quasi-state agencies; and clarifying the roles and responsibilities of these new organizations in relation to the ministry of health, ministry of finance and local governments.

The second group has had less comprehensive and smaller-scale reforms. Payroll taxes have been introduced as a complementary mechanism of resource mobilization, but general tax revenue still predominates. The effects of an inherited fragmentation of public-sector pooling and resource allocation mechanisms has become a key issue. At the same time, out-of-pocket payments – both formal and informal – have become a more significant revenue source than in the first group, with a parallel erosion in financial protection and equity despite legal entitlements to universal coverage.

Finally, in the third group, out-of-pocket payments have become the predominant mode of health financing, amounting to 50–80 per cent of total health revenue. This has severely reduced financial protection against the cost of illness. For these countries, rebuilding a system of resource mobilization from prepaid sources is a key reform priority.

In this chapter, we explore the factors that have led to the emergence of these three groups of countries and describe the health financing reforms adopted. In the next section, we present the analytical framework and key concepts. Next, we describe the macroeconomic context and give a detailed description of health financing reforms. We then discuss critical institutional issues that have supported or undermined the implementation of the envisioned new financing mechanisms. Finally, we present trends in indicators of health system performance and our conclusions.

Analytical framework

This chapter analyses health care financing in 16 CEE and FSU countries from the early 1990s, based on country-specific studies published by the World Health Organization (WHO) and the World Bank, the academic literature and cross-sectional data on health care expenditure.

'Health financing' is an imprecise term, encompassing several sub-functions related to the flow of resources through the health system. We discuss two aspects of health financing in detail: the mechanism for mobilizing resources and the pooling of various revenue sources. The third element of health care financing – allocating resources to (or purchasing services from) providers – is referred to in this framework but is not our focus. (This topic will be treated in greater detail in a forthcoming World Bank publication on resource allocation and purchasing in developing countries (Langenbrunner *et al.*, 2001).)

Table 4.1 illustrates the key characteristics used to describe each of these three sub-functions of health care financing. In terms of resource mobilization, prepaid revenue sources are contrasted with those collected by providers at the point of service, and whether payment of prepaid sources is compulsory or voluntary. Under pooling, this analytical framework emphasizes the fragmentation or integration of multiple revenue pools and their size as the critical determinants of the financial sustainability of health financing. Purchasing and resource allocation include the level and mix of services purchased, the population group covered, the providers of services and the payment mechanism adopted. The organizational and institutional issues related to the

Table 4.1 Analytical framework for improving the performance of health systems

	Raising resources	*Pooling and allocating resources*	*Purchasing*
Key characteristics	• Compulsory versus voluntary	• Fragmented versus integrated pools	• What to buy? • How much to buy?
	• Prepaid versus point of service	• Size of the pool	• For whom? • From whom? • How to pay?
Organizational and institutional variables	• Organizational form • Organizational incentives • Vertical and horizontal links		
Impact on performance	• Health, equity and financial protection and efficiency		

Source: adapted from WHO (2000)

sub-functions are also assessed. Finally, the framework takes into account the impact of changes in health financing on health, equity, financial protection and efficiency.

Macroeconomic context

All CEE and FSU countries experienced moderate to severe disruption in economic activity during the transition period. The closure of unproductive enterprises and industrial sectors and the collapse of previously established trade patterns – exacerbated in some cases by civil war – led to substantial declines in economic output in most countries. In the 16 countries reviewed, gross domestic product (GDP) declined in all but two in real terms between 1990 and 1997 (Table 4.2). The most serious decline (50–70 per cent) was experienced in the FSU countries. More broadly, the economic crisis that has swept CEE and FSU countries translated into declining real wages and increasing income inequality and poverty.

Parallel to these events, the tax base has been severely constrained by a decline in the formal economic sector, expanding activity in the informal sector and weak administrative capacity to enforce tax collection in the new market context. As a result, governments' ability to collect revenue and the total tax receipts needed to finance the social sectors have declined markedly in many of the countries examined. At the same time, expenditure pressure has grown because of increasing prices (especially for imported pharmaceuticals and medical equipment), demands for higher wages, technological developments in health care during the 1990s and increased expectations from people newly exposed to western European standards.

In this context, it is easy to understand why many health care policy-makers have looked for extra-budgetary sources of revenue while trying to maintain financial protection against the cost of illness and improve value for money (allocative efficiency) of scarce health care resources.

Key characteristics of health financing

During the socialist era, revenue for health care was generated mainly from the revenue of state-owned enterprises, and private sources were negligible except as informal payments to providers. Health expenditure was determined through the political bargaining process, in which the health sector competed with other claims on the government budget. Throughout the 1970s and 1980s, the health sector – as one of the economy's 'non-productive' sectors – received low priority in terms of overall public spending. Despite this relatively low level of spending, most countries offered their population a comprehensive range of services, ranging from ambulatory care to inpatient hospital care to population-based public health services. This low level of spending reflected the distorted prices characteristic of socialist economies.

In this section, we review two key dimensions of health financing in these countries: the sources of revenue and the pooling and resource allocation to purchasers.

Table 4.2 Trends in GDP and health expenditure in 16 CEE and FSU countries

	Per-capita GDP[a] (purchasing power parity in US$) 1997	Percentage change in real GDP[a] 1990–97	Per-capita health expenditure[b] (purchasing power parity in US$)				Total health expenditure as a percentage of GDP[b]		Real public health spending as a percentage of 1990 spending[b] 1997
			Total 1997	Public 1997	Private 1997	% Private	1990	1997	
Cluster A									
Croatia	6 735	−18	481.1	402.2	78.9	16.4	10.5	8.4	68.5
Czech Republic	12 930	−9	758.3	695.3	62.9	8.3	5.4	7.2	115.8
Estonia	7 504	−21	241.2	209.1	32.1	13.3	1.9	5.7	186.8
Hungary	9 914	−6	510.4	417.4	93.5	18.3	5.7	7.1	95.7
Slovakia	9 526	−2	617.6	498.4	119.2	19.3	5.4	7.8	113.3
Slovenia	14 032	4	897.0	802.8	94.2	10.5	5.6	7.6	149.2
Average, cluster A	10 107	−9	584.3	504.2	80.1	14.4	5.7	7.3	121.6
Cluster B									
Albania	2 683	−11	58.0	44.5	13.5	23.3	4.4	3.3	46.5
Kazakhstan	4 513	−40	123.7	83.5	40.2	32.5	3.3	4.1	57.9
Latvia	5 609	−45	195.4	151.2	44.2	22.6	2.5	4.5	77.8
Poland	7 438	27	413.9	315.4	98.5	23.8	4.6	6.5	132.1
Romania	6 209	−13	78.5	54.9	23.5	30.0	2.7	4.2	93.5
Russian Federation	7 031	−40	228.2	175.5	52.7	23.1	2.3	5.2	121.9
Average, cluster B	5 581	−20	182.9	137.5	45.4	25.9	3.3	4.6	88.3
Cluster C									
Azerbaijan	2 039	−57	64.5	11.9	52.5	81.5	2.6	7.4	21.8
Georgia	4 992	−68	34.6	4.3	30.3	87.5	3.2	4.6	28.9
Kyrgyzstan	2 310	−43	168.9	67.1	101.9	60.3	4.2	7.4	39.7
Republic of Moldova	2 175	−63	174.5	94.6	79.9	45.8	4.0	11.3	93.5
Average, cluster C	2 879	−58	110.6	63.1	62.0	60.2	3.5	7.7	46.0

Note: the averages are unweighted means for each cluster.

Sources: [a] World Bank (2000), World Development Indicators Central Database CD-ROM. [b] Authors' calculations based on published official figures and World Bank staff estimates and from household surveys where available. Detailed references are available from the authors on request

Figure 4.1 Percentage of total health expenditure financed by taxes and by social health insurance in 16 CEE and FSU countries, 1997 or latest available year

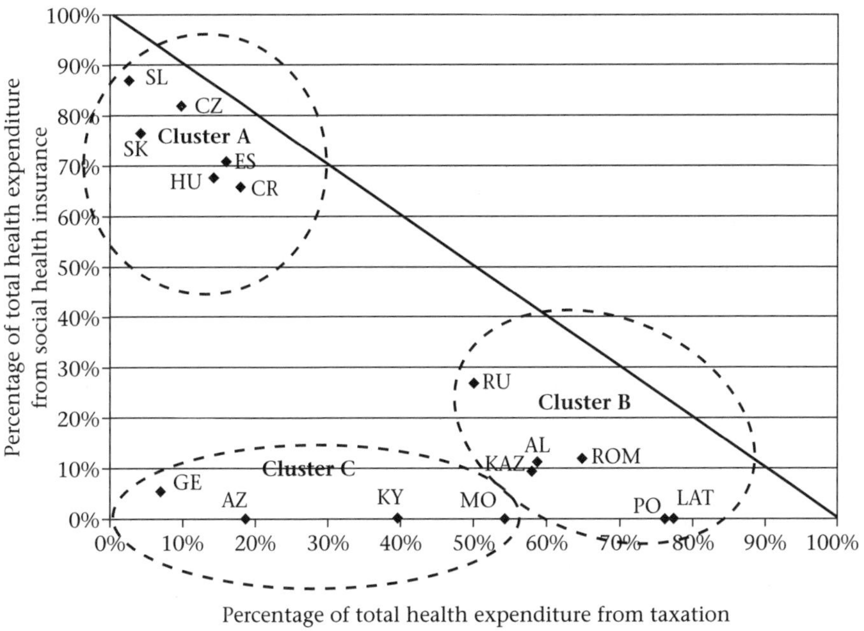

Percentage of total health expenditure from taxation

Key: AL, Albania; AZ, Azerbaijan; CR, Croatia; CZ, Czech Republic; ES, Estonia; GE, Georgia; HU, Hungary; KAZ, Kazakhstan; KY, Kyrgyzstan; LAT, Latvia; MO, Republic of Moldova; PO, Poland; ROM, Romania; RU, Russian Federation; SK, Slovakia; SL, Slovenia.

Source: Authors' calculations based on World Bank data. Details are available from the authors on request

Sources of revenue

One of the most important policy dimensions of revenue collection for the health sector is that adequate resources should be mobilized though prepayment in an equitable way. The more progressive the contribution plan (increasing contribution rates at increasing income levels), the more equitable the overall financing system. Out-of-pocket payments significantly reduce both financial protection against the cost of illness and the equity of the overall financing plan in terms of the burden of financing borne by poor people.

During transition, two new sources of funding emerged: payroll-based social health insurance and increased reliance on both informal out-of-pocket payments and official co-payments. Most countries have diversified health care financing sources, combining social health insurance, general tax revenue and private out-of-pocket payments. Private health insurance has not made strong inroads in any of the countries examined.

As Figure 4.1 illustrates, the relative proportion of these sources of financing separates the transition countries examined into three groups. Clusters A and B have maintained the predominance of prepaid revenue. The predominant source of financing in cluster A is social health insurance; cluster B continues to rely mostly on general tax revenue. Cluster C comprises countries in which prepayment has collapsed and the health system is now financed largely through direct out-of-pocket charges.[2]

A new revenue source: social insurance based on payroll taxes

Social health insurance based on payroll taxes has emerged as a standard part of a diversified source of health care financing in CEE and FSU countries, supplementing what is often dwindling general tax revenue. Of the 27 CEE and FSU countries, 14 have introduced payroll taxes – nine as a predominant mechanism of financing and five complementary to general tax revenue and out-of-pocket payments. In our sample of 16 countries, 14 have introduced payroll taxes – seven as a predominant source. This means that countries relying on general taxation as a predominant revenue source are under-represented in our sample and are factored into the assessment.

Contributions

The contribution rates for salaried employees are about 13 per cent in countries with social insurance as the predominant financing mechanism and between 2 and 4 per cent in countries in which it is a complementary source of revenue (Table 4.3). In most countries, the contribution rate between employers and employees is split equally. The contribution rate depends on such factors as the cost of the benefit package, the size of the covered population, the desirable level of redistribution towards non-employed people and other available sources of financing.

In most countries, the contribution rate was not calculated based on an actuarial analysis of expected cost and revenue for the insured population (Ensor 1999). Instead, the rate-setting process reflected a combination of optimistic eye-balling of desired revenue and guesses about the political acceptability of adding to the already heavy tax burden on employers and employees. In the mid-1990s, all social insurance taxes amounted to 30 per cent of total labour costs in a sample of 13 CEE and FSU countries, reaching as high as 40 per cent in some cases (Palacios and Palleres-Miralles 2000). This compares with 26 per cent in the high-income countries of the Organisation for Economic Co-operation and Development and under 20 per cent in the rest of the world (Table 4.3). Given the declining economic context, reducing high payroll taxes and thus labour costs were at the forefront of economic policies to jump-start growth. In response to the two opposing pressures of collecting more health revenue and reducing labour costs, the contribution rate has been adjusted frequently in most countries. For instance, the contribution rate in Croatia increased from 14 per cent in 1993 to 16 per cent in 1997 to 18 per cent in 1999. Conversely, Hungary reduced its payroll tax rate four times from a peak of 23.5 per cent in 1993 to 14 per cent (plus a flat fee) in 1997 (Table 4.3).

Most countries apply the same contribution rate to self-employed people (individual entrepreneurs and agricultural workers) as to salaried employees.

Table 4.3 Characteristics of health insurance contribution revenue in 16 CEE and FSU countries

	Year introduced	Payroll tax rate for health (1999)			Total social insurance taxes (mid-1990s)	
		Salaried (employer : employee)	Self-employed	Non-employed	As a % of gross wage	As a % of total labour cost
Cluster A						
Croatia	1993	18% (18% : 0%)	18% of declared income	18% of gross pension and other benefits plus central budget	43.0	36.0
Czech Republic	1993	13.5% (9% : 4.5%)	13.5% of 35% of net pretax income	Central budget transfer 13.5% of 80% of statutory minimum wage	48.5	35.9
Estonia	1992	13% (13% : 0%)	13% of declared income	Central budget transfer	33.0	24.8
Hungary	1990	14% (11% : 3%) plus hypothecated tax of US$170 per employed person	14% of declared income but at least the minimum; wage plus hypothecated tax of US$170 per person	Central budget; per-capita amount of transfer is not specified	60.5	40.6
Slovakia	1994	13.7% (10.0% : 3.7%)	13.7% of declared income	Central budget; per-capita amount of transfer specified as the contribution rate applied to 73% of the statutory minimum wage	46.0	34.1
Slovenia	1993	13.25%	13.25% of declared income	Central budget	45.8	37.2
Cluster B						
Albania	1995	Public: 3.4% (1.7% : 1.7%) Private: 3–5%	7% of statutory minimum wage	Central budget	42.5	32.1
Kazakhstan	1996	3% (3% : 0%)	3% of declared income	Per-capita oblast contribution for non-employed people	32.0	Not available
Latvia	1998	28.4% of personal income tax	28.4% of personal income tax	General budget transfer	38.0	27.7

Table 4.3   (*cont'd*)

		Payroll tax rate for health (1999)			Total social insurance taxes (mid-1990s)	
	Year introduced	Salaried (employer : employee)	Self-employed	Non-employed	As a % of gross wage	As a % of total labour cost
Poland	1999	7.5%	7.5% of declared income	7.5% of gross benefits	48.0	32.4
Romania	1999	14% (7% : 7%)	7% of declared income	7% income tax based on gross benefits	33.5	Not available
Russian Federation	1993	3.6% (3.6% : 0%)	3.6% of declared income	Central budget; per-capita amount of transfer is not specified	40.0	28.8
Cluster C						
Azerbaijan	No payroll tax for health				Not available	Not available
Georgia	1995	4% (3% : 1%)	4% income tax	Central budget, but amount unspecified	41.0	29.3
Kyrgyzstan	1997	2% (2% : 0%)	2% of declared income	Oblast region contribution of undetermined level	43.5	31.0
Republic of Moldova	No payroll tax for health				39.0	28.3

Sources: Palacios and Pallares-Miralles (2000) for overall social insurance rates and authors' compilations

Defining the contribution base for self-employed people is, however, a challenging task, as their income is irregular, often not in cash and difficult to verify. Some countries narrowly define the contribution base as the net income from selling personal services and goods; others rely on a broader definition that includes incomes such as royalties, revenue from patents and capital gains. Most countries have opted to introduce a required minimum contribution and a contribution ceiling, contributing to the regressive nature of this form of health care financing. In Hungary, for example, self-employed people must pay 14 per cent of their declared income or 14 per cent of the statutory minimum wage, whichever is higher. The government also introduced a flat per-capita fee, undifferentiated by income.

The third population group covered under health insurance encompasses non-employed population groups such as pensioners, children and other family dependants, officially registered unemployed people and poor people. Countries have used various mechanisms to cover their incurred expenditure. They may be covered indirectly through the contributions made by active population groups whose expected expenditure is less than their contributions. Second, they may be covered by explicit transfers from other public revenue sources such as central or local government budgets. Finally, the people covered may contribute directly by paying a premium levied on their cash benefits such as their pension or unemployment benefit.

When the source of funding for the non-employed population is a central or local government budget, the subsidy often does not fully cover the cost of care provided for the target population in question. This is especially true for pensioners, who use health services more than other segments of the population and whose care is often the most expensive because of the seriousness of their illnesses. Thus, the transfers are often notional and bear little relation to costs. In other cases, the transfer is not linked to the benefit group at all. For example, in the Russian Federation, the health insurance law mandates that the local government budget contribute to the mandatory fund on behalf of the non-employed population, although neither the level of such contributions nor the mechanism for enforcing this obligation has been defined. Not surprisingly, local government contributions have not always been forthcoming, and a distinct gap often remains between local budget resources and the revenue needs of the insurance funds. Furthermore, the different territories vary significantly in executing these financing responsibilities (World Bank 1997; Sheiman 1999).

Payroll taxes have yielded less revenue for the health sector than had been anticipated. First, the contribution base has continued to decline in many transition countries for several reasons: an increasing dependency ratio caused by the ageing of the population and unemployment; a decline in real incomes; arrears from bankrupt formerly state-owned and new private enterprises; and tax evasion in both the shrinking formal sector and growing informal sector. Evasion can take several forms: under-reporting private-sector earnings, especially by self-employed people; increased use of non-taxable forms of employee remuneration such as food, clothing and fuel allowances; and under-reporting of income by formal-sector employers and hiring staff on a short-term or contractual basis (Ellena *et al.* 1998). The high contribution rates in many transition countries created incentives to shift economic activity into the informal sector, at least during the initial years of transition when tax administration systems were weak.

Second, most CEE and FSU countries are under strong pressure to reduce the total fiscal burden (general and payroll taxes) in an attempt to stimulate the private sector, international competitiveness and economic growth. This has led many policy-makers to lower the payroll tax contribution rate, even when such a cut would lead to deficit financing. The expectation that downward pressure on the revenue side would lead to improved expenditure control has not materialized. Third, when health revenue is collected by a central collection agency that also collects other employment-related revenue, the money dedicated for health may be used to informally cross-subsidize expenditure for other benefits.

Population coverage

In principle, population coverage has remained universal, since most countries have retained the inherited legal safeguards to free access. In practice, however, the social insurance countries (cluster A and some countries in cluster B) have passed overriding health insurance legislation, tying active contribution status to eligibility. Nevertheless, this legislative effort has had little practical implication, since the contribution status of most individuals is not known when they contact service providers. The lack of effective information technology has prevented governments from addressing the missing link between contributions and benefits because the system does not allow them to explicitly identify those not current in their contributions. As better information technology becomes available, the eligibility status of those with a poor contribution record will become apparent. This will also reveal the issues not yet addressed of the eligibility of millions of workers in the agricultural sector and of those working increasingly under contractual as opposed to salaried arrangements. This will force policy-makers to explicitly address the problem of social exclusion of certain population groups in these countries.

Countries that have remained with general taxation have also not explicitly reduced the population coverage. As the decline in public resources was greater than in cluster A countries, there has been a loss of overall social protection for the whole population. Although some countries have had discussions to reorient public resources to cover only poor people and other vulnerable groups (such as Armenia), no effective policies have yet been implemented.

Social insurance benefits

In terms of benefits of social insurance programmes, the difference between the predominantly social insurance countries (cluster A) and the rest is pronounced. Cluster A countries have a comprehensive benefit package, and only the Czech Republic has chosen to explicitly define a benefit package with a list of services to be covered from public sources of financing (World Bank 1999b). In the other countries, services have been excluded at the margin in such areas as dental care, cosmetic surgery and non-curative services, such as treatment in sanatoriums, health spas and various forms of home care. For example, Croatia, the Czech Republic, Hungary and Poland have excluded (or introduced official co-payments for) high-frequency, low-cost services such as dental care, drugs, glasses, hearing aids and allied health services (Goldstein et al. 1996; Gaal et al. 1999; Karski et al. 1999; Vulic and Healy 1999). As the resulting loss of financial protection is not significant, the public absorbed these measures as a necessary price for the transition to a market economy. In contrast, the exclusion of low-frequency, high-cost interventions and setting priorities based on cost-effectiveness have been met by strong opposition both from the public and physicians and have had limited implementation.

Social health insurance in clusters B and C covers a limited range of benefits. In these countries, payroll taxes are a complementary revenue source to general taxes and out-of-pocket payments. In Albania, the social insurance benefit package finances primary care and pharmaceuticals, whereas the central budget pays for outpatient specialist and inpatient care (Nuri and Healy 1999). In Kyrgyzstan, social insurance only covers inpatient pharmaceuticals and, recently, a limited list of outpatient drugs (Kutzin 2000). In Georgia, social insurance initially covered only nine federally selected programmes chosen for their cost-effectiveness and epidemiological significance. By 1998, this list was increased to 28 through an increasingly politicized rather than evidence-based process (World Bank 1998a). In the Russian Federation, health insurance programmes typically pay for salaries, food and medicine for acute care services.

Most countries have opted to ration services by not making any explicit decisions regarding the scope and range of services. In these countries, non-specific broad expenditure control has pushed rationing decisions to the level of providers. Unfortunately, providers faced with enormous expectations and demand from the population often find it easier to allow the quality of services to deteriorate – through drug shortages, equipment breakdowns, depreciation of capital stock and lowering of hygiene standards – than to make politically and ethically difficult rationing decisions (Staines 1999; Alizade and Ho 2000). Also, providers in this context appear to ration the supply of services based on the ability and willingness of patients to pay for them, often through informal charges (see Chapter 8).

Increasing reliance on out-of-pocket payments

A second major change in health care financing has been the increase in out-of-pocket payments. Before transition, most CEE and FSU countries guaranteed free health care to their citizens. Official fees for services were rare during the socialist era and co-payments for drugs were low, although by the late 1980s informal charges had already become widespread in some of the former socialist countries.

Economic decline, together with fiscal and political reforms, during the transition changed this situation dramatically. The emerging paradox was how to achieve the objectives of economic and political liberalization while preserving the social protection the population had come to expect after decades of a cradle-to-grave welfare system. The emphasis on individual responsibility reduced state paternalism, and reducing the tax burden became a central part of fiscal and social policy throughout the region. Nevertheless, the population in most countries has reacted negatively to attempts to roll back social benefits and charge user fees for previously free services such as health care. The democratic process has offered an outlet for expressing discontent with unpopular reforms, leading to frequent changes in government and shifts in policy direction.

Few countries have reached a sustainable and coherent balance between these opposing forces. In cluster A countries, health services continue to be officially free in the Czech Republic, Hungary, Poland and Slovakia. In these countries, official co-payments (if any) are low, and reducing the range and scope of benefits, even at the margin, has been politically difficult. Reducing excess capacity through closing beds and labour adjustments has also been difficult. Exposure to western European practices of health care and increasing consumerism in other parts of the economy has fed expectations of higher consumer quality and a broader range of services. This has led to a greater willingness to pay for higher-quality health care through informal payments. These informal payments have provided a powerful incentive for providers working in public facilities to provide benefits that are not part of the government's official programme, and they often undermine official policy, as the willingness to 'buy' better health care through informal payments has other objectives (see Chapter 8). Nevertheless, although informal payments have increased, the previous mentality of universal entitlement to free health care restrained the growth of out-of-pocket payments, as did the ability of these governments to continue to fund health care services.

By contrast, in many cluster B and C countries – which suffered the most severe economic decline – the significant reduction in government revenue and in the size of the formal labour market has led to a collapse in prepaid financing for the health sector. Out-of-pocket spending – both formal and informal – as a proportion of total health expenditure amounts to 87 per cent in Georgia, 82 per cent in Azerbaijan, 60 per cent in Kyrgyzstan and 46 per cent in the Republic of Moldova (Figure 4.2, Table 4.2). To compensate

Figure 4.2 Percentage of health expenditure that is prepaid versus paid at the point of service in 16 CEE and FSU countries, 1997 or latest available year

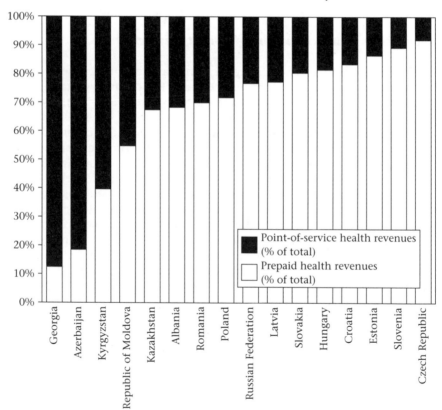

Source: Authors' calculations based on World Bank data. Details are available from the authors on request

for the loss of public revenue, most governments have introduced user charges, based on an official fee schedule, to raise additional resources. However, the official fee schedules often apply to a limited group of services that are part of the publicly funded benefit package. Physicians are free to charge for all other services. Moreover, physicians often forego charging official fees that would benefit the hospital and public services, since this cuts into the informal payment that they keep. Although some countries have subsidy programmes to exempt poor people from official charges, these arrangements have not worked well and do not cover informal payments.

In Georgia, the Ministry of Health regulates the official fees that hospitals can charge for services included in the publicly financed benefit package. Hospitals are required to post fee schedules in visible places. Nevertheless, only 3 per cent of total out-of-pocket expenditure is officially regulated fees. Twenty-four per cent of out-of-pocket expenditure is illegal gratuities for services covered by government programmes. The rest of out-of-pocket expenditure (73 per cent) is for goods and services not covered by government programmes. Over-the-counter pharmaceuticals, a major expenditure item, are not covered by exemptions and place an especially high financial burden on very poor people (World Bank 1998c).

Azerbaijan's experience is similar. Revenue from prepaid sources declined by 79 per cent in real terms between 1992 and 1997 and currently make up less than 20 per cent of total health revenue. At the republican level, the Ministry of Health made most hospitals and research institutes self-financing. The government introduced an official fee schedule for point-of-service payments but exempts half the population, based on categorical targeting, to protect poor people (MacFarquhar 1998). Many hospitals do not observe this exemption, and the government does not cover their cost through a subsidy. In contrast to Azerbaijan and Georgia, the Republic of Moldova did not introduce official out-of-pocket payments, yet private payments contribute to nearly half of total health care resources (UNICEF 1997).

Continued role of general taxes

Despite the introduction of social health insurance and an increase in out-of-pocket expenditure, general tax revenue remains a significant, although not predominant, source of financing in CEE and FSU countries. In cluster B and C countries, general tax revenue is the predominant public (compulsory) revenue-raising mechanism. In these countries (mostly FSU countries), tax revenue comprises a combination of national and local government taxes. In FSU countries, resources for health care are raised at the national (federal/ republican) level, at the regional (*oblast*) level and the district (*rayon*) level. The amount each level of government allocates for health care depends on local priorities. In most cases, the level of government collecting the revenue determines the proportion of general tax to be allocated for the health sector. Only two countries – Georgia and Romania – have earmarked taxes levied on tobacco and alcohol for health care.

Only a few countries rely on explicit equalizing mechanisms to the sub-national level to compensate for the differential revenue-raising ability of local governments. As a result, health care financing is very geographically inequitable in these countries.

In the Russian Federation – despite its payroll tax – general taxation remains the dominant source of revenue for the sector. The amount of available resources still depends on the prevailing budget-allocation process under which health often does not receive priority (Sheiman 1999). Furthermore, local authorities have dramatically decreased their participation in funding health care. The share of local budgets allocated to health slid from 18 per cent in 1993 to 12 per cent in 1998, making the central budget allocation even more important as the largest source of financing for health.

In Kazakhstan, the state budget funds mainly give priority to vertical programmes such as preventing and controlling HIV infection and AIDS, tuberculosis and vaccine programmes and health promotion programmes. By 1998, the republican government was financing less than 10 per cent of total health expenditure. Local budgets are used to fund 314 specific programmes, which include local specialty hospitals, institutions for tuberculosis and AIDS, vaccination and blood banks. Once again, without equalization transfers among the regions, this makes health care financing extremely inequitable.

The Republic of Moldova is one of the few countries examined that relies on general taxes as the only mechanism for prepaid revenue. Local governments cover about two-thirds of public expenditure for health and the central government one-third. Local governments are responsible for essentially all outpatient care facilities, local (*rayon* and rural) hospitals and emergency care (such as ambulances). The central government covers specialized care provided by a group of 17 large national hospitals and specialized national programmes (such as tuberculosis control and preventing HIV infection and AIDS) and part of sanitary-epidemiological and health education expenditure. Once again, local government spending varies widely, creating significant inequity across the country (although average per-capita expenditure was 87 lei in 1997, per-capita spending varied from 9 lei to 153 lei). Overall public spending on health also varied significantly between 1997 and 1998 – some regions experienced no change, whereas others declined more than 50 per cent in public resources (World Bank 1999a).

Pooling and resource allocation to purchasers

The second important function of health care financing is to pool the resources' collected from various sources and to allocate these resources to the organizations that directly pay providers. The two most important policy dimensions in pooling and resource allocation are the extent to which resources are transferred from rich to poor people (income redistribution) and from healthy to sick people (risk-sharing). Pooling and resource allocation are important instruments in achieving appropriate risk protection, equity and allocative efficiency.

Raising resources from one predominant source – such as general taxes – does not in itself ensure any of the above objectives if these resources are raised regressively at different administrative levels or are allocated to the healthy and richer segments of the population (see Chapter 2). The two important aspects of a well-designed pooling function are the extent to which multiple revenue channels are integrated or fragmented and the size of the population for which purchasing decisions are made.

Fragmentation in pooling

In many CEE countries and in the FSU countries in particular, the multiple revenue channels are not pooled. These fragmented revenue sources are often further splintered during the budget allocation process to multiple purchasers and providers. A single purchaser may receive revenue from one or several insurers, the national budget through the ministry of health, one or more local budgets through various levels of local government and patients' out-of-pocket payments. Each of these purchasers, although technically in a monopsony situation, is still prevented from realizing the potential benefits of its purchasing power because of overlaps in coverage, unclear specification of the benefit package, fragmentation of the revenue pool during the budget allocation process to the individual providers associated with ('owned by') each level of government, and the rigid rules and inherited practices governing the allocation of resources to providers.

In the Russian Federation, facilities receive funds from several sources, including the regional health insurance fund, the regional budget, local budgets, the Ministry of Health budget as well as private out-of-pocket payments (World Bank 1997). Allocation of budgetary revenue – be it local government or the Ministry of Health – is still based on inputs and reflects a lack of proactive purchasing. These budget transfers, based on capacity-linked normative standards (staff and beds), offer providers incentives to maintain as large an infrastructure as possible to maximize their income even if it increases the unit cost of treating the population.

In Kyrgyzstan, as in the Russian Federation, pooling of public budget funding for health care is organized at the level of government that owns the health facilities for which the funds are provided. Hence, the national Ministry of Health pools funds for national health facilities, each oblast health department pools funds for oblast health facilities and, similarly, each rayon (district) and municipality pools funds for its facilities. Because rayons and municipalities exist within oblasts, and because most national facilities are located in the capital of Bishkek, the pools and the catchment populations served overlap significantly (Kutzin 2000).

In the smaller countries predominantly funded by social insurance (Croatia, Hungary, Slovenia and others), revenue channels are less fragmented. In these countries, payroll taxes for social health insurance are allocated mostly for operational expenditure, but even there pooling remains an issue for two reasons. First, operational expenditure is not pooled with capital expenditure. Operational expenditure is typically funded from social insurance revenue, whereas capital investment is funded from budgetary (central and local) sources. This creates moral hazard for those making capital investment decisions (such as local governments), as they will not have to bear the operating expenditure of their decisions. This is a particular problem for the allocation of foreign aid resources. Second, tertiary facilities such as university clinics and national institutes receive funding for operational expenditure through social insurance, but also receive funding from central budget sources for teaching and research. Thus, these flagship facilities are more shielded from the impact of declining health revenue than other providers and can put off painful adjustment decisions. For instance, in a profiling review of debt-making, hospitals in Hungary university clinics topped the list.

Decentralization

A further complication in pooling has occurred through decentralization – that is, the transfer of state functions to local political and administrative levels. This process of decentralization originated outside the health sector and was motivated by a political rationale. Nevertheless, the health sector was affected in many ways, such as a change in the ownership of providers and the transfer of revenue-raising rights to local levels. The resulting institutional structure, however, often created rather than solved problems. In principle, decentralization offers a chance to bring health services closer to local needs and improve accountability. In practice, decentralization often further fragments the revenue pool and exacerbates geographical inequity. As a result of some of the negative consequences experienced, the pendulum has begun to swing back the other way, and some countries are beginning to recentralize. For example, in Estonia, the former 17 purchasing pools have been merged into eight pools and, in Hungary, the 19 county regional health insurance branches have been merged into the single national fund with most administrative functions centralized.

Institutional issues in health financing

During the socialist era, the organizational arrangement for health care financing in most countries was as an integrated part of the public bureaucracy (Yugoslavia, a notable exception, used payroll taxes even in the pre-transition period). In most cases, funds were transferred directly from the ministries of finance to the ministries of health, which were in charge of health financing, resource allocation, governance of providers and stewardship of the sector. This mechanism was somewhat more complicated in federal states such as the Russian Federation and countries with regional allocation mechanisms. Following the transition, the countries that switched to payroll tax revenue for a large share of health care financing established semi-autonomous quasi-state agencies to perform this function. These new social health insurance organizations often become involved in raising revenue, allocating resources, governing providers and sometimes even in providing stewardship. In this section, we review the predominant organizational forms that have emerged in health financing, the related organizational incentive structures and issues related to horizontal and vertical links.

Figure 4.3 Organizational forms for the relationships among transacting parties in health care

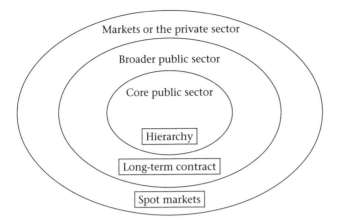

Organizational forms

Following the categorization of Williamson *et al.* (1991), there are three organizational forms for the relationship among transacting parties: hierarchies, long-term contracts and spot markets (Figure 4.3). These three organizational forms can also be applied to the health sector and give some interesting insight into some of the reforms that have taken place in transition.

In CEE and FSU countries, the three organizational forms happen to coincide with the three sources of funding discussed previously. Funding through general revenue by the ministry of finance is part of the hierarchical public bureaucracy. Payroll taxes are administered by social health insurance organizations that are quasi-state agencies with a long-term contract (explicit or implicit) to perform the financing function on behalf of the core public sector. Out-of-pocket expenditure allows direct spot-market transactions between patients and providers. The three organizational forms co-exist within any one country, but their relative weight corresponds to our earlier categories: in cluster A countries, the predominant organizational form is long-term contracts, cluster B countries rely on hierarchies and, to varying extents, spot markets have become the predominant organizational form in cluster C countries.

In general, the sources of funding and the organizational form of the financing function are not inherently linked. In other words, financing through general tax revenue can be organized through long-term contract arrangements. However, such arrangements are rare because public finance laws constrain the use of budgetary resources. In general, there is more legal flexibility for using payroll taxes administered as extra-budgetary funds.

Hierarchies

Following the transition, some countries maintained a hierarchical organization in health care financing. This organizational form is most typical in countries where general tax is the predominant source of funding, such as Albania and the Russian Federation. The core public sector collects revenue, allocates resources and provides services through a hierarchical bureaucracy. Although such command-economy organizational arrangements should, in principle, augment governments' strategic control over the health care system, in practice it stifles innovation, is unresponsive to the population's changing needs and is often associated with capture by political interests. As a result, in the countries that have maintained this system of health care financing, the ministry of health still governs by fiat instead of incentives or rational criteria based on equity considerations, efficiency, cost-effectiveness of services and quality of providers.

Long-term contracts

The shift from general revenue to payroll taxes has been associated with the creation of a new organizational form – social health insurance organizations. These new organizations are in reality quasi-state agencies mandated to carry out the financing function for government through an implicit long-term contract (in some cases, this contract is explicit). The creation of these organizations was often motivated by a belief that it would increase transparency and accountability, send a signal to the people that health services were not free and make the decision-making process less politicized. Some of these objectives were achieved; others were not. Payroll taxes have made it painfully clear to both employers and employees that health care is not free. But obscure governance arrangements and the lack of explicit contracts between government and health insurance organizations have clouded transparency and accountability. The decision-making process has remained highly politicized.

Spot markets

Finally, spot-market transactions between patients and providers are now common throughout CEE and FSU countries, in response to the liberalization of providers and the inability of the public sector to match expectations with sufficient public resources. These transactions often occur in the growing informal health sector and are not sanctioned by the government. Although this organizational form has become very prevalent, it undermines financial protection against the cost of illness, and the incentives to providers often conflict with officially promoted government policies. As a result, hierarchies and long-term contracts remain the preferred organizational form, and policy-makers in most of the countries examined are actively trying to control and reduce such spot-market transactions. Policy-makers, however, do not control the feasibility of these efforts directly, and it may take a while to do anything about it except for creating private pre-payment schemes.

Organizational incentives

Experience from other sectors and organizational reforms of providers indicates that the shift from reliance on hierarchies to long-term contracts as a predominant organizational form requires major parallel shifts in the incentive

Table 4.4 Organizational incentives for health systems according to form of organization

	Hierarchy		Long-term contract		Spot market
	Ministries of health or finance	Local governments	Social security organizations	Community financing schemes	Private insurance
Decision rights (autonomy)	Limited		Moderate	High	High
Market exposure	None		Variable (depends on market structure)	High	High
Financial responsibility	Limited		Limited	High	High
Accountability	Government, voters		Government, board	Community	Owners
Social functions	Implicit mandates		Variable	None	None or explicit

Source: adapted from WHO (2000)

regime of the organization in question if it is to avoid creating dysfunctional organizations (Jakab *et al.* 2001). The following five incentives are examined briefly: decision rights, accountability, residual claimant status (financial responsibility), market exposure and explicit coverage of social functions (Table 4.4). As in the hospital sector, a key failing of the semi-autonomous social health insurance agencies introduced in the region has been the frequent inconsistency in the way these five incentives were designed and implemented.

Decision rights

In many of the countries that have established social health insurance funds, the new agencies have been granted extensive but unclear decision rights over a wide range of activities: personnel, financial management, revenue collection and even modifications in the contribution rate and policy content of the benefit package. This has often brought the new agencies into conflict with the ministries of finance, which are anxious to control contribution and spending at times of fiscal constraints. It has created tension with the ministries of health, which want to retain overall control over health policy. Few countries have found an appropriate balance between the often conflicting objectives of the health insurance agencies exercising their decision rights and the core ministries wanting to retain control over activities that were explicitly transferred to these agencies.

Accountability

In the pre-transition era, accountability was ensured by hierarchical direct administrative control exercised by the ministries of health and finance. This control consisted of sanitary inspections by the public health network and financial inspections to ensure resource spending according to the budget line items. With the creation of semi-autonomous health insurance funds, new accountability instruments were also introduced. In most countries, the parliament is the ultimate accountability forum for health insurance organizations. The budget of health insurance organizations is tabled and discussed in the parliament, together with an official audit by the state audit agency of the previous year's financial performance.

However, additional accountability instruments such as performance monitoring, community involvement, explicit long-term contracts and market discipline were often missing, and the ministries of finance and health often lost control over core decisions. This has led to widespread suspicion of fraud and corruption. In Hungary, this has led to a recentralization of some of the core functions, such as revenue collection, rate-setting and benefit-package definition. The National Health Insurance Fund was eventually brought back under the direct control of the Ministry of Finance.

Residual claimant status

Residual claimant status refers to an organization's ability to keep the savings it generates and accept responsibility for financial losses. Core ministries of health during the socialist era were not true residual claimants, since unspent resources had to be returned to the ministries of finance, and deficits were usually written off at the beginning of the next fiscal year. Theoretically, the new health insurance agencies were supposed to have true residual claimant status. In practice, deficits in anticipated income from contribution collection have been offset by subsidies from the state budget. In many countries examined, a cross-subsidy from the contributing population was expected to cover the cost of the non-contributing population without making this subsidy explicit and without giving the agencies a chance to increase revenue or control expenditure policies. The ministry of finance usually kept overall control over the contribution base and rate, and the ministry of health controlled expenditure policies.

In the Russian Federation, for example, the Health Insurance Law passed in 1993 established one federal and 88 regional off-budget insurance funds. By March 1999, the Minister for Health reported that arrears to medical workers totalled 3.5 trillion roubles (US$615 million). The total debts of the compulsory health-insurance system were about 17 trillion roubles (US$3 billion) in 1997, including unpaid state contributions on behalf of non-employed people (Alizade and Ho 2000). The Russian Federation is an extreme example because of the magnitude of its deficit, but it is not a lone example. In Croatia and Hungary, the health insurance system experienced chronic structural deficits that reoccurred annually, although lower than those in the Russian Federation.

Market exposure

In other sectors of the economy, agency creation is usually associated with some sort of market exposure, and market discipline is one of the mechanisms used to replace hierarchical control. In the health sector, the need for financial protection against the cost of illness and the adverse selection that often occurs in competitive insurance markets have led many countries to deliberately avoid market exposure in social health insurance. Only two CEE and FSU countries – the Czech Republic and Slovakia – have chosen to move to competing health insurers as the predominant mechanism to raise and allocate resources for health care. In both countries, contributions remain income-based, and co-payments for health services are not officially allowed. Both the fee schedule and the benefit package are prescribed by law. Competition among insurers is, therefore, severely limited, and the cost of such competition – higher administrative costs – may outweigh its benefits (Massaro *et al.* 1994; World Bank 1999b).

Explicit coverage of social functions

When public agencies that provide social services are made autonomous or privatized, policy-makers have to ensure that concern for the bottom line and market exposure do not lead to the exclusion of low-income and other vulnerable groups. During the transition in the health sector, in addition to budget transfers, one of the most common ways used to achieve this objective has been to cross-subsidize the cost of covering non-employed population groups through higher contributions by the actively contributing population. As described earlier, in most countries the actual cost of care for the non-employed population (especially elderly people) has been higher than these two sources of income. Throughout CEE and FSU countries, this has led to structural deficits that created a no-win situation for both government and social health insurance agencies. This is a catch-22 situation: most agencies must maintain a balanced budget, but their income is almost always less than the expenditure they are required to make. The net effect is that the state ends up subsidizing the deficit instead of the non-employed population groups they could have explicitly covered in the first place. This undermines the financial discipline and accountability objectives for which these agencies were created.

Horizontal and vertical links

As the institutional environment has seen a proliferation of actors and transfer of functions and responsibilities, the links among the new and old actors can improve or stifle the policy-making process. In horizontal links, some countries fully separate revenue collection and purchasing. The tax collection agency collects all revenue, including payroll tax. The collected payroll tax earmarked for the health sector is transferred in its entirety to the purchaser. Georgia, Hungary, Latvia and the Russian Federation recently adopted this approach. In other social insurance countries, the purchaser is also responsible for collecting payroll taxes, and the tax collection agency transfers resources on behalf of non-contributors. Examples include Croatia, the Czech Republic and Estonia. In other countries with social insurance, a social insurance agency that collects all payroll taxes for social benefits (such as pensions) collects all payroll taxes for health insurance but is separate from the government agency responsible for collecting general tax revenue. The social insurance agency is responsible for allocating its revenue to the various social programmes, including health. Examples include Kyrgyzstan and probably several others.

In CEE and FSU countries as elsewhere, there is still active debate on the relative merits of having separate agencies to collect social health insurance premiums. The proponents for an administrative integration between general tax collection and the collection of social health insurance argue that it improves contribution compliance, since it forces everyone who pays taxes to contribute, it avoids duplication in administrative costs and it provides better overall fiscal control over public revenue. Those who favour separate collection systems argue that moving from a universal to contribution-based entitlement may actually improve compliance with paying contributions – especially given a growing informal sector – since contributors are more motivated when paying for something with tangible benefits. With current technology, it is easy to cross-check contribution compliance between the general tax system and social health insurance system. They also argue that having separate collection systems allows social health insurance agencies to collect, track and monitor information much more closely than is possible when the general tax system collects the premiums (most tax systems only track such data in the aggregate on a yearly basis). Finally, they argue that expenditure control has little to do with collecting revenue and is often performed better by social insurance agencies than the poorly managed economic departments of ministries of health. Unfortunately, good evidence to support either of these claims is lacking and is beyond the scope of this chapter.

A separate but related issue relates to vertical integration between collecting revenue, pooling, purchasing and delivering services. Many countries have recently experimented with a provider–purchaser split. No CEE or FSU country has experimented with a health plan like that in the United States (which creates a split between the collection of revenue and the purchasers), so little evidence is available on the relative merits or disadvantages of this approach.

Impact on performance

The health financing system in most transition economies has changed significantly, either because of explicit and directed reform efforts or because of the indirect impact of macroeconomic shocks. The key changes that have taken place include diversification of the revenue base (mainly the introduction of social health insurance and growth in out-of-pocket expenditure), multiplication of the revenue channels and a variety of organizational and institutional changes. In this section, we examine how these changes have affected three broad indicators of health system performance: health expenditure, equity and financial protection, and efficiency. We do not include their impact on health outcomes here. Although population health has changed significantly in these countries, the origins of these changes are attributable to many economic and social factors and probably only to a very limited extent, if at all, to changes in health financing. Any such changes are more likely to be caused by the level of health financing rather than changes in the system of health financing.

Trends in health spending

Table 4.2 illustrates the marked differences in the trend and level of health expenditure among the three clusters of CEE and FSU countries since the early 1990s. As the three clusters differ not only in the nature of their health financing reforms but also in macroeconomic trends, delineating whether alternative forms of financing have yielded better results is impossible. In other words, the countries that have moved to social insurance (cluster A) are the ones with higher initial incomes and less severe macroeconomic declines. The ones labelled cluster C started the transition with the lowest per-capita income and experienced the most severe and prolonged economic shocks. This lack of a natural experiment in CEE and FSU countries makes it difficult to create a counterfactual case and allows only for speculation about what would have happened if the higher-income countries had continued to finance health care predominantly from general taxes.

On the positive side, payroll taxes have generated a non-arbitrary revenue source for the health sector that is not subject to the political bargaining process at the time of tabling the annual government budget. On the negative side, however, payroll tax revenue is subject to socioeconomic factors equally outside the control of health policy-makers. All countries implementing social insurance based on payroll taxes experienced more difficulty than expected with this new revenue source. Rising unemployment, an ageing population, growth of the informal sector and increased liberalization of employment arrangements in the formal sector all contributed to a shrinking revenue base and dwindling contribution revenue. This should send a word of caution to policy-makers in countries with high dependency ratios, large informal sectors in urban areas and significant rural populations: shifting from general revenue to payroll tax may not yield significantly greater health revenue while increasing labour costs.

Of the six countries in cluster A, four recorded substantial increases in their public health care resources between 1990 and 1997 in real terms, and two registered declines. The 1997 level of public spending in real terms for the group was 22 per cent higher than in 1990. This suggests that, despite an overall decline in economic output during the transition period (only Slovenia surpassed its real GDP level in 1990), the health sector was partly shielded from the total overall loss in government revenue. The total payroll tax rates (including health, pensions and other) in cluster A countries are now similar to many western European countries, causing concerns about the impact of this development on labour costs, growth of informal market activities and international competitiveness.

By contrast, both prepaid and total revenue have declined in real terms in most countries in clusters B and C. By 1997, on average, public expenditure had dropped by 18 per cent in cluster B countries and by 54 per cent in cluster C countries. Most concerning is the dramatic decline in the lowest-income countries – a 78 per cent real decline in public expenditure for Azerbaijan, 71 per cent for Georgia and 60 per cent for Kyrgyzstan.

The share of private out-of-pocket expenditure shows a reverse trend. Where the decline in public resources was the most significant, private out-of-pocket expenditure has become a more significant source of health care financing. Both on a per-capita basis and as a share of GDP, out-of-pocket expenditure was greater in cluster C countries than in cluster B countries. This suggests primarily inadequate public expenditure and public authorities' difficulty in controlling direct out-of-pocket expenditure, even in countries that have laws and constitutions that say that health care is free of charge at the point of use.

In terms of health spending as a share of GDP, cluster A and C countries spend about 7 and 8 per cent of GDP, respectively, approaching western European spending levels relative to GDP. This is a significant increase from the 1990 spending level of 6 and 4 per cent, respectively. In cluster A countries, social insurance mobilized increased resources; in cluster C countries, this occurred through increased out-of-pocket payments. In cluster B, total health expenditure as a share of GDP increased to a lesser extent.

Trends in financial protection and equity

In most transition countries, health financing has become less equitable since the early 1990s for two reasons. First, out-of-pocket expenditure, which affects low-income groups the most even when subsidy programmes are in place, has increased significantly. Payroll taxes, which are typically proportional and have a ceiling, are usually less progressive than general taxation (Wagstaff et al. 1999). In very low-income countries that have shifted to direct consumption taxes as a major source of general revenue and have large informal sectors that do not contribute to formal taxation, this generalization is not true, and proportional contributory programmes may be more progressive than general tax financing.

Second, in cluster C countries, out-of-pocket expenditure has become the main source of financing for health care and, in cluster B countries, such direct charges have increased significantly. In both cases, this has eroded financial protection against the cost of illness. Available national household surveys increasingly report that the increase in out-of-pocket expenditure has affected poor people more than other people, becoming a significant risk factor for poverty in the lower-income countries (UNICEF 1997; World Bank 1999a,b,c). Two examples of these effects follow.

First, access for poor people has been reduced. Based on national surveys in Azerbaijan and Georgia, about 50 per cent of survey respondents reported that they did not seek treatment when ill for financial reasons (World Bank 1998b,c). In the Republic of Moldova, 30 per cent of all respondents did not seek care when ill because of a lack of financing. Lack of resources was a major reason for not seeking care for the lowest three income quintiles (33, 56 and 36 per cent, respectively) versus only 14 per cent in the second highest income quintile and 0 per cent in the highest (UNICEF 1997). Such situations occur even in cluster B countries. In the Russian Federation, among households earning less than 400,000 roubles (about US$70) in 1997 (roughly the lowest income quintile), 18 per cent did not seek inpatient care when ill and 36 per cent did not seek outpatient care (Feeley et al. 1998).

Figure 4.4 Infant mortality rates (< 1 year) and child mortality rates (< 5 years) among the population quintile with the lowest income (left columns) and highest income (right columns) in Kyrgyzstan and Kazakhstan, 1997

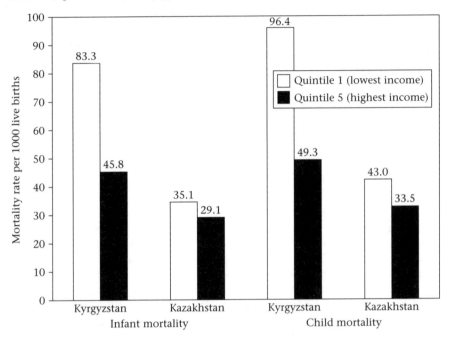

Sources: Gwatkin *et al.* (2000a,b)

Second, the cost of illness is a risk factor for poverty. The cost of one episode of hospitalization is often several times the average monthly household earnings. Many individuals are depleting their savings, selling their assets (including productive assets such as cattle and land) and going into debt to pay for health care in some of the poorest countries where out-of-pocket expenditure is highest. In Georgia, of those who were hospitalized, poor people on average paid 70 per cent of their monthly household earnings for health care. In the poorest quintile, 40 per cent of the households reported having to borrow funds or sell property to finance health expenditure (World Bank 1998a). In the Republic of Moldova, more than 30 per cent of respondents in the two lowest income quintiles reported having to borrow funds to meet the unexpected costs of illness. In the higher-income groups, respondents coped with unexpected health expenditure by relying on family income and savings (UNICEF 1997).

The emerging evidence on whether these trends have had a differential impact on the health status of poor people and on equality in health outcomes is not comprehensive and is to be interpreted with caution. For instance, in Kyrgyzstan, infant and under-5 mortality rates in the lowest income quintile are nearly twice the rates in the highest income quintile (Figure 4.4). This ratio is significantly smaller in Kazakhstan, which has higher per-capita income than Kyrgyzstan.

The available figures for health services utilization by quintile, however, do not show the same pattern. For both immunization and deliveries attended by trained staff, utilization rates do not differ across income quintiles (Gwatkin *et al.* 2000a,b). If these two services are indicative of utilization trends of general health services, it means that the observed trend in health equity can be attributed to either trends outside the health sector or systematic differences in the quality of care received by rich people and poor people. Given the findings of utilization surveys from other countries (see above) that suggest that equity in access declined significantly, the utilization trends of these two services might not be an appropriate reflection of trends in general health services. In other words, deliveries and immunization are priority services that are less likely to be affected by the decline in public resources than health services in general and thus access remained more protected.

Efficiency

Improving efficiency was an explicit objective of most health care financing reforms in the countries examined. Improvement in technical efficiency is expected by improving incentives and management practices and improvement in allocative efficiency by reorienting care from hospital to outpatient, primary and social care. However, these have little to do with the source of revenue, although user fees might alter the behaviour of some providers. When health financing mechanisms are compared, comparing the administrative efficiency of various financing arrangements would be helpful, but these costs are difficult to isolate systematically. Even for multiple collection systems that clearly increase the overall administrative cost of collecting revenue, determining whether the accompanying improved access to information actually improves overall efficiency is difficult. Many CEE and FSU countries are reversing earlier policies that established separate collection agencies, leaving only the purchasing function to the social insurance funds. More research is needed to determine whether this will improve the overall efficiency of the collection of revenue to pay for health care.

Conclusions

The CEE and FSU countries have been a fascinating social laboratory for reform in health care financing since the early 1990s.

- In the higher-income countries, social insurance appears to be an effective part of mobilizing resources for the health sector. However, in countries with lower incomes, less institutional capacity and little formal employment, payroll taxes are not necessarily a viable alternative to general taxation.
- Without strong strategic purchasing, social insurance cannot be automatically associated with improved expenditure control and administrative efficiency, nor is there evidence that it directly affects health outcomes or the quality of the service delivery system.

- Changing the source of financing for the health sector has significant implications for equity: financial protection risks deteriorate when policy-makers allow out-of-pocket expenditure to grow in an uncontrolled manner as a major source of revenue for the health sector; and social insurance is often more regressive than general taxation.
- Finally, shifting revenue collection from the central hierarchy to quasi-state agencies has created significant tensions among the different loci of stewardship of the health system. This issue still needs to be resolved in most countries.

This study has pointed to several unresolved issues that require further investigation. One key issue relates to the administrative efficiency of separating (or integrating) the collection of health insurance premiums from the collection of general taxes or a broader array of payroll taxes. Much more work is needed to unravel this issue and ensure that the transaction cost of change does not exceed the potential gains.

Finally, experience in the CEE and FSU countries seems to indicate that the creation of semi-autonomous agencies to perform the function of collecting and pooling revenue for the health sector is highly vulnerable to capture by vested stakeholders, whose motives may be very different from overall societal objectives. Countries that proceed down this route need to better balance increases in decision rights and market exposure with more effective accountability mechanisms, financial responsibility and social functions.

Notes

1 The chapter greatly benefited from the insights of a country case study on the Russian Federation by Igor Sheiman (1999) and one on the Czech Republic by Martin Dlouhy (1999).
2 These constructed clusters are heterogeneous. For instance, some cluster C countries had a more extreme transition (such as Azerbaijan) than others (such as Kyrgyzstan).

References

Alizade, N. and Ho, T. (2000) *Hospital Restructuring*. Washington, DC: Human Development Unit, Europe and Central Asia, World Bank.

Dlouhy, M. (1999) *Czech Republic – Case Study*, unpublished manuscript. Prague: VSE.

Ellena, G., Orosz, E. and Jakab, M. (1998) Reforming the health care system: the unfinished agenda, in L. Bokros and J-J. Dethier (eds) *Public Finance Reform During the Transition*. Washington, DC: World Bank.

Ensor, T. (1999) Developing health insurance in transitional Asia, *Social Science and Medicine*, 48: 871–9.

Feeley, F.G., Boikov, V.E. and Sheiman, I.M. (1998) *Russian Household Expenditures on Drugs and Medical Care*, unpublished manuscript. Boston, MA: Boston University.

Gaal, P., Rekassy, B. and Healy, J. (1999) *Health Care Systems in Transition: Hungary.* Copenhagen: European Observatory on Health Care Systems.

Goldstein, E., Preker, A., Adeyi, O. and Chellaraj, G. (1996) *Trends in Health Status, Services, and Finance*, World Bank Technical Paper No. 341. Washington, DC: World Bank.

Gwatkin, D.R., Rutstein, S., Johnson, K., Pande, R. and Wagstaff, A. (2000a) *Socioeconomic Differences in Health, Nutrition and Population in Kazakhstan.* Washington, DC: HNP/Poverty Thematic Group, World Bank.

Gwatkin, D.R., Rutstein, S., Johnson, K., Pande, R. and Wagstaff, A. (2000b) *Socio-economic Differences in Health, Nutrition and Population in Kyrgyzstan*. Washington, DC: HNP/Poverty Thematic Group, World Bank.

Jakab, M., Preker, A. and Harding, A. (2001) Hospital reform in transition economies, in A. Preker and A. Harding (eds) *Innovations in Health Services. Vol. 1: The Corporatization of Public Hospitals*. Baltimore, MD: Johns Hopkins University Press.

Karski, J.B., Koronkiewicz, A. and Healy, J. (1999) *Health Care Systems in Transition: Poland*. Copenhagen: European Observatory on Health Care Systems.

Kutzin, J. (2000) *Review of Kyrgyz Social Expenditures*. London: Institute for Health Sector Development.

Langenbrunner, J., Preker, A. and Jakab, M. (2001) *Resource Allocation and Purchasing of Health Services in Developing Countries*. Washington, DC: World Bank.

MacFarquhar, R. (1998) *Health and Education Financing in the Republic of Azerbaijan*. Washington, DC: Human Development Unit, Europe and Central Asia, World Bank.

Massaro, T.A., Nemec, J. and Kalman, I. (1994) Health system reform in the Czech Republic: policy lessons from the initial experience of the general health insurance company, *Journal of the American Medical Association*, 271(23): 1870–4.

Nuri, B. and Healy, J. (1999) *Health Care Systems in Transition: Albania*. Copenhagen: European Observatory on Health Care Systems.

Palacios, R. and Pallares-Miralles, M. (2000) *International Patterns of Pension Provision*, Social Protection Discussion Paper No. 0009. Washington, DC: World Bank.

Sheiman, I. (1997) From Beverige to Bismarck: health finance in the Russian Federation, in G. Sheiber (ed.) *Innovations in Health Care Financing*, World Bank Discussion Paper No. 365. Washington, DC: World Bank.

Sheiman, I. (1999) Health care funding in Russia: transition to health insurance model, unpublished manuscript. Moscow: Boston University.

Staines, V. (1999) *A Health Sector Strategy for the Europe and Central Asia Region*, Health Nutrition Population Series. Washington, DC: World Bank.

UNICEF (1997) Accessibility of health services and evaluation of expenditures on health in the Republic of Moldova, unpublished manuscript. New York, UNICEF.

Vulic, S. and Healy, J. (1999) *Health Care Systems in Transition: Croatia*. Copenhagen: European Observatory on Health Care Systems.

Wagstaff, A., van Doorslaer, E., van der Burg, H. *et al.* (1999) Equity in the finance of health care: some further international comparisons, *Journal of Health Economics*, 18(3): 263–90.

WHO (2000) *The World Health Report 2000. Health Systems: Improving Performance*. Geneva: World Health Organization.

Williamson, O.E., Winter, S.G. and Coase, R.H. (1991) *The Nature of the Firm: Origins, Evolution, and Development*. Oxford: Oxford University Press.

World Bank (1997) *Health Sector Support Strategy: Russia*. Washington, DC: World Bank.

World Bank (1998a) *Georgia Project Concept Document: Health II*. Washington, DC: World Bank.

World Bank (1998b) *Azerbaijan Poverty Assessment*. Washington, DC: World Bank.

World Bank (1998c) *Georgia Poverty Assessment*. Washington, DC: World Bank.

World Bank (1999a) *Health Expenditure Review: Republic of Moldova*. Washington, DC: World Bank.

World Bank (1999b) *Social Sector Development in Transition in Czech Republic – Toward EU Accession*, World Bank Country Report Series. Washington, DC: World Bank.

World Bank (1999c) *Azerbaijan Poverty Assessment Report*. Washington, DC: World Bank.

World Bank (2000) *World Development Indicators Central Database CD-ROM*. Washington, DC: World Bank.

chapter five

Private health insurance and medical savings accounts: theory and experience

Alan Maynard and Anna Dixon

Introduction

In this chapter, we focus on two private mechanisms for funding health care – private health insurance and medical savings accounts. We refer specifically to countries outside the European Union (EU). Chapter 6 analyses the role of voluntary health insurance within EU countries.

In the first section, we consider the potential advantages of private health insurance and discuss its traditional failures. Then we appraise the performance of private insurance systems in relation to the policy objectives of equity in financing and access, macroeconomic efficiency and allocative, technical and administrative efficiency. Next, we present case studies analysing the experience of private health insurance in the United States, Switzerland, Australia and Chile. These examples demonstrate that the challenges of private insurance are common across countries and are generally tackled similarly. Finally, we focus on medical savings accounts, with particular reference to their implementation in Singapore and more briefly in the United States. We argue that private health insurance without adequate regulation fails to meet society's policy objectives. Even with heavy regulation, it is not an efficient or equitable way of funding health care.

The market for private health insurance

Neo-liberalist economists believe that the market can optimally allocate resources. However, this is based on the assumption of perfect competition. In

Table 5.1 Market failures in health care financing

Market failure	Consequences	Measures used to correct failures	Empirical outcomes
Adverse selection	Little risk-pooling, no insurance market, only some people insured	Educating people to take out insurance	Ineffective
		Tax subsidy	Ineffective
		Compulsory universal coverage	Effective
		Lifetime enrolment	Effective
Risk selection	No insurance for disabled, sick, poor and elderly people	Open enrolment	Moderately effective
		Community rating	Moderately effective
		Risk-adjusted premiums for individuals	Technically unfeasible
Monopoly or insurance cartel	Excess profit, poor quality products and underproduction	Anti-trust laws	Effective
Moral hazard	Overuse of services by patients	Deductibles or co-insurance	Moderately effective
		Gatekeepers	Patient dissatisfaction
		Waiting lists	Patient dissatisfaction

Source: Hsiao (1995a)

health care, with several specific market failures, regulation may be advocated to overcome them (Table 5.1) (Hsiao 1995a). Generally, an unregulated health insurance market does not work efficiently for the following reasons:

- Individuals may have knowledge about their health that can be concealed from the insurer (adverse selection).
- Ill health is highly probable for people with pre-existing conditions or hereditary or chronic diseases and elderly people, making them 'uninsurable'.
- The insurer lacks information about the current and future health status of the individual, which makes estimating future claims and calculating a risk-rated premium difficult.[1]
- Once insured, individuals may participate in risk-taking behaviour or affect their need for services (moral hazard). This 'risk' is often excluded from private health insurance at the time of enrolment.
- The probability of falling ill is not always independent of the probability of someone else falling ill because some diseases are communicable.

Potential advantages and disadvantages of private health insurance

Private health insurance as a means of funding health care may have several advantages in practice:

- enabling the demands of relatively affluent people to be self-financed, leaving the government to target (limited) public resources on delivering health care for poor and disadvantaged people without access to private health insurance;
- mobilizing additional resources for infrastructure that may benefit poor and rich people alike;
- encouraging innovation and efficiency, which may catalyse the reform of the public sector, because of its flexibility and the profit motive (Chollet and Lewis, 1997); and
- increasing choice for the consumer.

Such potential advantages may or may not be realized: how private health insurance performs depends on its design and regulation and how it interfaces with the public sector. Private health insurance also has potential problems in practice. The analysis here is limited to information problems related to defining the benefits package and setting premiums.

Defining the benefits package

For competition to operate in the health insurance market, people must be able to compare the benefit packages of different plans. If a standard minimum package is not regulated, the potentially positive role of competition based on consumer choice is greatly diminished.

Consumers are likely to be uncertain about the health care benefits being offered when they purchase private insurance in most countries. Regulators worldwide are seeking to reduce this uncertainty by pressing for the definition of a basic benefits package – the size and content of what is available to consumers (Ellwood *et al.* 1992). For example, the Office of Fair Trading (1998) in the United Kingdom recommended that insurers should create a benchmark or core term product. Such a basic package would facilitate comparison of differing products by consumers. However, insurers typically are loathe to comply. Until a core or basic package is defined, consumers will be very uncertain about what their insurance purchase will provide for them as compared with what they would get from other insurers.

Setting premiums

Premiums can be risk rated (based on an individual assessment of the future risk of ill health), community rated (based on the average risk in a defined group or population) or group rated (based on the average risk of employees in a firm). Because people who know they are likely to need care are more likely to purchase health insurance (adverse selection), competing health insurers usually adopt risk rating and charge higher premiums to individuals likely to be at greater risk of using care. As a result, private health insurance tends to discriminate in favour of healthy, young adults who use little health care. Because of the potential for spreading financial risk across several people, many private insurers only market their plans to groups (usually of employees). Purchasing individual insurance, therefore, tends to be very expensive, and poorer people (with a risk of ill health that is higher than average) have great difficulty purchasing health insurance (Chollet and Lewis 1997). Although government subsidies for poor people to purchase insurance have been widely discussed (Ellwood *et al*. 1992), such schemes have been difficult to implement successfully.

Because older people need relatively more health care, private insurance coverage tends to be available only at a very high premium after retirement. Thus in South Africa and Chile, retirees 'drop out' of the private sector (Medical Aid Societies and the ISAPRES) into the public sector (van den Heever 1998). Furthermore, insurers may exclude specific conditions from coverage, shifting the costs of care for these to the public system. If government forces insurers to insure sick people ('poor risks'), who are often elderly, the insurers may leave the market.

Community rating is often developed based on a concern for equity and solidarity. In the context of voluntary purchase of insurance, however, good risks (relatively healthy people) may consider the community-rated premium too expensive and exit the pool to self-insure, leaving the less good risks to drive up the community-rated premium and gradually make insurance less affordable.

Unless there is a single pool consisting of the entire population of a country (such as a national health service), regulators have to define the rules governing pooling. Without appropriate regulation, there will be market segmentation, cream-skimming and exclusion of vulnerable groups, which may be inconsistent with social objectives. In particular, solidarity principles may be undermined, as can be seen in the export of private health insurance to Latin America (Perez-Stable 1999; Stocker *et al*. 1999). For instance, in Mexico, in an effort to improve the efficiency of the public sector, it was proposed that more affluent people should be allowed to opt out of social security and transfer their contributions to private insurers (in a way similar to that created by the Pinochet regime in Chile). This was resisted in Mexico because it was seen that the migration of these 'good risks' to the private sector would leave the state with the 'poor risks', and the average cost of provision would rise.

In the United States, most insurance is group rated and employer plans cover 90 per cent of the people who are privately insured (Gruber 1998). The greater purchasing power of large employers and generous tax incentives mean that group-rated insurance among large employers is better value than either individually purchased insurance or group-rated insurance for small employers. Many of the people without any insurance are low-income workers and employees of small firms. In 1998, employers' health plans covered 47 per cent of the employees of firms with less than 200 workers. Average premiums among small firms were about 10 per cent higher than the average premiums of large firms and usually offered fewer benefits with higher deductibles (Gabel *et al*. 1999). The group rating of premiums benefits those in large employee pools but leaves employees of small firms and self-employed people with high risk-rated premiums.

The complexity of market regulation

Regulating markets is an element in making competition work: using resources efficiently and controlling costs. However, private health insurance markets are often not regulated adequately.

In an effort to create such a regulatory framework for the United States, a group of academics, insurers and providers met at Jackson Hole in Wyoming (Ellwood *et al.* 1992). Their efforts demonstrate the complexity of regulation required to create and sustain a competitive health care market anywhere in the world. The architects of these proposals identified six causes of market failure in the United States health insurance market:

- *Cost-unconscious demand*: with the third party (insurer) paying passively for benefits, neither providers nor consumers have an incentive to economize.
- *Biased risk selection as a source of profit*: insurers can garner profits by product differentiation and cream-skimming.
- *Market segmentation to minimize price competition*: large numbers of complex heterogeneous benefit packages segment the market, making comparison difficult and choice based on price practically impossible.
- *Lack of information on outcomes relative to cost*: little outcome measurement and a reluctance to focus such investments on care packages rather than particular events.
- *Little choice for members of small groups*: half the employed people in the United States are in groups of less than 100 and have little choice of health plan.
- *Perverse public subsidies*:[2] tax breaks benefit rich employees – the richer the insuree, the greater the subsidy. Subsidies might be better targeted at poor people to facilitate their sustained membership of plans.

Market characteristics such as these are ubiquitous and require careful regulation. To remedy these market failures in the United States, the Jackson Hole Group proposed an elaborate and complex regulation framework. The major elements of the proposals were:

- *Universal access*: federal legislation would ensure everyone has access to at least a minimum benefit package, financed through a combination of obligatory employer contributions, government subsidies and individual resources.
- *Choice of packages*: at least one collective purchaser acting on behalf of small employers (health insurance purchase cooperative) would be created in each state that could pool risks across employer groups and exploit economies of scale in financing and purchasing.
- *National regulation*: three standard-setting boards would be established to ensure uniform definitions and uniform standards of performance, to ensure clinical effectiveness information and to ensure the market worked efficiently.

These plans were described as a 'blueprint without a real life counterpart' (Reinhardt 1993): the regulation was in principle correct but in practice could not be implemented. The Jackson Hole proposals were ambitious, complex and resource intensive. They suggest that, for a health financing system characterized by managed care similar to that in the United States to work efficiently, a complex and coordinated set of regulations and incentives is needed to encourage private markets to serve the public interest.

Performance of private health insurance

In this section, we focus on health policy objectives that recur in reform debates around the world (Hsiao 1995b; Maynard and Bloor 1995). Those especially relevant to an analysis of private health insurance are equity in financing and access, macroeconomic efficiency and allocative, technical and administrative efficiency.

Equity in financing and access

Wagstaff *et al.* (1999) and van Doorslaer *et al.* (1999) conclude that private health insurance contributes to the regressivity of health care financing in the United States and Switzerland. However, in Germany and the Netherlands, mainly affluent people purchase private insurance, and it therefore contributes to the progressivity of the financing system. The same effect, but to a lesser extent, is seen in England and Portugal, where the purchase of private health insurance is concentrated among affluent people (Wagstaff *et al.* 1999). Drawing conclusions about the impact of private health insurance on equity in different contexts requires an assessment of the overall effect on equity (combining an analysis of the distribution of cost and benefits). In terms of equity on the delivery side, private health insurance creates access based on a willingness and ability to pay and typically discriminates against poor, ill and elderly people. Such discrimination creates inequality in access to services and may ultimately widen the gap in inequality in health outcomes.

Equitable access to health care has been further undermined as a result of greater sophistication in risk rating, which enables insurers to select preferred risks. The result is that a growing number of people in the United States lack private health insurance. The export of private health insurance to many Latin American countries has threatened solidarity because of private incentives to 'skim' the market, leaving poor risks and elderly people in the state system. Such effects can be seen in Chile and elsewhere, but have been resisted to date in Mexico (Perez-Stable 1999; Stocker *et al.* 1999).

Macroeconomic efficiency

The policy discussion of macroeconomic efficiency tends to focus either on concerns about how health expenditure 'crowds out' other forms of public and private expenditure or how it affects wage costs and international competitiveness.

The argument that public expenditure crowds out private expenditure on health care has no substantial empirical support. Research into whether the expansion of Medicare is 'crowding out' private health insurance in the United

States seems to show that, because of the income definition of Medicare, it is unlikely that people can substitute between the two (Shore Sheppard *et al.* 2000).

United States economists argue that private health costs do not affect competitiveness under the present health system. They argue that private health insurance costs do not raise overall labour costs but simply change the composition of labour costs from wages to benefits. There is no knock-on effect on prices and the ability to sell products overseas, therefore, remains unaffected. Even if labour costs increased, other studies have suggested that this would affect the value of the dollar and not international competitiveness (Glied 1997). However, because insurance is often provided by employers, it reduces the flexibility of the labour market: employees are reluctant to move jobs due to transitional loss of access to benefits (Gruber 1998).

The desire to have macroeconomic cost control of health care expenditure is well articulated by finance ministries around the world. Two main schools of thought currently inform decisions as to how expenditure control can best be achieved: market competition or cash-limited budgets.

Some people who advocate market competition as a means of controlling costs recognize that extensive regulation would be needed for this purpose (Ellwood *et al.* 1992). Others advocate the market without any government intervention, including tax subsidies (Friedman 1962).[3] The evidence base for such advocacy is limited, as in most areas of health care policy there is continuous reform (social experimentation) but little evaluation.

Private health insurance is usually one of several sources of revenue. Even in the United States, where everyone who can afford to do so should voluntarily purchase insurance, government financing of health services accounts for a significant share of total health expenditure. Multiple sources of funding are more difficult to control than a single source. Furthermore, where multiple sources exist, an effort to reduce the flow of funds down one 'pipe' (such as tax-funded expenditure) can lead to compensatory increases in funding down other pipes (such as private insurance). Although the evidence base is incomplete, a consensus appears to exist that, if the goal is cost containment, single-pipe tax-financed systems are superior to multiple-pipe insurance systems in macroeconomic cost control.

Allocative efficiency

In an ideal world, the market is supposed to allocate resources optimally. In practice, the resource allocation process in the private insurance sector (as in the public sector) is unclear. Neither the public nor the private sector can fund all the health care demanded by users.[4] A crucial policy issue, therefore, is how access to care will be rationed or priorities set[5] to allocate health care resources efficiently. The issue, for both the public and private sectors, is which criteria should determine access to care. There is no obvious criterion in the private sector apart from willingness and ability to pay. This leaves open the question – willingness and ability to pay for what?

If clinical effectiveness alone were to drive private-sector reimbursement, many insurees would be given what is inefficient but clinically effective. If user preferences (as determined perhaps by provider preferences because of supplier-induced demand) determine the contents of the benefits package, again the system could be clinically effective but inefficient (Maynard 1997a).

In most countries, private insurers compete with or complement the state system. If the state allocates based on ability to benefit (cost-effectiveness), the private sector will be left with a residue (such as what is inefficient and costly). Private health insurance may also cover cost-effective services because the public sector does not deliver them because of mismanagement, such as hip and knee replacements and cataract removal in the National Health Service in the United Kingdom. Private health insurance may cover more rapid access to services or the costs of amenities (such as private hospital rooms) not covered in the public insurance benefit package.

Technical efficiency

Achieving technical efficiency depends on several factors, not all of which are directly related to the source of funding. However, how purchasing is organized can have a significant influence on the ability of a system to achieve technical efficiency. A system predominantly funded by voluntary contributions to private insurance companies has a fragmented funding pool and purchasing function. The monopsonistic purchasing present in most publicly financed systems[6] does not exist if there are multiple private insurers;[7] the insurers tend to be price takers rather than price makers. Only since the early 1990s, with the creation and export of managed care (in particular, the introduction of vertical integration between insurer and provider or contracts between an insurer and selected providers), have private insurers strengthened their leverage over providers and begun to define and enforce contracts with providers more vigorously. However, even when individual insurers function as quite active purchasers, the nature of a private insurance market fragments and dilutes this purchasing power at the level of the health care system.

Anti-trust legislation has been one obstacle to developing the insurers' purchasing potential. In principle, insurers using their power separately or in collaboration to affect service delivery in terms of price, quantity and quality can be construed as using monopolistic market power.[8]

Administrative efficiency

Transaction costs may be systematically higher in a health system with competing insurers than in a monopsonistic system because of the costs associated with marketing, promotion and underwriting. In addition, if private insurers operate on a for-profit basis, further revenue needs to be generated to pay shareholders' dividends (see Chapter 6).

Private health insurance in practice

In this section, we present the experience with private health insurance of four countries outside the European Union. These case studies have been chosen because, in each, private health insurance has been promoted as the main source of revenue and coverage for the population (or a significant group within the population). The first study reviews the private health insurance market in the United States, emphasizing in particular the changes resulting from the shift to managed care. Although many purchasers are controlling providers more strictly, private health insurance has failed to attain the objectives of cost control and efficiency at the system level. In both Australia and Switzerland, private health insurance was promoted as the main form of coverage in the past. Concerns about solidarity and cost control led to policy reversals with the introduction of tax-financed universal insurance in Australia in 1984 (Medicare) and mandated purchase of health insurance in Switzerland in 1996. The final case study on Chile shows how private health insurance has been implemented in one middle-income country and the implications for the public sector.

The United States

In the United States, private health insurance is the sole form of coverage for the people not eligible for federal and state programmes such as Medicare (for elderly people), Medicaid (for some poor people, inside and outside the labour force) and the Veterans Administration (for former and current members of the armed forces). Insurance is mainly organized by employment groups (group rated), with the employer determining the choice of available insurers. This means that, in practice, employees have little or no choice of insurance carrier.

The private health insurance market in the United States was dominated in the mid-1980s by a system of indemnity insurers that paid providers on a fee-for-service basis. The system was the epitome of a price-taking market in which insurers paid providers with little questioning of price, quantity and quality. Fees for hospital and physician payments were determined based on their being 'usual, customary and reasonable'. Table 5.2 illustrates some of the features of this transition from indemnity insurance to managed care. Iglehart (1995) and Rivo *et al.* (1996) have reviewed the specific organizational forms and methods of managed care.

Before managed care, the fee-for-service system combined with federal subsidies led to over-insurance and cost inflation two or three times the rate of growth in the consumer price index. Managed care reduced the rate of inflation, and the percentage of gross domestic product (GDP) spent on health care stabilized at about 13.6 per cent from 1992 to 1996. Nevertheless, the denominator was growing and hence total spending increased even in these years (Levit *et al.* 1998). However, since 1997, inflation has re-emerged and premiums are increasing at twice the rate of the consumer price index.

Table 5.2 Private-sector paradigms in the 1980s and 1990s in the United States that are emerging elsewhere

1980s	1990s
Fee-for-service payments to providers ('usual, customary and reasonable charges')	Capitation payments to providers
Passive purchasers (insurers are price-takers)	Aggressive, organized purchasers (insurers are price-makers)
Open choice of many plans	Limited choice of plans
Managed care (health maintenance organizations) was marginal	Managed care (health maintenance organizations) was dominant
Free (open) choice of providers	Restricted choice: closed panels and primary care gatekeepers
Independent physicians (solo or small groups)	Managed physicians in group practice
Independent hospitals and facilities	Larger integrated systems of hospitals and facilities
Little attempt to control utilization	Tighter utilization management with problems of arbitrary guidelines and a poor evidence base

Managed care, which now covers over 80 per cent of employees, gave temporary palliation but no sustained control of cost inflation (Maynard and Bloor 1998). Although efficiency may have increased somewhat (at least technical efficiency, even if not preferred by many consumers!) measured at the level of some individual insurers, managed care has failed to contain costs at the system level in the medium term. The reason may be that care is managed at the level of individual insurers; there has been no system-wide remedy such as proposed by the Jackson Hole Group. Thus, despite the innovative managed-care techniques, the health system remains fragmented and the actions of individual insurers can do little to affect the aggregate performance of the system.

There is also evidence that inequity is increasing; for example, about 250,000 people per year are giving up insurance for cost reasons, even though the economy has been prospering and employment has grown.

Many advocates of managed care believe that it has not failed but it has not been designed efficiently with an appropriate regulatory framework. However, the legislative effort required to remedy regulatory deficiencies by, for instance, a Jackson Hole regulatory framework seems as difficult to implement in the United States as a national health insurance scheme. The stalemate is unlikely to be resolved unless economic downturn and loss of benefit act as a political catalyst for some kind of reform.

Switzerland

Until 1996, purchasing health insurance in Switzerland was a voluntary and individual act. Premiums were individually risk rated, but because Switzerland is relatively affluent and premiums are relatively low (supported by general tax subsidies), 98 per cent of the population was insured (Minder *et al.* 2000). The proportion of subsidies in relation to expenditure declined from the mid-1970s, undermining the solidarity of the system, with insurers exerting pressure on the insurees (through higher premiums) rather than on the suppliers (Theurl 1999). Further cost escalation in health care in the 1980s drove up the cost of premiums, making insurance less affordable. As a result, increasing numbers of people, especially those with pre-existing conditions and elderly people, found it difficult to purchase health insurance. The desire to control costs and promote solidarity led to a policy reversal in 1996.

The Health Insurance Act of 1996 established a system of compulsory health insurance for all residents of Switzerland. Insurance is provided by companies and funds, which are prevented from making a profit from their compulsory health insurance activities. Premiums are community rated (for all subscribers to one company within a canton or sub-region of a canton), and tax-financed means-tested subsidies are targeted at individuals (Minder *et al.* 2000).

The transition from an unregulated market for voluntary health insurance to a highly regulated system of compulsory health insurance has ensured universal coverage but has failed to contain costs: Switzerland still has one of the highest shares of GDP spent on health care (10 per cent) as well as a very high GDP (OECD 1999).

Several reasons may explain this: supply-side pressures, especially physician power and the adoption of unproven, high-technology interventions; expansion of the benefits package; fragmentation of purchasers reducing leverage over providers; and continuation of fee-for-service reimbursement of providers. Thus, the health care system continues to lack cost control and microeconomic efficiency. The source of funds (or changes to these) appears to have had little influence on these objectives. However, residents are now guaranteed coverage for a comprehensive range of benefits.

Australia

For four decades, the focus of the policy debate in Australia has been the public–private mix for health care, with Labour governments reducing its role and National governments fostering its development. Premiums have been community rated since 1953 with the aim of ensuring equitable access to health insurance regardless of risk. The purchase of private health insurance despite community rating has been concentrated in the wealthiest households (Schofield 1997; Hall *et al.* 1999). At its peak in 1970, before the introduction of universal public health insurance, 80 per cent of the population had private health insurance (Australian Institute of Health and Welfare 1999). Universal tax-financed health insurance was first introduced in 1975, but its role has been altered frequently since. Since Medicare was established in 1984, the proportion of the population with private insurance has declined from about 50 per cent to 30 per cent. Under Medicare, everyone has free access to medical care in public hospitals, thus reducing demand for private health insurance. Further disincentives to the purchase of private health insurance include the escalating cost of premiums and the largely unexpected out-of-pocket payments faced by privately insured people.

The current (National) government, honouring election commitments, has introduced extensive new subsidies. From July 1997, single people earning less than A\$35,000 and couples earning less than A\$70,000 annually were offered a part rebate on private insurance premiums (the annual average income at that time was A\$32,700). In January 1999, a 30 per cent tax rebate on health insurance premiums was introduced. In July 2000, a Lifetime Healthcover programme was introduced to encourage young people to purchase insurance coverage by allowing the premium to rise over the life cycle in relation to the age at which coverage was first purchased. The opportunity cost of these subsidies is considerable, some A\$2.19 billion (Duckett and Jackson 2000).

The chequered history of private health insurance in Australia reflects the political ideology of the ruling parties as much as its success or failure. Since 1996, a political consensus has favoured the continued existence of Medicare (Harris and Harris 1998), but this has not silenced debate on the role of private funding. Since Medicare was introduced, the role of private health insurance has been ambiguous (Hall *et al.* 1999). The massive public subsidies, which currently benefit wealthy people, are justified (rhetorically) on the grounds that private funding is essential to the sustainability of the public sector (Duckett and Jackson 2000).

Such policy interventions are familiar worldwide. The Australian policies, however, are more radical and comprehensive and, therefore, undermine equity and generously subsidize relatively well off people.

Chile[9]

The economic restructuring by the Pinochet regime separated the public and private sectors. All workers pay a mandatory health care contribution of 7 per cent of their earnings. All contributors have a choice: they can elect to direct their contribution to a private insurer (ISAPRE) or to the state scheme (FONASA). Their decision is determined by the value of the contribution and the cost of the available benefit packages. In general, young, affluent and healthy people purchase private insurance and old, poor and unhealthy people use the public sector. In 1998, FONASA served two-thirds of the population and spent about US\$200 per capita (of which administration was 4 per cent) and private insurers served one-third, spending US\$300 per capita with administrative costs of 20 per cent. The private sector has 15 insurers. There is no community rating and over 3000 benefit packages are available. The private insurance market in Chile is regulated by a Superintendency, a model emulated in Argentina and Peru. However, the regulatory capacity of the Superintendency is limited by legislation and focused on financial probity. The Superintendency has no power to monitor and evaluate the capacity of the ISAPREs to act as cost-effective purchasers of care for their members. Furthermore, the consumer movement in Chile is in its infancy, and consumer protection from benefit packages of poor value is therefore practically absent.

The extent to which the public sector deals with insurees at public expense is also poorly monitored, in part because FONASA is not permitted to charge back to the private sector the care provided for private insurees (Kifmann 1998).

About one-third of the population had private insurance throughout the early and mid-1990s. Cost inflation has fuelled inflation in premiums. Membership fell in the recent economic downturn as capacity to contribute was undermined by unemployment.

Summary

These case studies illustrate that private health insurance tends to control costs poorly, experiences most of the efficiency problems common to the public sector and creates inequity in access, which may increase inequity in health status. These problems create a rationale and a need to regulate the private insurance market. However, another more radical alternative to voluntary health insurance has been proposed and tested in Singapore and the United States.

A radical alternative: medical savings accounts

One alternative form of prepayment that is meant to address perceived demand-driven cost escalation caused by moral hazard has been the introduction of medical savings accounts. Medical savings accounts evolved first in Singapore. They are based on the principle of self-reliance and individual accountability. Citizens are required to save a proportion of their income every month in an earmarked account, specifically for meeting health care costs. The idea is that medical savings accounts overcome some of the problems inherent in health insurance markets, including adverse selection (because there is no risk-pooling), moral hazard, third-party payer problems and the high administrative costs (Ham 1996). Unlike most forms of private health insurance (except for Switzerland), medical savings accounts (as they function in Singapore) constitute a form of compulsory contribution for health care.

Since they were introduced in 1984, the medical savings accounts (known as Medisave in Singapore) have been supplemented by an insurance element and protection for people with low income. Thus, Singapore's health care system has three parts.

- Medisave requires each working person to deposit 6–8 per cent of tax-deductible income into a Medisave account to pay for hospital services

and costly outpatient procedures. At death, any account balance can be bequeathed to relatives. The account holders have free choice of provider.
- Medishield is catastrophic illness insurance created in 1990. Premiums are deducted from medical savings accounts and there are high deductibles, co-insurance and lifetime limits to reduce moral hazard.
- Medifund is an endowment fund created in 1993. Interest can be used to fund care for poor people based on means tests. Care is only available in open wards, and only 3 per cent of patients used this in 1993. Government subsidizes public hospital beds and outpatient facilities on a scale that diminishes in relation to 'luxury'.

The apparent success of medical savings accounts in Singapore, with a take-up of 95 per cent of working Singaporeans by 1992 and a total account value of US$9 billion, must be seen in context. Singapore is a small country of 3 million Chinese emigrants that has experienced rapid economic growth in recent decades, based in part on adopting high-technology medicine and an extraordinarily high savings rate (over 40 per cent of income is saved).

In evaluating medical savings accounts, Hsiao (1995b) concluded that this 'ingenious financing mechanism combined with a well crafted system of publicly subsidized primary and hospital services assured that everyone had reasonable access to basic medical care'. Thus, the system achieves basic equity. Hsiao cites data on productivity per staff member and consumer survey results to argue that the system is also efficient.

Nevertheless, Singapore's health care system has no price competition. The care delivered is characterized by very high technology, and this 'quality' competition has inflated costs. Medical savings accounts and related demand-side financing methods have not constrained supplier-induced demand. Indeed, these methods have fuelled price inflation. This inflation led to a government white paper, which concluded that: 'Market forces alone will not suffice to hold down medical costs to the minimum. The health care system is an example of market failure. The government has to intervene directly to structure and regulate the health care system' (quoted in Hsiao 1995a: 265).

More libertarian economists such as Massaro and Wong (1995) and policy analysts have advocated medical savings accounts as a remedy for cost inflation and inefficiency in the United States, despite its performance in Singapore. In addition, to the extent that catastrophic insurance coverage costs less than traditional alternatives, medical savings accounts are seen as a way of reducing insurance costs (Eichner *et al.* 1997) and encouraging uninsured people to purchase insurance.

Medical savings accounts were introduced in the United States under the Health Insurance Portability and Availability Act of 1996, also known as the Kennedy–Kassenbaum legislation. As an incentive for people to save, the accounts are tax-free. This means that medical savings accounts benefit high-rate taxpayers, people with surplus income to save and those with a low risk of ill health. Thus in the United States, where medical savings accounts operate in parallel with traditional private health insurance, they may concentrate the risks in the health insurance market, increase premiums and lead to more uninsured people (Jefferson 1999). Various simulations applied to the economics of health in the United States have demonstrated that equity might be impaired further and that the accounts would have little impact on cost (Chollet 1995; Keeler *et al.* 1996; Zabinski *et al.* 1999).

Other studies have also shown that the appeal of plans with a high deductible to younger and healthier workers will split the insurance market. Premiums for traditional plans would rise, forcing more people to lose insurance coverage (Moon *et al.* 1996). Medical savings accounts would only provide a very limited impetus to businesses that do not currently provide insurance for their employees (Goldman *et al.* 2000).

There is limited evidence of the effect of medical savings accounts on health care expenditure in the United States, since they have only been in operation since 1997. However, simulations carried out before the introduction suggested that a cross-section of non-elderly adults switching from indemnity insurance to medical savings accounts (plus catastrophic insurance) would reduce health care spending by between 0 and 15 per cent (Nichols *et al.* 1996; Ozanne 1996; Eichner *et al.* 1997; Kendix and Lubitz 1999). Despite tax subsidies, medical savings accounts cannot solve the problem of over-insurance caused by unlimited tax subsidies in the group insurance market (Keeler *et al.* 1996).

Despite the apparent failure of Singapore's experiment with medical savings accounts, they continue to be advocated. Even policy analysts in the United Kingdom have considered its applicability (Ham 1996). This advocacy is the product of the pro-market libertarians who find the individual reliance aspects of medical savings accounts attractive. Such values must not be dismissed in democratic societies, but their effects in terms of cost inflation, inefficiency and inequity should not be lost.

Conclusions

The policy process involves identifying and setting priorities among objectives and recognizing that choices between objectives involve trade-offs and opportunity costs. Decision-makers – public and private – are often reluctant to be explicit about their objectives.

Consumer and pro-competition groups in all countries with a private health insurance market advocate clearly defining the benefit package, especially exclusions, and accrediting and better regulating providers to improve patient safety. Private health insurers have been regulated in part, focusing largely on issues of financial probity. Only recently have regulators begun to consider defining the benefit package, pooling rules and the exercise of purchasing power. These issues are fundamental if private insurance is to facilitate controlling costs and promoting efficiency and equity. However, with or without regulation, the private sector has had limited success in controlling costs and improving efficiency in nearly all countries.

Private insurance can undermine equity in financing and access to care because individual and even group-rated premiums for 'poor risks', such as elderly people and people with chronic illnesses, are very high. Community rating may mitigate this, as in Switzerland, but does not eliminate the problem entirely unless risk adjustment is appropriate.

Concerns for people without insurance and the lack of solidarity in the system led Australia and Switzerland to adopt universal systems of insurance. In Australia, private health insurance continues to receive large public subsidies – no longer justified when private insurance is purely supplementary.

Medical savings accounts clearly appeal to politicians who value individual responsibility and the free market. However, medical savings accounts do not allow any risk-pooling and there is no purchasing leverage over providers, which results in a lack of cost control and allocative and technical efficiency. Competition is based on high-technology equipment and hotel facilities rather than clinical quality or price, as patients (the purchasers) lack adequate information to make informed decisions. When medical savings accounts complement private health insurance, they segment the market, attracting young and healthy people away from traditional plans.

The choice of funding mechanism reflects social values and policy goals. This choice alters through time as decision-makers grapple with the manifest deficiencies of the public and private sectors in health care. All too often policy is driven by beliefs with no evidence base. There are no magic bullets (Hsiao 1994), but logic and evidence offer much to those who wish to create better institutions for rich and poor people in the health care sector. Unfortunately, logic and evidence are often overwhelmed by ideology and political self-interest.

Notes

1 Genetic testing will swing the balance in favour of the insurer and will lead to the further exclusion of insurees who are genetically disposed to develop a certain disease.
2 Perverse financial incentives caused by tax-expenditure subsidies are not strictly a market failure but a failure of government tax policy.
3 In the United States and other countries, health care insurance is subsidized by tax deductions against income tax. Such subsidies induce over-insurance, over-consumption and cost inflation (see Chapter 2).
4 Different reasons for having to limit the provision of services may apply. For example, global budgets and resistance to contribution increases in the public sector and caps on annual expenditure and the high cost of premiums in the private sector.
5 Rationing occurs 'when someone is denied (or simply not offered) an intervention which everyone agrees would do them some good and which they would like to have' (Maynard and Bloor 1999).
6 Even in competitive social insurance systems, collective negotiation takes place between associations or groups of sickness funds and associations or groups of providers, who therefore have the equivalent purchasing power of a monopsonist. If purchasing is devolved to regional or local authorities, these agents will normally operate within a defined geographical area and thus have the power of a monopsony purchaser in relation to local service providers, who may find it difficult to contract with purchasers in different areas.
7 Legislation that prohibits monopolies and cartels in the insurance market also restricts insurers from becoming monopsonies.
8 Such anti-trust legislation does not apply to social health insurance funds if associations of sickness funds and associations of providers contract collectively.
9 Much of the material in this section is drawn from annual reports on the private health insurance sector in Chile (Maynard 1997b, 1998, 1999).

References

Australian Institute of Health and Welfare (1999) *Health Expenditure Bulletin*. Canberra: Australian Institute of Health and Welfare.

Chollet, D. (1995) Why the Pauly/Goodman proposal won't work, *Health Affairs*, 7(4): 273–7.

Chollet, D.J. and Lewis, M. (1997) Private insurance: principles and practice, in G.J. Schieber (ed.) *Innovations in Health Care Financing: Proceedings of a World Bank Conference*, 10–11 March 1997. Washington, DC: World Bank.

Duckett, S.J. and Jackson, T.J. (2000) The new health insurance rebate: an inefficient way of assisting public hospitals, *Medical Journal of Australia*, 172: 439–42.

Eichner, M.J., McClellan, M.B. and Wise, D.A. (1997) Health expenditure persistence and the feasibility of medical savings accounts, in J.M. Poterba (ed.) *Tax Policy and the Economy*, Vol. 11. Cambridge, MA: MIT Press.

Ellwood, P.M., Enthoven, A.C. and Etheridge, L. (1992) The Jackson Hole initiatives for the twenty-first century American health care system, *Health Economics*, 1(3): 149–68.

Friedman, M. (1962) *Capitalism and Freedom*. Chicago, IL: Chicago University Press.

Gabel, J., Hurst, K., Whitmore, H. *et al.* (1999) *Health Benefits of Small Employers in 1998*. Menlo Park, CA: Henry J. Kaiser Family Foundation.

Glied, S. (1997) *Chronic Condition: Why Health Reform Fails*. Cambridge, MA: Harvard University Press.

Goldman, D.P., Buchanan, J.L. and Keeler, E.B. (2000) Simulating the impact of medical savings accounts on small business, *Health Services Research*, 35(1(Part 1)): 53–75.

Gruber, J. (1998) *Health Insurance and the Labor Market*. Cambridge, MA: National Bureau of Economic Research.

Ham, C. (1996) Learning from the tigers: stakeholder health care, *Lancet*, 347: 951–3.

Hall, J., De Abreu Lourenco, R. and Viney, R. (1999) Carrots and sticks: the fall and fall of private insurance in Australia, *Health Economics*, 8(8): 653–60.

Harris, M.G. and Harris, R.D. (1998) The Australian health system: continuity and change, *Journal of Health and Human Services Administration*, 20(4): 442–67.

Hsiao, W. (1994) Marketisation: the illusory magic pill, *Health Economics*, 3(6): 351–8.

Hsiao, W.C. (1995a) Abnormal economics in the health sector, in P.A. Berman (ed.) *Health Sector Reform in Developing Countries: Making Health Development Sustainable*. Boston, MA: Harvard University Press.

Hsiao, W. (1995b) Medical savings accounts: lessons from Singapore, *Health Affairs*, 7(4): 260–6.

Iglehart, J. (1995) Physicians and the growth of managed care, *New England Journal of Medicine*, 331: 1167–71.

Jefferson, R.T. (1999) Medical savings accounts: windfalls for the healthy, wealthy and wise, *Catholic University Law Review*, 48(3): 685–723.

Keeler, E.B., Malkin, J.D., Goldman, D.P. *et al.* (1996) Can medical savings accounts for the nonelderly reduce health care costs?, *Journal of the American Medical Association*, 275(21): 1666–71.

Kendix, M. and Lubitz, J.D. (1999) The impact of medical savings accounts on Medicare program costs, *Inquiry – the Journal of Health Care Organization Provision and Financing*, 36(3): 280–90.

Kifmann, M. (1998) Private health insurance in Chile: basic or complementary insurance for outpatient services?, *International Social Security Review*, 51(1): 137–52.

Levit, K.R., Lazenby, J.C., Braden, B.R. and the National Accounts Team (1998) National health spending trends in 1996, *Health Affairs*, 17(1): 35–51.

Massaro, T.A. and Wong, Y-N. (1995) Positive experience with medical savings accounts in Singapore, *Health Affairs* (*Millwood*), 14(2): 267–72, 277–9.

Maynard, A. (1997a) Evidence based medicine: an incomplete method for informing treatment choices, *Lancet*, 349: 126–8.

Maynard, A. (1997b) *The Chilean Health Care System, the Reform of Private Sector Regulation*. London: Institute of Health Sector Development.

Maynard, A. (1998) *The Chilean Health Care System, the Reform of Private Sector Regulation*. London: Institute of Health Sector Development.

Maynard, A. (1999) *The Chilean Health Care System, the Reform of Private Sector Regulation*. London: Institute of Health Sector Development.

Maynard, A. and Bloor, K. (1995) Health care reform: informing difficult choices, *International Journal of Health Planning and Management*, 10(4): 247–64.

Maynard, A. and Bloor, K. (1998) *Managed Care: Palliative or Panacea*, Occasional Papers in Health Economics No. 8. London: Nuffield Trust.

Maynard, A. and Bloor, K. (1999) *Our Certain Fate: Rationing in Health Care*. London: Office of Health Economics.

Minder, A., Schoenholzer, H. and Amiet, M. (2000) *Health Care Systems in Transition: Switzerland*. Copenhagen: European Observatory on Health Care Systems.

Moon, M., Nichols, L.M. and Wall, S. (1996) *Medical Savings Accounts: A Policy Analysis*. Washington, DC: Urban Institute. http://www.urban.org/pubs/HINSURE/MSA.htm (accessed 25 February 2001).

Nichols, L.M., Moon, M. and Wall, S. (1996) *Tax-preferred Medical Savings Accounts and Catastrophic Health Insurance Plans: A Numerical Analysis of Winners and Losers*. Washington, DC: Urban Institute. http://www.urban.org/pubs/hinsure/winlose.htm (accessed 25 February 2001).

OECD (1999) *OECD Health Data 99: A Comparative Analysis of 29 Countries*. Paris: Organisation for Economic Co-operation and Development.

Office of Fair Trading (1998) *Health Insurance*, OFT Report No. 230. London: Office of Fair Trading.

Ozanne, L. (1996) How will medical savings accounts affect medical spending?, *Inquiry*, 33(3): 225–36.

Perez-Stable, E.J. (1999) Managed care arrives in Latin America, *New England Journal of Medicine*, 340(14): 1110–12.

Reinhardt, U.E. (1993) Comments on the Jackson Hole initiatives, *Health Economics*, 2(1): 7–14.

Rivo, M.L., Mayns, H.I., Katzoff, J. and Kindig, D.A. (1996) Managed care: implications for physician workforce and education, *Journal of the American Medical Association*, 274: 712–15.

Schofield, D. (1997) *The Distribution and Determinants of Private Health Insurance in Australia, 1990*. Canberra: National Centre for Social and Economic Modelling, University of Canberra. http://www.natsem.canberra.edu.au/pubs/dps/dp17/dp17.html (accessed 25 February 2001).

Shore Sheppard, L., Buchmueller, T.C. and Jensen, G.A. (2000) Medicaid and crowding out of private insurance: a re-examination using firm level data, *Journal of Health Economics*, 19(1): 61–91.

Stocker, K., Waitzkin, H. and Iriart, C. (1999) The exportation of managed care to Latin America, *New England Journal of Medicine*, 340(14): 1131–5.

Theurl, E. (1999) Some aspects of the reform of the health care systems in Austria, Germany and Switzerland, *Health Care Analysis*, 7(4): 331–54.

van den Heever, A.M. (1998) Private sector health reform in South Africa, *Health Economics*, 7(4): 281–9.

van Doorslaer, E., Wagstaff, A., van der Burg, H. *et al.* (1999) The redistributive effect of health care finance in twelve OECD countries, *Journal of Health Economics*, 18(3): 291–314.

Wagstaff, A., van Doorslaer, E., van der Burg, H. *et al.* (1999) Equity in the finance of health care: some further international comparisons, *Journal of Health Economics*, 18(3): 263–90.

Zabinski, D., Seldon, T.M., Moeller, J.F. and Banthin, J.S. (1999) Medical savings accounts: microsimulation results from a model with adverse selection, *Journal of Health Economics*, 18(2): 195–218.

Voluntary health insurance in the European Union

Elias Mossialos and Sarah M.S. Thomson

Introduction

Private health insurance[1] does not play a dominant role in funding health care in the European Union, as it does in the United States, Australia and Switzerland. For largely historical reasons, governments in European Union (EU) member states have aimed to preserve the principle of health care funded by the state or social insurance and made available to every citizen, regardless of ability to pay. This has led to the development of health care systems broadly characterized by high public expenditure, almost universal coverage, mandatory participation and the provision of comprehensive benefits. As a result, voluntary health insurance has had little scope to play anything other than a marginal role in funding health care in the EU.[2]

It is not our intention in this chapter to discuss the advantages and disadvantages of voluntary health insurance as a means of funding health care; these have been widely assessed elsewhere (see, for example, Chapter 5 and Barr 1998). However, very few studies have considered the workings of the market for voluntary health insurance in the EU. Our aims here, therefore, are to examine the characteristics of voluntary health insurance[3] and the nature of the market for voluntary health insurance in the EU. The framework we use is based on a simplified version of the structure–conduct–performance model of industrial analysis, although our use of the model does not necessarily imply a causal relationship between these three elements; rather, we use it as an analytical tool to examine the potential interaction between structure, conduct and performance in the market for voluntary health insurance (Mason 1939; Bain 1956). The chapter is structured as follows. After setting out the characteristics of voluntary health insurance in the EU, we discuss the implications of public policy in the form of national tax incentives and EU regulation. We then assess the demand for voluntary health insurance in the EU, based on information regarding subscriber characteristics. The following three sections outline market structure (the type of product on offer, the number and type of insurers in the market, barriers to entry, subscriber characteristics and information asymmetry), examine market conduct (defining benefits, setting premiums, the extent to which insurers cream-skim low-risk individuals, financial equalization between insurers and measures taken by insurers to address moral hazard) and assess market performance (levels of coverage, the price of premiums, health service costs, administrative costs, insurers' profit ratios, impact on the health care system as a whole and equity implications). In the final section, we present our conclusions.

The characteristics of voluntary health insurance in the EU

A classification of types of voluntary health insurance

The literature on voluntary health insurance distinguishes between insurance that duplicates statutory insurance and insurance that constitutes the main means of protection for sections of the population (Couffinhal 1999). In the context of the EU, however, it may be more accurate to classify insurance according to whether it substitutes for the statutory health care system, provides complementary coverage for services excluded or not fully covered by the state, or provides supplementary coverage for faster access and increased consumer choice. It should be noted that the distinction between complementary and supplementary voluntary health insurance is not always clear and there may be significant cross-over between them. Due to recent changes in EU regulation of the voluntary health insurance market (see later), some of the issues we raise regarding structure, conduct and performance will be more relevant to the market for complementary and supplementary voluntary health insurance, which is largely unregulated, than to the market for substitutive voluntary health insurance, in which greater government intervention is permitted.

Substitutive voluntary health insurance

Health care systems in the EU are mainly financed through taxation or contributions from employers and employees. This means that participation in the statutory health care system is usually mandatory. In Germany, the Netherlands and Spain, however, certain groups of people are either not covered by the statutory health care system or allowed to opt out of it, leaving them free to purchase voluntary health insurance as a substitute for statutory protection.

Germany is unique both in restricting substitutive voluntary health insurance to high-income employees, self-employed people and civil servants and in prohibiting these individuals from returning to the statutory health care system once they have left it. Civil servants and self-employed people are only eligible to remain under statutory protection if they have been members of the statutory health insurance scheme for a specific length of time. Individuals earning above a certain amount can choose to opt out of the statutory health insurance scheme and purchase substitutive voluntary health insurance. Because German voluntary health insurers compete directly with the public sector, substitutive voluntary health insurance policies cover more than one type of insurance and may result in improved amenities, faster access and greater choice of provider.

The health care system in the Netherlands operates on three levels. The first level is a universal statutory scheme for exceptional medical expenses (known as AWBZ) that provides coverage in kind to all residents of the Netherlands for expensive, uninsurable, long-term care such as nursing care in hospitals (after the first 365 days) and nursing homes, mental health care and care for disabled people (Ministry of Health, Welfare and Sport 2000). This scheme is implemented by public health insurance funds and voluntary health insurers. The second level of the health care system (known as ZFW) comes under the Health Insurance Act, which automatically insures resident employees up to the age of 65 earning less than €29,300, residents living on state benefits and some self-employed people. Those who are covered when they reach 65 years can remain covered under the 'stay where you are' principle, whereas those who are not can join it on a voluntary basis if their annual household income is below a certain level. High earners are not covered by the statutory health insurance scheme and can choose to take up substitutive voluntary health insurance, which most of them do.[4] The ZFW covers the first year of hospital care, physician services, prescription drugs and some physiotherapy and basic dental care (again, in kind). Level three of the health care system consists of voluntary complementary and supplementary health insurance.

Spanish public-sector workers are allowed to opt out of the statutory health care system (run by the national social security agency INSALUD) and join a government-subsidized health insurance scheme (MUFACE), which also covers their dependants; about 85 per cent choose to do so (95 per cent in the Ministry of Health). Legislation in Portugal in 1990 gave individuals the right to opt out of the statutory system, but this aspect of the law has never been implemented (Dixon and Mossialos 2000). During the 1990s, the Italian government also considered an opt-out clause.

Complementary voluntary health insurance

In contrast to substitutive voluntary health insurance, complementary voluntary health insurance provides full or partial cover for services that are excluded or not fully covered by the statutory health care system. It is available to the whole population, albeit in varying forms, in every EU member state. Some insurers restrict benefits to hospital treatment, but where cover is available for non-hospital treatment, it may include a significant part of the costs of primary care practitioners, specialists, nursing staff, drugs, tests, medical appliances, transport costs, glasses, dental care, maternity care and alternative treatment. Levels of reimbursement vary from country to country and may also vary according to the insurance package chosen.

Complementary voluntary health insurance also provides cover for the reimbursement of co-payments in Belgium, Denmark (pharmaceuticals only), France (ambulatory care), Ireland (outpatient care) and Luxembourg (hospital co-payments). As a result of reform in Italy, Italian mutual associations will soon be allowed to cover co-payments and the costs of services excluded from the statutory benefit package funded by the national health service (SSN) (Taroni 2000). With the exception of France, the market for voluntary health insurance to cover co-payments is not substantial in the EU, probably because it is not particularly profitable.

Patients can purchase complementary voluntary health insurance to cover outpatient costs in Austria (in conjunction with a more comprehensive health insurance package), Belgium, France, Ireland, Italy, Portugal and Spain. Although statutory health care systems increasingly exclude dental care, the voluntary health insurance market for dental care in the EU is not as large as might be expected. The reasons for this are not clear. Some cover for dental care is available in Belgium (for self-employed people), Denmark, France, Luxembourg, Germany, the Netherlands and the United Kingdom.

Supplementary or choice-increasing voluntary health insurance

Supplementary voluntary health insurance increases consumer choice and access to different health services, traditionally guaranteeing superior accommodation and amenities and, crucially, faster access to treatment, especially in areas of health care with long waiting lists, such as surgery. In some cases, supplementary voluntary health insurance increases the choice of provider and benefits. Supplementary voluntary health insurance is sometimes referred to as 'double coverage' and is especially prevalent in EU member states with national health service systems such as Greece, Italy, Portugal, Spain and the United Kingdom.

Levels of voluntary health insurance expenditure and coverage

Although the last 20 years have seen a general decline in public expenditure on health care in the EU, particularly in member states where public expenditure was high as a proportion of total spending on health care, this has not led to sustained growth in the demand for voluntary health insurance (see Table 6.1), partly because the state continues to provide comprehensive benefits (and participation is mandatory in most EU member states) and partly because governments have tended to rely on other methods of shifting health care costs onto consumers, such as user charges, rather than promoting and subsidizing voluntary health insurance. Consequently, out-of-pocket payments make up the bulk of private expenditure on health care in all EU member states except France and the Netherlands (OECD 2000). In 1998, voluntary health insurance accounted for a very small fraction of private spending on health care in Greece, Italy and Portugal and for less than 25 per cent in Austria,

Table 6.1 Voluntary health insurance expenditure as a percentage of total expenditure on health in the EU, 1980–98

Country	1980	1985	1990	1995	1998
Austria	7.6	9.8	9.0	7.8	7.1
Belgium	0.8	1.2	1.6	1.9	2.0*
Denmark (not-for-profit)	0.8	0.8	1.3	1.2	1.5
Finland total	1.4	1.8	2.2	2.4	2.7
for-profit	0.8	1.2	1.7	2.0	2.2
not-for-profit	0.6	0.6	0.5	0.4	0.5
France total	NA	5.8	11.2	11.7	12.2
for-profit	NA	NA	4.4	4.2	4.4
not-for-profit	NA	5.8	6.8	7.5	7.8
Germany	5.9	6.5	7.2	6.7	6.9**
Greece	NA	NA	0.9	NA	NA
Ireland (not-for-profit)	NA	NA	NA	NA	9.4
Italy	0.2	0.5	0.9	1.3	1.3**
Luxembourg (not-for-profit)	NA	1.6	1.4	1.4	1.6**
Netherlands total	NA	11.2	12.1	NA	17.7
for-profit	NA	11.2	12.1	NA	11.7
not-for-profit	NA	NA	NA	NA	6.0
Portugal	NA	0.2	0.8	1.4	1.7**
Spain	3.2	3.7	3.7	5.2	1.5**
Sweden	NA	NA	NA	NA	NA
UK	1.3	2.5	3.3	3.2	3.5

* 1996, ** 1997. NA = not available

Source: OECD (2000)

Belgium, Denmark, Finland, Luxembourg, Spain and the United Kingdom (OECD 2000). Voluntary health insurance has a much bigger share of private expenditure on health care in EU member states offering substitutive voluntary health insurance (29.9 per cent in Germany and 70 per cent in the Netherlands), and in France (51.7 per cent), where there is extensive coverage of co-payments (OECD 2000).

European Union data suggest that, even where governments have pursued a deliberate and explicit policy of encouraging people into the private sector, the results, in terms of voluntary health insurance coverage, have been mixed (see Table 6.2).[5] For example, the relatively small size of voluntary health insurance markets in Denmark, Finland and Sweden is traditionally attributed to the generosity of public benefits, but recent increases in cost-sharing have not had much impact on voluntary health insurance coverage. Conversely, increases in cost-sharing have succeeded in stimulating growth in France, causing coverage for the reimbursement of co-payments to rise from 69 per cent of the population in 1980 to 85 per cent in 1999 (INSEE 2000). However, France is very much an outlier in this respect. Voluntary health insurance coverage remains low in southern member states such as Greece, in spite of

Table 6.2 Voluntary health insurance coverage in the EU in 1998

Country	Per cent population covered
Austria	13 (hospital expenses)
	21 (hospital cash payments)
Belgium	30
Denmark	28
Finland	33 (children)
	10 (adults)
France	85 (co-payments)
	20 (other types of voluntary health insurance)
Germany	8.9*
Greece	10
Ireland	42
Italy	5
Luxembourg	75 (active population)
Netherlands	28.9*
Portugal	10
Spain	17.6 (including 6.8 with substitutive VHI)
Sweden	0.5
UK	11.5

* Figures for Germany and the Netherlands are for substitutive voluntary health insurance.

Source: Mossialos and Le Grand (1999), updated using *Health Care Systems in Transition* country profiles from the European Observatory on Health Care Systems

the fact that individuals in Greece often make high direct payments to providers (Mossialos and Le Grand 1999). One reason for this may be a reluctance to pay a third party. When people are used to paying their doctor or hospital directly, the transferral of money to a third party may be seen as an unnecessary erosion of the patient–doctor relationship. The implications of this cultural element for the expansion of voluntary health insurance in other countries with a high level of direct or unofficial payments, such as some central and eastern European states, should not be underestimated. In Germany, where voluntary health insurance coverage is not as high as might be expected, it is not clear whether this is because public expenditure is high (and statutory benefits are comprehensive) or because voluntary health insurance is expensive, offering relatively poor value for money. For more detailed information on levels of coverage and the price of premiums, see pp. 147–9.

Tax incentives and regulation of the market

Tax incentives to encourage the take-up of voluntary health insurance in the EU

National tax laws are a form of public policy that can provide consumers with significant incentives to take up voluntary health insurance, usually in the form of tax relief on premiums. Tax laws can also influence the behaviour of insurers, either by making premiums deductible from corporate tax (an incentive) or by imposing a tax on premium income (a disincentive).

Tax relief for voluntary health insurance premiums does feature in the EU, although the last 10 years have seen efforts to reduce this type of incentive in many member states. Tax laws also vary considerably between member states. For example, there is currently no tax relief for voluntary health insurance in Belgium, Denmark, Finland, France, Spain, Sweden and the United Kingdom and only very limited tax relief in Germany and the Netherlands, while in recent years the Austrian and Spanish governments have taken steps to cut tax relief (Bennett *et al.* 1993; Freire 1999). Ireland and Portugal are major exceptions to this trend.

Ireland still provides a substantial public subsidy to voluntary health insurance through generous tax relief, which costs the government €79 million a year at the standard rate of income tax of 27 per cent (equal to 2.5 per cent of public expenditure on health in 1997). Withdrawing this subsidy would increase the net cost of premiums by 32 per cent (Department of Health and Children 1999). Until 1999, tax relief in Portugal was capped at about US$329 for all types of insurance premiums, but since then the government has established a tax-deductible amount exclusively for voluntary health insurance premiums (Dixon and Mossialos 2000).

The industry argues that increased demand for voluntary health insurance will reduce demand for statutory health services and that tax incentives therefore work in the public's interest, but this argument could be challenged for several reasons (Davies 1999). Tax relief for voluntary health insurance is, in effect, a government subsidy to subscribers of voluntary health insurance, who tend to be high earners (see p. 136), and is regressive in terms of finance because the value of the relief is greater for those who have a higher marginal tax rate. It is administratively complex, which generates additional transaction costs. It can also distort price signals and may create opportunities for fraud and tax evasion.

Perhaps the most effective argument against tax relief is that it does not appear to be particularly successful in encouraging people to subscribe to voluntary health insurance. In the United Kingdom, for example, the incoming Labour government of 1997 abolished the tax relief on voluntary health insurance premiums for individuals aged 60 and over (introduced in 1990 by the Conservative government), because research showed that, in spite of annual public spending of £140 million on these incentives, the number of voluntary health insurance subscribers rose by only 50,000 in 7 years (an increase of 1.6 per cent) (Department of Health 2000). In spite of industry claims to the contrary, it is also unlikely that the cost of this subsidy to voluntary health insurance would be less than the National Health Service (NHS) expenditure saved. Recent estimates conclude that at least an additional 1.8 million individuals would have to take out voluntary health insurance (equivalent to a 28 per cent growth in coverage) for a subsidy to all adults, equal to the basic rate of income tax, to be self-financing (that is, for the NHS expenditure saved to equal the subsidy) (Emmerson *et al.* 2000). However, if the health care provided by the NHS actually costs less than the health care provided by voluntary health insurance (and Department of Health figures suggest that NHS costs for treatment such as cataract extraction and hip replacement are approximately a third less than the same treatment in the private sector), then an additional 3.1 million voluntary health insurance subscribers would be needed to make the tax subsidy self financing (Emmerson *et al.* 2001).

In some EU member states, tax laws are used to influence market structure by favouring certain types of insurers over others or certain types of contract over others. French, Belgian and Italian tax laws favour mutual associations over for-profit insurers, although in France's case this may contravene EU regulation (European Commission 2000). Tax laws can also affect market structure by encouraging the purchase of group rather than individual contracts and vice versa (Freire 1999; Datamonitor 2000).

The trend towards removing or reducing tax relief on voluntary health insurance premiums in the EU suggests that governments have found tax incentives for consumers to be expensive, regressive and largely unsuccessful in stimulating demand.

The EU regulatory framework

In recent years, the EU regulatory framework has become an increasingly important aspect of public policy towards voluntary health insurance. This is largely the result of European Commission directives leading to the creation of a single market for life and non-life insurance in the EU.

According to the European Commission, the ultimate objectives of a single market are to provide consumers with a greater choice of insurance products and to increase competition between insurance companies (European Commission 1997). The third non-life insurance directive (European Commission 1992), adopted by national law on 1 July 1994 (European Commission 1997), gives insurance companies the freedom to establish a branch or agency anywhere in the EU, to sell their products without a branch presence and to compete on price, products and service. More importantly, it has abolished national controls on premium prices and prior notification of policy conditions. Under certain conditions, a country may invoke 'the general good' to justify national regulation, but in practice this only applies to substitutive voluntary health insurance; complementary and supplementary voluntary health insurance are no longer subject to national regulatory controls. For this reason, some of the issues we raise in this chapter are more relevant to the market for complementary and supplementary voluntary health insurance, which has been largely unregulated since 1994, than to the market for substitutive voluntary health insurance, in which greater government intervention is permitted.

The EU's current approach to the creation of a single market, based on liberalization and substantial deregulation, appears to demonstrate more concern for the financial viability of voluntary health insurers than for consumer protection. Given the market failures inherent in voluntary health insurance (see Barr 1998), it could be argued that relying primarily on market mechanisms may not be the best way of delivering cost-effective and competitively priced voluntary health insurance products. Our analysis suggests that further regulatory developments will be necessary to ensure that the EU market for voluntary health insurance works efficiently and allocates resources in a more equitable manner.

The demand for voluntary health insurance in the EU

The existence of a market for voluntary health insurance depends on three conditions: positive demand (some individuals must be averse to risk), insurance supplied at a price the individual is prepared to pay (the individual's risk aversion must be sufficient to cover the insurer's administrative costs and normal profit) and supplying insurance must be technically possible (Barr 1998). In addition to risk aversion, the demand for voluntary health insurance is likely to be influenced by some or all of the following factors: the probability of illness, the magnitude of the loss that illness might incur, the price of insurance, the level of taxes and subsidies, income and education. However, the influence of each factor varies from country to country, and some factors may be harder to measure than others. The level of public expenditure on health care, the institutional rules that apply to the statutory health care system and the amount and distribution of satisfaction with the statutory health care system may also determine the demand for, and scope of, voluntary health insurance.

Evidence from the United States shows that the demand for voluntary health insurance is price inelastic.[6] Empirical studies reveal price elasticity values ranging from –0.03 (Marquis and Long 1995) to –0.54 (Manning and Marquis 1989) and a relatively small income effect (0.15 and 0.07, respectively). This may in part result from the high tax subsidies for voluntary health insurance in the United States and the fact that most voluntary health insurance is purchased by an employment group rather than individually.[7] A recent study estimated the price elasticity of voluntary health insurance in the United Kingdom to be in the range of –0.003 to –0.004 (that is, highly price inelastic) (Emmerson 2001). The much smaller effect of price on voluntary health insurance shown in this study may be due to the fact that in the United Kingdom it is mostly purchased by high earners. Unfortunately, very few similar studies have been conducted in the EU and there is, therefore, little direct evidence on the price or income elasticity of voluntary health insurance in the EU. Most information concerns the characteristics of those who subscribe to voluntary health insurance.

The distribution of coverage for voluntary health insurance in many EU member states is heavily skewed in favour of people with high incomes. Subscribers in the United Kingdom are typically middle-aged professionals, employers and managers based in London and the southern region (ABI 2000; Laing and Buisson 2000). Voluntary health insurance coverage in Germany varies considerably, favouring men, younger people, professionals and those living in western Germany (PKV 1994). The French system also appears to discriminate against people on lower incomes, foreigners, young people aged between 20 and 24 and those over 70 years old, all of whom are less likely to be covered by voluntary health insurance. Furthermore, poorer people tend to have lower-quality coverage than richer people (Blanpain and Pan Ké Shon 1997). Coverage in Ireland, Italy and Spain is similarly dominated by high-earning individuals (Mossialos and Thomson 2001).

Long waiting lists for NHS treatment are often cited as a major determinant of the demand for voluntary health insurance in the United Kingdom (Besley *et al.* 1998, 1999). However, the evidence regarding waiting lists and voluntary health insurance is inconclusive, and links between them may be tenuous given that waiting lists have continued to rise while voluntary health insurance coverage has declined (King and Mossialos 2001). One possible explanation for the decline in coverage is that premiums are extremely expensive and have consistently risen above the rate of inflation (see p. 148).

In Germany, 16 per cent of GKV (statutory health insurance) subscribers are voluntary members who are eligible to opt out of the statutory system, because they have earnings above the statutory income threshold, but have chosen not to do so (Busse 2000). In fact, less than one-quarter of the people with earnings above the statutory income threshold choose to purchase substitutive voluntary health insurance, largely because the GKV continues to provide comprehensive benefits, but also because people 55 years or older who opt for voluntary health insurance cannot return to the statutory system, even if their earnings fall below the statutory ceiling (CEA 2000), and because voluntary health insurers do not automatically cover dependants or offer family policies (unlike the GKV). Substitutive voluntary health insurance subscribers must pay separate premiums for spouses and children, making voluntary health insurance more attractive to single people and double-income couples (Busse 2000). This leaves the statutory scheme to insure a higher proportion of elderly people, large families and people in poor health (Rupprecht *et al.* 2000). The main marketing strategy of voluntary health insurers is to highlight the better facilities they provide, but many people regard substitutive voluntary health insurance as expensive compared with the GKV (Natarajan 1996).

The structure of the voluntary health insurance market

In this section, we outline several market features, including the number and type of voluntary health insurers in the EU, barriers to entry, subscriber characteristics (that is, whether voluntary health insurance contracts are purchased by individuals or groups) and information asymmetry.

Types of insurers

Voluntary health insurance in the EU shows great diversity in terms of the type of institutions offering health insurance, the amount of competition between them, the extent of market penetration, the range of benefits on offer, the price of premiums, the existence of incentives to take up insurance and the characteristics of national regulatory frameworks. Some companies offer life insurance alongside health insurance or combined coverage to protect against accident and ill health. Products can also be classified in more than one insurance category (medical expenses, loss of earnings, cash benefits or long-term care), which can make separating data for each function impossible. Germany is the largest market for voluntary health insurance in the EU, worth €19.5 billion in 1998 (CEA 1999). France is the second largest market, followed by the Netherlands and the United Kingdom.

Commercial insurers are present in most EU member states, although for largely historical reasons mutual associations (not-for-profit organizations) dominate the market in many member states, including Belgium, Denmark, France, Germany, Luxembourg, the Netherlands and the United Kingdom. However, the dominance of mutual associations may change in future, with commercial (for-profit) insurers gaining an increasing share of the market.

Voluntary health insurance in the EU is dominated by a relatively small number of players. In 1998, 54.9 per cent of all voluntary health insurance premiums in Europe were written or earned by as few as 25 companies, 17 of which were German (four of the top five) (Datamonitor 2000). The United Kingdom's BUPA is the fourth largest insurer in the EU (Datamonitor 2000). There is considerable variation in the number of insurers operating in each member state (from nine in Austria to 142 in France) and significant mergers in some EU member states have led to a reduction in the overall number of insurers (OECD 1998). The ratio of specialist to non-specialist companies varies from no specialist insurers in Austria to one-third in the United Kingdom, just under half in the Netherlands and all in Germany (Natarajan 1996; CEA 2000). In future it seems likely that there will be further consolidation of the market, and commercial (for-profit) and non-specialist insurers may increase their market share.

The risk borne by insurers also varies in different member states. Insurers in the Netherlands, for example, bear relatively little risk because the universal statutory scheme for exceptional medical expenses (AWBZ) covers nursing care in hospital after the first 365 days, mental health care and care for disabled people and therefore picks up a substantial proportion of the costs of voluntarily insured individuals. The AWBZ also covers the costs of care in nursing homes, thereby creating a significant incentive to treat high-cost patients in nursing homes rather than in hospital. In Spain, 85 per cent of the insurance scheme for civil servants (MUFACE) is carried out by voluntary health insurers and the rest by the national social security agency (INSALUD), but both types of insurer are publicly funded by a flat capitation fee (equal to INSALUD's per-capita health care expenditure); MUFACE does not, therefore, bear much financial risk (Pellisé 1994).

Barriers to entry

Since the creation of a single EU market for insurance, in theory there have been no significant barriers to entry for voluntary health insurers. A key aim of the third non-life insurance directive was to prevent national regulators from erecting barriers to the entry of insurers from other member states (Rees *et al.* 1999). In practice, however, substantial barriers do remain to the successful achievement of a single market, including the extent to which individual member states have decided to comply with the directives, the high costs of technical investment and differential tax treatment of national and foreign insurers. For example, mutual associations in France enjoy a preferential tax status, which means that foreign insurers may be unable to enter the French market on the same terms as domestic mutual insurers (Datamonitor 2000). So far, the single market has failed in its attempt to encourage consumers to purchase insurance products in member states other than their own. The growth of internet-based insurance may promote cross-border sales in future, but the lack of tax harmonization will continue to pose problems in this respect. It would appear that market expansion has mostly occurred through the purchase of foreign insurance companies rather than through increases in cross-border sales or the establishment of branches in other member states.

Individual versus group contracts

A key factor in both the distribution and the extent of voluntary health insurance coverage is the extent to which insurance is purchased individually or through employment-based group schemes. Group schemes are popular with voluntary health insurers because they generally have a lower unit cost and provide high volumes of business without a correspondingly large market outlay (BMI 2000). The distinction between individually and group purchased voluntary health insurance is important from the subscriber's perspective too, partly because group premiums are often group rated, whereas individual premiums are more likely to be adjusted for risk, and partly because they are usually substantially cheaper. Offering reduced premiums and favourable conditions to groups means that insurers automatically cover a younger, healthier, more homogeneous population.

Group contracts providing different types of voluntary health insurance expanded rapidly in the 1980s and now account for almost all voluntary health insurance policies in Portugal (Dixon 1999), a very high proportion in Greece (Sissouras *et al.* 1999), well over two-thirds in Belgium, Ireland and Italy and over half in France and the Netherlands (CEA 2000). Insurers in Ireland and the Netherlands attract employers by offering them discounted premiums (Hermesse and Lewalle 1995; CEA 2000). Much of the growth in voluntary health insurance in the United Kingdom in the 1980s resulted from the expansion of employment-based company schemes providing voluntary health insurance as an employee benefit (ABI 2000). Companies purchased about 59 per cent of voluntary health insurance subscriptions in 1998 versus 48 per cent in 1993 (Youngman 1994; Robinson and Dixon 1999). In 1999, the number of people with voluntary health insurance cover fell by 4.5 per cent, with the fall in demand concentrated solely in individually purchased policies (Laing and Buisson 2000). This is almost certainly linked to British insurers' pricing strategy; not only are group premiums in the United Kingdom much cheaper than individual premiums, their annual increases have also been much smaller (Papworth 2000).

Information asymmetry

Information is vital to both buyers and sellers in a competitive insurance market. The absence of clear information about the price, quality and conditions of voluntary health insurance policies is a type of market failure that prevents subscribers from making informed comparisons between different products and puts them at a competitive disadvantage in the marketplace. Information asymmetry in the EU is likely to be more problematic in the market for complementary and supplementary than substitutive voluntary health insurance, as the third non-life insurance directive abolished national product controls for complementary and supplementary voluntary health insurance in July 1994. Since then, the market has been awash with different health insurance products, giving the appearance of fierce competition. In practice, however, subscribers do not have adequate access to clear information. A recent report by the European Parliament's Committee on Employment and Social Affairs concluded that not only were subscribers unlikely to find policies easy to grasp, but variation between policies made them difficult to compare in terms of value for money (Rocard 2000). Although the European Commission expected the creation of a single market to encourage competition, little effort has been made to address the problem of information at an EU level and, as a result of deregulation, insurers have no incentive to reduce subscriber confusion and increase transparency by introducing standardized terms or 'core' benefits packages.

The exclusions of voluntary health insurance policies in the United Kingdom are numerous and often difficult to assess. The profusion of voluntary health insurance products means that both subscribers and brokers are easily confused (Calnan et al. 1993; Youngman 1994). In 1996 and 1997, the Office of Fair Trading in the United Kingdom launched enquiries into the voluntary health insurance sector to identify consumer detriment and information gaps (Davey 1998). Although the Office of Fair Trading (1999) finally cleared the industry of major competition problems, it highlighted the need for much greater clarity and accuracy in the information available to policy-holders, describing the information provided by BUPA and PPP Healthcare as unsatisfactory. Since then, the industry does not appear to have succeeded in reducing confusion; a 50-year-old man considering buying a policy from PPP Healthcare still has to choose from 90 different monthly premium options ranging from £28.67 per month (£344.04 per year) to £363.82 per month (£4365.84 per year) (CareHealth 2000).

Where insurers have more information than subscribers, they may be able to cream-skim low-risk individuals and deny coverage to high-risk individuals (see p. 142 for an analysis of the implications of cream-skimming). However, if subscribers have more information about their own level of risk than insurers, the latter will find it difficult to distinguish between high-risk individuals and those who are merely risk averse. This type of information failure can lead to adverse selection. One way of avoiding adverse selection is to adjust premiums according to an individual's level of risk (risk rating or adjustment), although this is not always straightforward and can be expensive (see p. 143). Although the literature makes much of adverse selection, it does not seem to pose particular problems in the EU market for voluntary health insurance. In the Netherlands and Germany, the only member states in which it is really possible to test for adverse selection (because it is not compulsory for individuals to be insured), very few individuals are uninsured. According to the Public Information Office of the Dutch Ministry of Health, Welfare and Sport, only 1.25 per cent of the population did not have any insurance coverage in 1999 and most of these uninsured people were homeless, while a few refused to insure themselves for reasons of principle (Ministry of Health, Welfare and Sport 2000).

The conduct of the voluntary health insurance industry

In this section, we examine the conduct of voluntary health insurers in the EU in terms of their pricing behaviour (setting premiums), product strategy (defining benefits and cream-skimming), financial equalization between insurers and the extent to which they address supply-side and demand-side moral hazard.

Setting premiums

Insurance premiums can be based on a community (or group) rating or on individual risk rating. Community (group)-rated premiums are the same for all subscribers (or for a group) in a given community or firm, whereas individual risk-rated premiums differ according to several factors, including age, gender, occupation, family history of disease, past health care utilization and claims experience – but insurers typically rate premiums on the basis of age and pre-existing conditions alone rather than using more detailed information.

Thanks to the abolition of national price and product controls, insurers offering complementary and supplementary voluntary health insurance are free to rate premiums on any basis they choose, while insurers offering substitutive voluntary health insurance are generally subject to some regulation regarding the price of premiums and policy conditions. Most individual complementary or supplementary voluntary health insurance premiums are therefore rated according to individual risk, although group contracts often benefit from group-rated premiums. The key exception to this trend is Ireland, where insurers are still obliged to offer community-rated premiums, open enrolment and lifetime cover. However, preserving community rating in the face of competition has been problematic, as Ireland's experience with BUPA demonstrates.[8] Although the Irish government successfully opposed BUPA's plans to offer a risk-rated cash policy in November 1996 (Mossialos and Le Grand 1999), the European Court of Justice may challenge its stance in supporting community rating in future.

Defining benefits

Voluntary health insurance in the EU covers a wide range of health services and offers a variety of benefit options, from total reimbursement of hospital costs to payment for cosmetic surgery or alternative treatment. Substitutive voluntary health insurance schemes offer the most comprehensive packages, largely as a result of strict government regulation, providing benefits similar to those covered by statutory health insurance. But the benefits arising from complementary and supplementary voluntary health insurance are unregulated, leaving insurers free to determine the size and scope of the packages they offer. This has led to a proliferation of complementary and supplementary voluntary health insurance products; individuals may be able to choose from a wide selection of packages with differences in levels of coverage, payment mechanisms, reimbursement (in kind or cash) and the extent of cost-sharing through co-payments, deductibles and ceilings on expenditure.

Numerous benefits may be excluded from supplementary coverage. In the United Kingdom, for example, voluntary health insurance does not usually cover pre-existing or chronic conditions (such as diabetes, multiple sclerosis and asthma), accident and emergency admission, normal pregnancy and childbirth, kidney dialysis, organ transplants, HIV/AIDS, outpatient drugs and dressings, infertility, preventive treatment, drug abuse, self-inflicted injuries, cosmetic surgery, gender reassignment, mobility aids, experimental treatment and drugs, war risks and injuries arising from hazardous pursuits (ABI 2000).

Over the last few years, in addition to emphasizing luxurious or upgraded accommodation, insurers in some EU member states have also offered budget plans with fixed cash payments. In the United Kingdom, an estimated 7.4 million people were covered by health cash plans at the end of 1999, up 2.5 per cent from the previous year (Papworth 2000).

Is there evidence of cream-skimming?

Cream-skimming (risk selection) is the process by which insurers seek to encourage custom from individuals with below-average risk and discourage or refuse custom from individuals with above-average risk. It is argued that cream-skimming is much more likely to take place under regulatory regimes that restrict insurers' freedom to rate premiums according to individual risk (that is, where insurers are paid a community or group-rated premium), therefore sophisticated risk adjustment may be the only means of successfully preventing insurers from cream-skimming (van de Ven et al. 2000). However, risk adjustment is expensive to administer and extremely difficult to carry out with accuracy, and while these problems may be mitigated if a central agency undertakes risk adjustment on behalf of all insurers, as in the Netherlands, risk adjustment mechanisms in other EU member states are limited in scope, with many insurers relying on crude indicators such as age, gender, occupation, family history of disease, health care utilization and claims experience. Crude risk adjustment may also give insurers strong incentives to cream-skim, to the detriment of both equity and efficiency (Puig-Junoy 1999).

A primary consequence of cream-skimming is that certain individuals will not have access to, or will be unable to afford, adequate cover. Cream-skimming not does not only pose serious equity problems; it may also lead to inefficiency, particularly where the financial advantages arising from risk selection outweigh potential gains from improvements in efficiency, leaving insurers with little incentive to compete on the basis of efficient management or quality (Gauthier *et al.* 1995). For example, in a competitive market, insurers may attempt to lower premiums by attracting low-risk individuals rather than by increasing efficiency, which reduces the optimal level of competition in the insurance market (Puig-Junoy 1999). BUPA's pricing trend in Ireland (premiums 10 per cent lower for people younger than 19 years and 20 per cent higher for people older than 54 years) suggests that it is following a policy of competition based on cream-skimming rather than on quality (Light 1998). Offering reduced premiums and favourable conditions for group insurance schemes has a similar effect – since people who are too ill or too old to work are excluded from the workplace, insurers automatically cover a younger, healthier, more homogeneous population.[9] Some voluntary health insurers use less explicit means to avoid covering potentially high-risk individuals. Physicians in Ireland have expressed concern about the possibility of reduced coverage for psychiatric patients under a competitive market system; recent reports indicate that BUPA Ireland's policy of insisting on detailed diagnostic information before admitting psychiatric patients, including the diagnosis, prognosis and expected date of discharge (a requirement that does not apply to any of its other patients), has led to serious delays in admission and has stigmatized individuals with mental disorders (Payne 2000). A report on the Austrian health care system noted that private hospital administrators increasingly inform physicians that no beds are available for patients who are likely to be resource-intensive, such as elderly people or people requiring total hip replacement (Bennett *et al.* 1993).

Cream-skimming is highly likely to occur when insurers are able to reject applications, exclude pre-existing conditions and cancel contracts, and when there is no standard or core package of benefits available. Insurers' incentives to cream-skim can, therefore, be addressed to some extent by guaranteeing access to coverage and automatic renewal of contracts, by limiting exclusions for pre-existing conditions and by requiring insurers to offer a standardized package of benefits. But since the third non-life insurance directive abolished product controls in 1994, thereby largely exempting insurers from regulation, governments in EU member states can only take this type of preventive action where substitutive voluntary health insurance is concerned. During the 1970s and 1980s in the Netherlands and the early 1990s in Germany, for example, cream-skimming in the substitutive voluntary health insurance sector led to steep rises in premiums for high-risk individuals, particularly elderly people, forcing the government in both member states to intervene (Wasem 1995). In contrast to government intervention in substitutive voluntary health insurance in Germany and the Netherlands, complementary and supplementary voluntary health insurance coverage can be offered as a short-term (non-life) contract or on a long-term (life) basis. Premiums are used to finance both current year costs and to build reserves for increasing age, although short-term (usually annual) contracts are the norm. The exceptions are Ireland, where insurers must provide lifetime coverage, and Greece, where individual voluntary health insurance contracts may be extended to lifetime coverage (CEA 1999). In the United Kingdom, coverage is provided on an annual basis. It is claimed that contracts are automatically renewed on a continuous basis (ABI 2000), but there is no evidence to indicate whether this happens in practice.

Financial equalization between voluntary health insurers

One way of avoiding cream-skimming is to set up a system of redistribution or financial equalization between insurers, which reduces their incentives to cream-skim in the long run. In fact, Swiss analysts suggest that financial equalization should be a permanent feature of a deregulated voluntary health insurance market (Beck and Zweifel 1998). At present, however, only two member states require financial equalization between insurers – Ireland and the Netherlands – and there are growing concerns that this type of government intervention may infringe EU legislation.

The Irish government is pursuing a policy of redistribution to support the operation of community rating, open enrolment and lifetime coverage in a competitive voluntary health insurance market. According to the Health Insurance (Amendment) Bill 2000, new insurers can choose to exempt themselves from participating in risk equalization arrangements for 3 years from the start of trading in Ireland (extended from the 18 months originally envisaged in a 1999 white paper on voluntary health insurance). Not surprisingly, risk equalization is extremely unpopular with BUPA Ireland (BUPA Ireland 2000).

Voluntary health insurers in the Netherlands are subject to a financial equalization scheme known as MOOZ, which spreads the risk of providing insurance to the disproportionately high number of older people insured under the statutory system (ZFW) by requiring each privately insured individual to make an annual contribution of €50 (0–19 years), €101 (20–64 years) or €81 (65 years or older) (Ministry of Health, Welfare and Sport 2000). Voluntary health insurers are also subject to financial equalization as a result of the WTZ scheme, which guarantees access to voluntary health insurance for elderly people and high-risk individuals. Because WTZ premiums only cover half the cost of providing standard coverage to elderly people and high-risk individuals, voluntary health insurers involved in the scheme receive full compensation from a central equalization fund financed by a mandatory surcharge on all other voluntary health insurance premiums, currently an annual flat-rate fee of €90 (0–19 years) or €180 (20–64 years) (Ministry of Health, Welfare and Sport 2000).

The creation of the single market has made it increasingly difficult for governments to justify this type of direct intervention, even in the interest of preserving health policy objectives such as accessibility and solidarity. A report produced by an independent government advisory body in the Netherlands argues that the government's equalization schemes contravene EU law;

the report's authors fear that confirmation of this by the European Court of Justice will undermine a fundamental element of health policy in the Netherlands (Raad voor de Volksgezondheid & Zorg 2000). The Dutch government is currently examining the extent to which the health care system is incompatible with EU regulation (van de Ven 2000). Compulsory redistribution in Ireland may also contravene EU law.

Addressing moral hazard in voluntary health insurance markets

Third-party payment incentives (or moral hazard) are inherent in any insurance market and may result in over-prescription of treatment by providers and over-consumption of health care by subscribers. Insurers can take several measures to reduce the risk of moral hazard on both the supply side (providers) and the demand side (subscribers).

Supply-side measures

Moral hazard can occur on the supply side when providers stand to gain financially from exploiting a subscriber's relative insensitivity to price. The resulting over-prescription of health care wastes resources and may expose the subscriber to unnecessary clinical risk. Insurers can address this problem by selectively contracting, adopting preferred provider networks or integrating with providers. Compared with insurers in the United States, however, EU insurers have done very little to tackle supply-side moral hazard, which is often seen as the state's responsibility. Integrated care still only plays a minor role in the EU, although there is a tendency towards vertical integration among the largest insurers in some EU member states, notably BUPA and PPP Healthcare in the United Kingdom and SANITAS in Spain (acquired by BUPA in the early 1990s), where insurers have traditionally been providers as well. Vertical integration also exists to some extent in Belgium and France, but is actually precluded by legislation in the Netherlands, at least for the time being (Ministry of Health, Welfare and Sport 2000).

The transition from indemnity insurance to integrated care is possible in countries with large voluntary health insurance markets (Chapter 5 shows this for the United States), but it is much harder to effect in smaller markets like the EU, where coverage is voluntary, there is double coverage and subscribers may object to any restriction in choice. Under these circumstances, insurers must strike a delicate balance between limiting preferred providers and maintaining subscriber choice, but recent experiments with integrated care systems in Belgium, France and Spain have had limited success (Mossialos and Thomson 2001).

For subscribers in the United Kingdom, the use of services outside BUPA's preferred network of providers is penalized with co-payments varying from about £65 for a minor operation to £575 for a major operation. Following complaints of anti-competitive practice, the Office of Fair Trading launched an inquiry into BUPA's and PPP Healthcare's development of preferred provider networks, vertical integration and negotiation of hospital charges. It did not uphold the complaints, but concluded that it would closely monitor any further moves towards vertical integration. It also demanded greater transparency and better information for subscribers (Office of Fair Trading 1999).

Demand-side measures

Demand-side measures work by restricting subscribers' access to health care. This can be achieved by introducing a referral system, by requesting prior authorization of treatment, by imposing cost-sharing or by reimbursing subscribers rather than providing benefits in kind. None of these measures is unique to voluntary health insurance; they can also occur under social health insurance and national health service systems.[10]

Voluntary health insurance policy-holders in the United Kingdom and the Netherlands still need a general practitioner referral before they can consult a specialist or receive inpatient treatment, although few insurers in the Netherlands conduct checks before reimbursing subscribers (Kulu-Glasgow *et al.* 1998). Some insurers in the United Kingdom encourage subscribers to obtain permission before undergoing treatment; others insist that subscribers contact them first to check that they are covered for the treatment they plan to undergo (ABI 2000).

Cost-sharing in the form of ceilings (usually annual caps), deductibles (excesses) and co-payments all seek to increase subscribers' awareness of the costs of health care. The extent to which subscribers are subject to cost-sharing varies considerably in different EU member states, but the trend is towards increasing reliance on cost-sharing as a means of securing income for voluntary health insurers (PPP Healthcare 2000). No-claims bonuses are a similar form of incentive, rewarding subscribers who make few or no claims. Some analysts argue that expanding the use of no-claims bonuses would be an effective means of containing costs; others have expressed concern about their potentially negative impact on beneficial health care utilization, as they may encourage subscribers to postpone treatment for as long as possible (Zweifel 1987).

Reimbursement requires subscribers to pay out of pocket and then claim back their expenses at a later date. This payment mechanism implicitly discourages and may even prevent some subscribers from using health services. It is the norm among voluntary health insurers in Belgium, Denmark, Germany and the Netherlands (although insurers in the Netherlands are increasingly paying providers directly) and takes place to a lesser extent in Austria, France and Spain.

The performance of voluntary health insurance

In this section, we assess the performance of voluntary health insurance in the EU in terms of coverage, the price of premiums, health service costs, administrative costs, insurers' profit ratios, impact on the health care system as a whole and equity implications.

Table 6.3 Annual increases in the average price of voluntary health insurance premiums in selected EU member states

Country	Per cent increase compounded annually (years)	Average annual growth rate of per-capita total expenditure on health measured in national currency units at current prices (%)
Germany	7.6 (1994–98)	4.5
Italy	6.5 (1994–98)	5.4
Spain	10.5 (1993–97)	5.5
United Kingdom		4.5
individual contracts	12.0 (1994–99)	
group contracts	< 3.0 (1994–99)	

Source: Datamonitor (2000) and OECD (2000)

Coverage

Levels of voluntary health insurance coverage vary substantially between EU member states and at first glance the figures can be misleading (see Table 6.2). France appears to have an extremely high coverage (85 per cent), but this is for the reimbursement of co-payments imposed by the statutory insurance scheme (see previously). Coverage for supplementary voluntary health insurance is much lower, at about 20 per cent of the population (CEA 1999).

It is also difficult to find reliable data on trends in voluntary health insurance coverage in the EU. Although trends in expenditure on voluntary health insurance as a proportion of total expenditure on health care could be used as an indirect measure of coverage levels (see Table 6.1), these data should be interpreted with caution. A recent report on European health insurance notes that, although the market for voluntary health insurance in the EU grew at a compound annual rate of 5.4 per cent in real terms between 1994 and 1999 (from €32,569 million to €42,423 million), a large proportion of this growth was caused by increases in the price of voluntary health insurance (rising premiums) rather than increases in coverage (see Table 6.3) (Datamonitor 2000).

Coverage remains low in many EU member states, even where people make substantial out-of-pocket payments to health care providers. Data published by the Comité Européen des Assurances (CEA 2000) show that, between 1992 and 1998, the proportion of insured individuals declined by −3.8 per cent in Austria and by −1.5% in the Netherlands, remained largely the same in the United Kingdom, and increased only slightly in Denmark, France, Portugal and Germany (by between 1.0 and 3.4 per cent). In 1999, however, the number of subscribers in the United Kingdom fell by 4.5 per cent (Laing and Buisson 2000). In Germany, less than a quarter of those individuals who can choose between statutory and substitutive voluntary health insurance have chosen the voluntary option, with approximately 77 per cent of them preferring to stay in the statutory health care system (Busse 2000). These findings are surprising, given that many of these member states, experienced sustained economic growth during the 1990s, but may be explained by the high cost of premiums in many EU member states (see the following section).

Costs

Premiums

Poor growth in the voluntary health insurance market in many EU member states may be attributed to expensive premiums and annual rises in premiums above the rate of inflation. A survey by a consumer analyst and research group in the United Kingdom found that 58 per cent of subscribers considered voluntary health insurance coverage to be too expensive (BBC 2000). Between 1991 and 1996, the real price of premiums rose at an average annual rate of nearly 5 per cent after inflation (Couchman 1999), with the average annual premium per subscriber rising from £323 (£373 for individual subscribers) in 1989 to £582 (£746) in 1998 (Laing and Buisson 2000). In 1988, the average individual premium was 15.5 per cent higher than the average group premium, but by 1998 it was 28.2 per cent more expensive (Laing and Buisson 2000). Not only are individual premiums much more expensive than group premiums, their annual increases have also been higher, typically over 10 per cent (Papworth 2000).

A comparison of the average amount paid per person covered by individual or employee paid voluntary health insurance in the United Kingdom with the average NHS per-capita expenditure for those aged 16–64 years shows just how expensive voluntary health insurance is, relative to the NHS, and its relative lack of value for money. In 1998–99 it cost the NHS in England on average £365.54 to provide all hospital and community health services (HCHS) for each individual aged 16–64 years (Department of Health 2000). During the same period, the average amount paid per person covered by individual or employee paid voluntary health insurance in the United Kingdom was £442.44 (Laing and Buisson 2000). The NHS figure of £365.54 not only covers treatment for most of the conditions typically excluded by voluntary health insurance in the United Kingdom, some of which are expensive to treat (for a full list of common exclusions, see the section above on defining benefits), it also covers mental health services, learning disability and other community health services. In 1995 these services and maternity care accounted for over 25 per cent of HCHS expenditure in England, while acute care accounted for approximately half (Department of Health 2000b, unpublished data). For the 50-year-old man buying a policy from PPP Healthcare in the United Kingdom, only the two lowest premium options, providing the least amount of cover and requiring the patient to pay the first £500 or £200 of any claim, are comparable to the NHS figure; the other 88 premium options rise well above it, with the most expensive costing as much as £4365 a year (CareHealth 2000). Some voluntary health insurance subscribers will also continue to make use of the NHS.

The proportion of spending on voluntary health insurance in Spain increased from 24 per cent of private expenditure in 1986 to 30 per cent in 1995, largely because of the rising cost of premiums (Lopez i Casasnovas 1999). The average premium more than doubled over the same period (rising from PTE23,670 in

Table 6.4 Voluntary health insurance profit ratios (premiums divided by benefits) in 11 EU member states in 1995 and 1998

Country	1995	1998
Austria	1.35	1.32
Belgium	1.33	1.35
Denmark	1.10	1.09
Finland	NA	1.44
France	1.29	1.27
Germany	1.25	1.42
Italy	1.35	1.28
Netherlands	1.14	1.12
Portugal	1.31	1.28
Spain	1.22	1.19
United Kingdom	1.22	1.20

Note: Profit ratios are obtained by dividing premium income by benefits paid.
NA = not available

Sources: authors' estimates based on CEA (1997, 2000)

1990 to PTE48,691 in 1997 in current prices) (Lopez i Casasnovas 1999). In the United Kingdom, the Office of Fair Trading (1996) recommended that subscribers should be given a comprehensive warning about the probable increase in voluntary health insurance premiums. The Social Health Insurance Reform Law of 2000 in Germany makes the same stipulation (CEA 2000). As Table 6.3 shows, the average price of premiums (for individual subscribers) in Germany, Italy, Spain and the United Kingdom rose by between 6.5 and 12.0 per cent a year during the second half of the 1990s, whereas the growth rate of per capita total expenditure on health was much lower, between 4.5 and 5.5 per cent a year.

Profit ratios

Between 1995 and 1998, voluntary health insurance premium income adjusted for inflation grew most in Belgium (14.8 per cent) and Portugal (14.4 per cent), followed by Spain (5.8 per cent) and the Netherlands (5.6 per cent); other EU member states, experienced growth of 3–4 per cent, whereas premium income actually declined in Austria (–2.6 per cent) and France (–1.8 per cent) (CEA 2000). During the same period, the growth in benefits paid exceeded the growth in premium income in some EU member states. Nevertheless, profit ratios[11] (obtained by dividing premium income by benefits paid) did not decline significantly between 1995 and 1998, and Germany's profit ratio actually increased substantially from 1.25 in 1995 to 1.42 in 1998 (Table 6.4).[12]

Health service costs

It is argued that high premium increases are caused by rising health service costs, but the extent of this causal relationship has not been established. It is also argued that increased competition in the voluntary health insurance market will improve efficiency by offering subscribers a wider range of options and prices, by controlling better the growth of health care costs and by forcing changes in the supply structures of health care providers. However, it is more likely that the cost of claims will increase in the long term because health service providers are unlikely to reduce their charges. In Ireland, for example, health service providers have consistently demanded increased payment without providing detailed evidence to justify their demands (Byrne 1997). Furthermore, it is estimated that charges to private patients in Dublin teaching hospitals are only half the average cost of beds in private hospitals, a public subsidy that costs the government €44 million (O'Shea 2000). Physicians in Germany are able to charge more for privately insured patients; consequently, cost increases in the private sector are almost two-thirds higher than in the statutory system – and twice as high for ambulatory care and pharmaceuticals (Busse 2000).

Administrative and marketing costs

Management and administration tend to be much more costly under a system of voluntary health insurance because of the extensive bureaucracy required to assess risk, set premiums, design complex benefit packages and review, pay or refuse claims. Voluntary health insurers also need to spend money on advertising, marketing and reinsurance. An estimated 14 per cent of voluntary health insurance benefits in the United States is spent on administrative costs, marketing expenses, profits and taxes, compared with 3 per cent in the publicly provided health insurance system and 1 per cent in Canada's provincial health plans (Woolhandler and Himmelstein 1991).

Data on the administrative costs of voluntary health insurance in the EU are limited, although the available evidence suggests that these costs are high. In Ireland, BUPA has struggled to compete with the Voluntary Health Insurance Board's low administration costs: only 2 per cent of premium income in 1996 versus BUPA's 12 per cent (Light 1998). By 1999, administrative costs had risen for both insurers, but the Voluntary Health Insurance Board's costs (4.7 per cent of premium income) were still considerably lower than those of BUPA (14.2 per cent) (BUPA 2000; Voluntary Health Insurance Board 2000). In 1998, the administrative costs of PPP Healthcare in the United Kingdom were even higher, at 16.9 per cent of premium income (AXA Sun Life 1999).

Economic theory suggests that high transaction costs are inefficient if they can be avoided under an alternative system of funding and providing health care (Barr 1998). However, some industry commentators in the United States argue that high transaction costs are justified by innovation (Danzon 1992), although this has been refuted by others (Barer and Evans 1992). Danzon claims that voluntary health insurers compete 'by devising ways to control moral hazard more effectively, including structured co-payments, utilization review, case management, selective contracting with preferred providers and provider targeted financial incentives such as capitation and other risk-sharing forms of prospective reimbursement' (Danzon 1992: 26). But this argument clearly cannot be applied to the EU, where most insurers do not, on the whole, adopt innovative strategies to attract subscribers; nor do they generally engage in the activities mentioned above to contain costs. Insurers in the EU tend to compete on the basis of risk selection rather than through purchasing, and their attempts to contain costs operate on the demand side rather than the supply side.

Impact on the health care system

We suggest that the market for voluntary health insurance may affect the statutory health care system in two ways. First, the existence of voluntary health insurance may be problematic where the boundaries between public and private health care are not clearly defined. Second, voluntary health insurance may undermine attempts to improve efficiency in the statutory health care system.

Boundaries between public and private health care

There is little evidence of the impact of double coverage on the efficiency and equity of health care systems in the EU, but it is reasonable to suppose that there may be negative consequences, particularly where voluntary health insurance gives rise to faster access. For example, faster access to private health care in some EU member states may mean that individuals undergo private consultations or receive private prescriptions which they then follow up in the public sector, leading to an increased burden on the public sector. If these individuals had received this treatment in the public sector, the public workload may have been the same, but the cost of that treatment to the individual would have differed substantially; and where doctors engage in both private and public practice, they may spend more time with private patients, leading to shorter treatment time or delayed treatment for public patients. Some insurers in the United Kingdom make cash payments to patients who opt to receive treatment in a public hospital (paid for by the NHS) instead of receiving treatment in a private hospital (paid for by the insurer).

Dual employment of physicians in both the public and the private sector may have an adverse effect on the quantity of care in the public sector. In the United Kingdom, the 25 per cent of specialists that performed the most private work, largely financed by voluntary health insurance and direct payments, carried out less NHS work than their colleagues (Audit Commission 1995).

Voluntary health insurance may undermine attempts to improve efficiency in the health care system

We have identified three areas in which voluntary health insurance might undermine a government's attempts to improve efficiency in the health care system: evidence-based health care, gatekeeping and co-payments to reduce demand. First, voluntary health insurers in the EU do not generally have incentives to promote evidence-based health care, although industry representatives in the United Kingdom claim that insurers are increasingly taking into account evidence-based guidelines and generally exclude treatments for which the evidence base is poor (Doyle and Bull 2000). It is true that some of the larger insurers in the United Kingdom have adopted evidence-based guidelines for treatments such as extraction of wisdom teeth, tonsillectomy and hysterectomy. At the same time, however, insurers are influenced by rising demand for alternative therapies such as acupuncture, homeopathy, osteopathy and chiropractic (currently among the areas of expenditure growing most rapidly for insurers in the United Kingdom). They therefore ultimately expand coverage of treatments for which there is little or no evidence base. It is questionable whether providing ineffective treatment to those who are willing to pay for it is a desirable policy objective. It could be argued that this is acceptable so long as the treatment provided is not actually harmful, but there may be cause for concern if patients are not well informed and are therefore vulnerable to over-charging or other exploitative practices.

In the Netherlands, weak gatekeeping in the private sector (leading to fewer general practitioner contacts for privately insured individuals) has negatively affected gatekeeping in the public sector. Until recently, individuals with statutory health insurance had to obtain a general practitioner referral before seeing a specialist or receiving treatment in hospital, but as a result of competition from voluntary health insurers, who do not insist on referral, some public sickness funds have decided to relax their gatekeeping requirements (Kulu-Glasgow *et al.* 1998).

In France, where insurers provide complementary cover for co-payments imposed by the statutory health care system, research shows that those with complementary voluntary health insurance consume more health care than those without, making 1.5 visits to a doctor in a 3 month period (compared to 1.1 visits for individuals without complementary voluntary health insurance) and seeking health care once every 73 days on average (compared to once every 100 days for those without this type of insurance) (Breuil-Genier 2000). There is also evidence that higher social classes in Germany use more specialist care than lower social classes; it is claimed that this reflects their voluntary health insurance coverage (Wysong and Abel 1990), although it may also be linked to information and educational levels.

Equity

There is a distinct lack of research on the equity implications of expanding voluntary health insurance in the EU. As we have shown, however, the fact that most subscribers are high earners suggests that any form of tax incentive to encourage the take-up of voluntary health insurance in the EU is likely to subsidize those who are already well off and will therefore be regressive in terms of funding health care. Voluntary health insurance is also likely to increase inequality in the provision of health care where it gives rise to faster access.

Wagstaff *et al.*'s (1999) analysis of vertical equity (that is, the extent to which individuals on unequal incomes are treated unequally)[13] in health care funding in 12 OECD countries in the early 1990s found voluntary health insurance to be regressive in France, Ireland and Spain, proportionate to income in Finland and progressive in Denmark, Germany, Italy, the Netherlands, Portugal and the United Kingdom (Wagstaff *et al.* 1999). The analysis also found that over time, voluntary health insurance had become less progressive in every country except Spain. The finding that voluntary health insurance was progressive in some countries can be attributed to the fact that only high earners are allowed to subscribe to it in Germany and the Netherlands, while most subscribers in the other countries come from high income groups, as we have shown.[14] An accompanying study attempted to measure horizontal equity (that is, the extent to which individuals on equal incomes are treated equally) in health care funding in the same set of countries. The study's analysis of the redistributive effect of health care funding among individuals with equal incomes found that voluntary health insurance caused income inequality in France and Ireland, had no redistributive effect in Denmark and had a very small redistributive effect in Germany and the Netherlands (van Doorslaer *et al.* 1999).

Borràs *et al.* (1999) suggest that the existence of voluntary health insurance may increase health inequity in Spain's health care system, with negative consequences for the health of poorer people. A further study of inequality in access to, and utilization of, health services in Catalonia according to social class found that, although double coverage did not influence the social pattern of visits to health services provided by the government, there was social inequality in the use of the health services provided only in part by the government (mostly dental care), and visits to a dentist were more frequent among those with complementary voluntary health insurance (Rajmil *et al.* 2000).

It is argued that an expansion of complementary and supplementary voluntary health insurance will not increase the regressivity of health care funding because individuals who take up these types of voluntary health insurance will be paying twice for their health care (Propper and Green 1999). According to this argument, double payment may even be beneficial because it reduces demand in the statutory health care system, enabling more resources to be spent on those without voluntary health insurance (Propper and Green 1999). Although this initially seems plausible, it may not happen in practice. For example, because both the public and the private sector in the United Kingdom depend on the same supply of doctors to provide medical treatment, an increase in private-sector activity *per se* may not lead to an increase in the public sector's capacity to tackle long waiting lists. Double payment or double coverage may have a negative effect on the delivery of health care where there is no clear boundary between public and private provision, as in the United Kingdom, and where some providers are paid by both sectors, which could lead to cost shifting from the private to the public sector. In such circumstances, the total equity effect of complementary and supplementary voluntary health insurance (taking into account both equity in finance and equity in the receipt of benefits) would be negative. It is also difficult to see how an expansion of complementary and supplementary voluntary health insurance would increase the redistributive effect of health care funding.

Conclusions

In this chapter we have classified voluntary health insurance in the EU accord-ing to whether it substitutes for the statutory health care system, provides complementary coverage for services excluded or not fully covered by the state or provides supplementary coverage for faster access and increased consumer choice (although the distinction between complementary and sup-plementary voluntary health insurance is not always clear and there may be significant cross-over between them).

On the whole we do not find evidence of EU member states favouring an expansion of voluntary health insurance. Statutory health care systems con-tinue to provide comprehensive benefits; governments have tended to reduce or remove tax incentives to encourage the take-up of voluntary health insur-ance, finding them to be expensive, regressive and largely unsuccessful in stimulating demand; and where private expenditure has increased in recent years, it has largely been due to the imposition of user charges.

In spite of sustained economic growth in several EU member states, levels of voluntary health insurance coverage only grew slightly or stagnated during the 1990s. Coverage remains low in many EU member states, even where people make substantial out-of-pocket payments to health care providers. Our analysis suggests that this is because the benefits provided by voluntary health insurance in the EU are expensive when compared to those provided by the statutory health care system. The cost of premiums in many EU member states has consistently risen above the rate of inflation and many people find pre-miums to be unaffordable. Rising demand for voluntary health insurance in the 1980s and early 1990s can largely be attributed to substantial growth in the group purchased voluntary health insurance sector, which expanded rapidly during the 1980s and still accounts for over half of all voluntary health insur-ance policies in several EU member states. Coverage through group contracts continues to rise faster than individual voluntary health insurance coverage, probably because group premiums are substantially lower than individual pre-miums and their annual increases are also much smaller.

Evidence regarding the distribution of voluntary health insurance coverage in the EU shows that the majority of subscribers are high earners, which is to be expected where substitutive voluntary health insurance is concerned, as eligibility for this type of insurance depends on income or occupation, but complementary and supplementary voluntary health insurance also show a strong bias in favour of high-income groups.

The EU market for voluntary health insurance is diverse in terms of the number and type of insurers in operation, although the number of insurance companies is falling and further market consolidation is likely to take place. For largely historical reasons, not-for-profit mutual or provident associations dominate the voluntary health insurance market in many EU member states, sometimes benefiting from differential tax treatment. This situation is unlikely to continue indefinitely, however, as differential treatment of mutual associ-ations in France may be challenged by the European Court of Justice. In future, for-profit commercial insurers are likely to gain an increasing share of the market.

The market for complementary and supplementary voluntary health insurance in the EU was liberalized and deregulated in 1994, but the expected benefits of deregulation (increased competition, leading to greater efficiency and improved consumer choice) have not materialized. A closer look at the EU market suggests that deregulation has actually exacerbated significant information failures that limit its potential for competition or efficiency gains and reduce equity. Deregulation has also stripped regulatory bodies of sufficient power to protect consumers.

Given the information failures inherent in any insurance market, it is generally acknowledged that privatization should be accompanied by strong government supervision, at least in terms of controlling information flows. However, since the abolition of price and product controls for complementary and supplementary voluntary health insurance in 1994, these markets have been awash with different insurance products. In the absence of clear information about price, quality and conditions, voluntary health insurance subscribers in the EU find it difficult to compare these products in terms of value for money, which puts them at a competitive disadvantage in the marketplace. In fact, it is questionable whether price and product competition is feasible in a market with multiple insurance products.

Vertical integration of insurers and providers of health care has not enjoyed much success in the EU, partly because the market is relatively small and partly because it exists to increase subscriber choice. Although evidence is limited, cream-skimming appears to be a feature of the voluntary health insurance market in some EU member states, where it may lead to gaps in coverage for those who are most likely to be vulnerable, such as elderly people. While financial equalization mechanisms can reduce insurers' incentives to cream-skim in the long term, they are only used in Ireland and the Netherlands, and there are fears that they may contravene existing EU legislation.

Where the boundaries between public and private health care are not clearly defined, voluntary health insurance may have a negative effect on the wider health care system. It may also undermine attempts to improve efficiency. Voluntary health insurance may increase inequality in terms of access to health care and there is some evidence to suggest that the existence of voluntary health insurance increases health inequity in some EU member states.

Notes

1 In the context of the European Union we use the term voluntary health insurance. We define voluntary health insurance as health insurance that is taken up and paid for at the discretion of individuals or employers on behalf of individuals. Voluntary health insurance can be offered by public or quasi-public bodies and by for-profit and not-for-profit private organizations.

2 With the exception of the Netherlands and, to a lesser extent, Germany.

3 We focus on voluntary health insurance for medical expenses. Voluntary health insurance in the EU also covers loss of earnings, cash benefits and long-term care, although in practice very few markets can be split up in such a detailed way.

4 Civil servants in the Netherlands are also obligated to leave the statutory system; they are covered through a special public health insurance scheme closely resembling the statutory scheme.

5 The figures we present on levels of coverage should be interpreted with some caution, as at first glance they can be misleading. For example, France appears to have an extremely high level of coverage (85 per cent), but this is for the reimbursement of co-payments imposed by the statutory insurance scheme. Coverage for supplementary voluntary health insurance is much lower, at about 20 per cent of the population (CEA 1999).

6 Price elasticity is a measurement of the change in demand for a good or service caused by a change in the price of that good or service. Income elasticity is a measurement of the change in demand for a good or service caused by a change in the income of the individual purchasing that good or service.

7 In 1998, tax expenditure on voluntary health insurance cost the United States government US$111.2 billion and mainly benefited the rich; families with incomes of US$100,000 or more (10 per cent of the population) accounted for 23.6 per cent of all tax subsidies for voluntary health insurance (Sheils and Hogan 1999).

8 BUPA Ireland is the only major insurer to have entered and remained in Ireland since the Irish market was opened to limited competition in 1994, in order to comply with the third non life insurance directive. The Irish market is dominated by the Voluntary Health Insurance Board, which was established in 1957 as a not-for-profit, quasi public but independent body. It is soon to be converted to a state owned public limited company with full commercial freedom (Department of Health and Children 1999).

9 Group insurance schemes also limit adverse selection by imposing compulsory coverage, thereby spreading risk across a wider pool of people (Gauthier *et al.* 1995; Deber *et al.* 1999).

10 When prior authorization is a feature of statutory health care systems, however, it usually only applies to treatment that must be taken abroad because it is not available in the home country.

11 In our estimation of profit ratios, we do not take into account any investment of revenue or profit.

12 Although many insurers in the EU have not-for-profit, mutual or provident status, their income may (and generally does) still exceed expenditure. The same applies to not-for-profit insurers in the United States.

13 In a regressive funding system the poor spend a greater proportion of their income on health care than the rich; in a proportionate funding system everybody spends the same proportion of their income; and a progressive funding system is one in which the rich spend a greater proportion of their income on health care than the poor.

14 Because access to substitutive voluntary health insurance is mainly determined by income, those covered by this type of insurance are expected to be high earners. The distribution of coverage for complementary and supplementary voluntary health insurance should show greater overall variation; in general it does, but it is also strongly biased in favour of high income groups.

References

ABI (2000) *The Private Medical Insurance Market*. London: Association of British Insurers.

Audit Commission (1995) *National Report. The Doctor's Tale: The Work of Hospital Doctors in England and Wales*. London: HMSO.

AXA Sun Life (1999) *Sun Life and Provincial Holdings Annual Report and Accounts for 1999*. Bristol: AXA Sun Life.

Bain, J. (1956) *Barriers to New Competition*. Cambridge, MA: Harvard University Press.

Barer, M. and Evans, R. (1992) Interpreting Canada: models, mind-sets and myths, *Health Affairs*, 11(1): 44–61.

Barr, N. (1998) *The Economics of the Welfare State*. Oxford: Oxford University Press.

BBC (2000) Private medical insurance 'too expensive', *BBC News*, 5 October 2000. http://news6.thdo.bbc.co.uk/hi/english/health/newsid%5F957000/957844.stm (accessed 25 February 2001).

Beck, K. and Zweifel, P. (1998) Cream-skimming in deregulated social health insurance: evidence from Switzerland, *Developments in Health Economics and Public Policy*, 6: 211–27.

Bennett, C.L., Schwarz, B. and Marberger, M. (1993) Health care in Austria: universal access, national health insurance and private health care, *Journal of the American Medical Association*, 269(21): 2789–94.

Besley, T., Hall, J. and Preston, I. (1998) Private and public health insurance in the UK, *European Economic Review*, 42(3–5): 491–7.

Besley, T., Hall, J. and Preston, I. (1999) The demand for private health insurance: do waiting lists matter?, *Journal of Public Economics*, 72: 155–81.

Blanpain, N. and Pan Ké Shon, J-L. (1997) L'assurance complémentaire maladie: une diffusion encore inégale [Complementary health insurance: an unequal distribution], *INSEE Première*, 523, June.

BMI (2000) *Medical Insurance*, London: BMI Europe Ltd. http://www.bmieurope.com/cover/medical.html (accessed 25 February 2001).

Borràs, J., Guillen, M., Sánchez, V., Juncà, S. and Vicente, R. (1999) Educational level, voluntary private health insurance and opportunistic cancer screening among women in Catalonia (Spain), *European Journal of Cancer Prevention*, 8: 427–34.

Breuil-Genier, P. (2000) Généraliste puis spécialiste: un parcours peu fréquent, *INSEE Première*, 709, April.

BUPA (2000) *Report and Accounts 1999*. London: BUPA.

BUPA Ireland (2000) *BUPA Ireland Chief Calls for Healthy Competition: Risk Equalisation 'Rigs the Market'*, Dublin: BUPA Ireland. http://www.bupaireland.ie/whatsnew/rigsthemarket.htm (accessed 25 February 2001).

Busse, R. (2000) *Health Care Systems in Transition: Germany*. Copenhagen: European Observatory on Health Care Systems.

Byrne, A. (1997) The Voluntary Health Insurance Board: prospects for survival in a competitive environment, *Administration*, 45(2): 59–79.

Calnan, M., Cant, S. and Gabe, J. (1993) *Going Private: Why People Pay for their Health Care*. Buckingham: Open University Press.

CareHealth (2000) *Criticisms of Private Medical Insurance by the Office of Fair Trading*, London: CareHealth. http://www.carehealth.co.uk/pmicrit.htm (accessed 25 February 2001).

CEA (1997) *Health Insurance in Europe 1997*. Paris: Comité Européen des Assurances.

CEA (1999) *Annual Report 1999*. Paris: Comité Européen des Assurances.

CEA (2000) *Health Insurance in Europe: 1998 Data*, CEA ECO 12, July. Paris: Comité Européen des Assurances.

Couchman, A. (1999) *UK Health and Welfare Insurance, Management Reports 1999*. London: Financial Times Finance.

Couffinhal, A. (1999) *Concurrence en assurance santé: entre efficacité et sélection [Competition in health insurance: between efficiency and selection]*. PhD thesis, Université Paris IX-Dauphine.

Danzon, P.M. (1992) Hidden overhead costs: is Canada's system really less expensive?, *Health Affairs*, 11: 21–43.

Datamonitor (2000) *European Health Insurance 2000: What's the Prognosis, Doctor?* London: Datamonitor.

Davey, B. (1998) The OFT's continuing work on health insurance, a *Speech to the Money Marketing Conference on Health Insurance*, 22 April, London: Office of Fair Trading. http://www.oft.gov.uk/html/rsearch/sp-arch/speech10.htm (accessed 25 February 2001).

Davies, P. (1999) The role of health insurance in New Zealand: health insurance in New Zealand, *Healthcare Review – Online*, 3(4 April 1999). http://www.enigma.co.nz/hcro_articles/9904/vol3no4_002.htm (accessed 25 February 2001).

Deber, R., Gildiner, A. and Baranek, P. (1999) Why not private health insurance? 1. Insurance made easy, *Canadian Medical Association Journal*, 161(5): 539–42.

Department of Health (2000) *The NHS Plan: A Plan for Investment, a Plan for Reform*. London: The Stationery Office.

Department of Health and Children (1999) *Private Health Insurance, White Paper*. Dublin: Government of Ireland.

Dixon, A. (1999) *Health Care Systems in Transition: Portugal*. Copenhagen: European Observatory on Health Care Systems.

Dixon, A. and Mossialos, E. (2000) Has the Portuguese NHS achieved its objectives of equity and efficiency?, *International Social Security Review*, 53(5): 49–78.

Doyle, Y. and Bull, A. (2000) Role of private sector in United Kingdom health care system, *British Medical Journal*, 321: 563–5.

Emmerson, C., Frayne, C. and Goodman, A. (2000) *Pressures in UK Healthcare: Challenges for the NHS*, Commentary 81. London: The Institute for Fiscal Studies.

Emmerson, C., Frayne, C. and Goodman, A. (2001) Should private medical insurance be subsidised?, *Health Care UK*, 51(4): 49–65.

European Commission (1992) Council Directive 92/49/EEC of 18 June 1992 on the coordination of laws, regulations and administrative provisions relating to direct insurance other than life assurance and amending Directives 73/239/EEC and 88/357/EEC (third non-life insurance Directive), *Official Journal of the European Communities*, L228(11/08): 1–23.

European Commission (1997) *Liberalisation of Insurance in the Single Market – an Update, 15 October 1997*. Brussels: European Commission. http://europa.eu.int/comm/internal_market/en/finances/insur/87.htm (accessed 25 February 2001).

European Commission (2000) *Insurance: Infringement Proceedings against France Concerning Mutual Societies and the Requirement of a Marketing Information Sheet*, 28 July. Brussels: The European Commission.

Freire, J. (1999) The new tax status of private health insurance, *Gaceta Sanitaria*, 13(3): 233–6.

Gauthier, A., Lamphere, J.A. and Barrand, N.L. (1995) Risk selection in the health care market: a workshop overview, *Inquiry*, 32: 14–22.

Hermesse, J. and Lewalle, H. (1995) Regulation of prices and services covered by complementary health schemes: *status quo* and future needs, in M. Schneider (ed.) *Complementary Health Schemes in the European Union*, European Commission Seminar, Prien am Chiemsee, Bavaria, 14–16 October 1992. Augsburg: BASYS.

INSEE (2000) *Tableaux de l'Economie Française 1999/2000* [Overview of the French Economy 1999/2000]. Paris: National Institute for Statistics and Economic Studies.

King, D. and Mossialos, E. (2001) *Determinants of the Demand for Private Medical Insurance in Britain*, LSE Health and Social Care Working Paper. London: LSE Health and Social Care.

Kulu-Glasgow, I., Delnoij, D. and de Bakker, D. (1998) Self-referral in a gatekeeping system: patients' reasons for skipping the general practitioner, *Health Policy*, 45: 221–38.

Laing and Buisson (2000) *Private Medical Insurance: UK Market Sector Report 2000*. London: Laing and Buisson.

Light, D. (1998) Keeping competition fair for health insurance: how the Irish beat back risk-rated policies, *American Journal of Public Health*, 88(5): 745–8.

Lopez i Casasnovas, G. (1999) Health care and cost containment in Spain, in E. Mossialos and J. Le Grand (eds) *Health Care and Cost Containment in the European Union.* Aldershot: Ashgate.

Manning, W.G. and Marquis, M.S. (1989) *Health Insurance: The Trade-off between Risk Pooling and Moral Hazard* (R-3729-NCHSR). Santa Monica, CA: RAND.

Marquis, M.S. and Long, S.H. (1995) Worker demand for health insurance in the non-group market, *Journal of Health Economics,* 14: 47–63.

Mason, E.S. (1939) Price and production policies of large-scale enterprise, *American Economic Review,* 29(suppl.): 61–74.

Ministry of Health, Welfare and Sport (2000) *Health Insurance in the Netherlands,* 5th edn. The Hague: Ministry of Health, Welfare and Sport.

Mossialos, E. and Le Grand, J. (1999) Cost containment in the EU: an overview, in E. Mossialos and J. Le Grand (eds) *Health Care and Cost Containment in the European Union.* Aldershot: Ashgate.

Mossialos, E. and Thomson, S.M.S. (2001) *Voluntary Health Insurance in the European Union,* LSE Health and Social Care Discussion Paper No. 19. London: LSE Health and Social Care.

Natarajan, K. (1996) *European Health Insurance Markets: Opportunity or False Dawn?* London: FT Financial Publishing/Pearson Professional Ltd.

OECD (1998) *Competition and Related Regulation Issues in the Insurance Industry.* Paris: Organisation for Economic Co-operation and Development.

OECD (2000) *OECD Health Data 2000: A Comparative Analysis of 29 Countries.* Paris: Organisation for Economic Co-operation and Development.

Office of Fair Trading (1996) *Health Insurance: A Report by the Office of Fair Trading.* London: Office of Fair Trading.

Office of Fair Trading (1999) *VHI and PMS Markets are Competitive Says OFT but Better Information for Policy Holders is Needed,* 5 November. London: Office of Fair Trading.

O'Shea, D. (2000) Private bed charges to increase by £35 million, *Irish Medical Times,* 34: 24.

Papworth, J. (2000) Take more care of yourself, *The Guardian,* 5 August.

Payne, D. (2000) Health insurer delays psychiatric admissions, *British Medical Journal,* 320: 1162.

Pellisé, L. (1994) Reimbursing insurance carriers: the case of 'MUFACE' in the Spanish health care system, *Health Economics,* 3: 243–53.

PKV (1994) *Private Health Insurance: Facts and Figures 1992/93.* Cologne: Verband der privaten Krankenversicherung e.V.

PPP Healthcare (2000) *PPP Healthcare Update – 09/11/1999,* Kent: PPP Healthcare. http://www.ppphealthcare.co.uk/html/siteplan/siteplan.htm (accessed 25 February 2001).

Propper, C. and Green, K. (1999) *A Larger Role for the Private Sector in Health Care? A Review of the Arguments,* CMPO Working Paper No. 99/009. Bristol: Centre for Market and Public Organization.

Puig-Junoy, J. (1999) Managing risk selection incentives in health sector reforms, *International Journal of Health Planning and Management,* 14: 287–311.

Raad voor de Volksgezondheid & Zorg (Council for Public Health and Healthcare) (2000) *Europe and Healthcare,* Zoetermeer: Raad voor de Volksgezondheid & Zorg. http://www.rvz.net/Samenvat/Werk99/europe.htm (accessed 25 February 2001).

Rajmil, L., Borrell, C., Starfield, B. *et al.* (2000) The quality of care and influence of double health care coverage in Catalonia (Spain), *Archives of Diseases in Childhood,* 83(3): 211–14.

Rees, R., Gravelle, H. and Warnbach, A. (1999) Regulation of insurance markets, *Geneva Papers on Risk and Insurance Theory,* 24: 55–68.

Robinson, R. and Dixon, A. (1999) *Health Care Systems in Transition: United Kingdom.* Copenhagen: European Observatory on Health Care Systems.

Rocard, M. (2000) *Report on Supplementary Health Insurance* (A5-0266/2000). Brussels: Committee on Employment and Social Affairs.

Rupprecht, F., Tissot, B. and Chatel, F. (2000) German health care system: promoting greater responsibility among all system players, *INSEE Studies*, 42(January): 1–23.

Santerre, R. and Neun, S. (2000) *Health Economics: Theories, Insights and Industry Studies*. Orlando, FL: The Dryden Press.

Schneider, M. (ed.) (1995) *Complementary Health Schemes in the European Union*, European Commission seminar, Prien am Chiemsee, Bavaria, 14–16 October 1992. Augsburg: BASYS.

Sheils, J. and Hogan, P. (1999) Cost of tax-exempt health benefits in 1998, *Health Affairs (Millwood)*, 18(2): 176–81.

Sissouras, A., Karokis, A. and Mossialos, E. (1999) Health care and cost containment in Greece, in E. Mossialos and J. Le Grand (eds) *Health Care and Cost Containment in the European Union*. Aldershot: Ashgate.

Taroni, F. (2000) Devolving responsibility for funding and delivering health care in Italy, *Euro Observer*, 2(1): 1–2.

van de Ven, W.P.M.M. (2000) The first decade of market oriented health care reforms in the Netherlands, presented at the First Meeting of the European Health Care Systems Discussion Group (EHCSDG), London School of Economics and Political Science, 14–15 September.

van Doorslaer, E., Wagstaff, A., van der Burg, H. *et al.* (1999) The redistributive effect of health care finance in twelve OECD countries, *Journal of Health Economics*, 18(3): 291–313.

van de Ven, W.P.M.M., van Vliet R.C.J.A., Schut, F.T., van Barneveld, E.M. (2000) Access to coverage for high-risks in a competitive individual health insurance market: via premium rate restrictions or risk-adjusted premium subsidies?, *Journal of Health Economics*, 19: 311–39.

Voluntary Health Insurance Board (2000) *Annual Report 2000*. Dublin: Voluntary Health Insurance Board.

Wagstaff, A., van Doorslaer, E., van der Burg, H. *et al.* (1999) Equity in the finance of health care: some further international comparisons, *Journal of Health Economics*, 18(3): 263–90.

Wasem, J. (1995) Regulating private health insurance markets, in K. Okma (ed.) *Four Country Conference on Health Care Reforms and Health Care Policies in the United States, Canada, Germany and the Netherlands*, Amsterdam, 23–25 February. The Hague: Ministry of Health, Welfare and Sport.

Woolhandler, S. and Himmelstein, D.U. (1991) The deteriorating administrative efficiency of the US health care system, *New England Journal of Medicine*, 324: 1253–8.

Wysong, J.A. and Abel, T. (1990) Universal health insurance and high-risk groups in West Germany: implications for US health policy, *The Milbank Quarterly*, 68(4): 527–60.

Youngman, I. (1994) *The Health Insurance Opportunity: A Worldwide Study of Private Medical Insurance Markets*. Dublin: Lafferty Publications.

Zweifel, P. (1987) Bonus systems in health insurance: a microeconomic analysis, *Health Policy*, 7(2): 273–88.

chapter seven

User charges for health care

Ray Robinson[1]

Introduction

The often high cost and uncertain demand for health care has meant that direct user charges comprise a small proportion of total health care expenditure in most European countries. Instead, several types of risk-pooling arrangements have been developed to cushion individuals from the financial effects of ill health. The United States, for example, has a large private insurance market. Most European countries, in contrast, place more emphasis on schemes that are publicly funded through social insurance contributions or general taxes. In publicly funded schemes, contributions are more closely related to the ability to pay than to personal risk status. But all insurance arrangements – both public and private – protect individuals from the full financial costs of the services they receive at the time of use. Instead, a third-party payer, either public or private, picks up all or most of the bill.

Although the nature of health care markets provides strong reasons for a third-party payer system, the absence of user charges is periodically criticized on the grounds that it encourages excessive demand for health services and thereby contributes to escalating expenditure. This is generally referred to as the problem of 'moral hazard'. It is argued that introducing or increasing user charges will make individuals more aware of the costs of health care services and will deter people from using services that are not really necessary: where the expected marginal private benefit is less than the marginal private cost or, at the societal level, where the marginal social benefit is less than the marginal social cost.

In addition to this argument, a separate case in support of user charges is that they provide additional revenue when governments are having difficulty in funding health care by taxation or social insurance contributions. This applies to several countries in central and eastern Europe (CEE) and the former

Soviet Union (FSU), in which low economic growth, falling levels of employment and wariness about government funding in the post-communist world have made relying on general taxation and social insurance contributions difficult. In these circumstances, cost-sharing does not aim to reduce demand: on the contrary, additional revenue is maximized when there is price-inelastic demand.

This chapter analyses these arguments for user charges. It provides an analytical framework for examining international evidence on user charges and for assessing their impact. An overview is also provided of the international evidence on the scope and scale of user charging in western and central and eastern Europe and some important trends are highlighted. This is followed by an assessment of the evidence on the impact of user charging in terms of the evaluation criteria of efficiency, equity and public acceptability. Finally, cost sharing is discussed and some tentative arguments are offered about the appeal of user charges to politicians and policy makers.

An analytical framework

User charges can take several different forms. Conceptually, these can be viewed as different positions on a continuum ranging from full third-party payment (zero cost-sharing) to full user charges (costs met completely by out-of-pocket payments). Rubin and Mendelson (1995) have conveniently summarized two ranges on this continuum by distinguishing between direct and indirect cost-sharing.

Direct cost-sharing includes co-payment (a flat fee or charge per service), co-insurance (a percentage of the total charge), deductible (a payment covering the first x dollars before insurance coverage begins) and balance billing (an additional fee the provider levies in addition to the payment received from the third-party payer). *Indirect* cost-sharing involves those policies that can result in out-of-pocket expenditure for patients even though charges are not directly imposed. According to Rubin and Mendelson, these policies include coverage exclusions (such as insurance contracts specifying services that will not be reimbursed, such as *in vitro* fertilization) and various forms of pharmaceutical regulatory mechanisms such as generic substitution and formularies (positive, negative and selected lists).

Here, most attention will focus on systems of direct cost-sharing, although some complicating factors need to be borne in mind. For example, at the empirical level, national data on out-of-pocket payments usually cover all user charges and fail to distinguish between direct and indirect cost-sharing. Furthermore, in some countries (such as France), people take out insurance to defray the costs of charges arising from cost-sharing. In such cases, direct costs are themselves met by third-party payments. Finally, in most CEE and FSU countries, informal payments represent an important source of direct cost-sharing, but their informal nature means that they fail to meet the standards of transparency met by formal systems, and the magnitude is largely unrecorded (see Chapter 8 for more discussion).

In analysing the impact of direct cost-sharing schemes, Chalkley and Robinson (1997) highlighted the importance of the payment profile faced by health service users. In particular, they point out the importance of marginal prices and their expected impact on behaviour. User-charging schemes take a variety of forms, including linear pricing (co-insurance), two-part tariffs, non-linear full marginal cost pricing (deductibles) and non-linear partial marginal cost pricing (balance billing or reference pricing). Each of these offers different financial incentives at the margin.

Attention to marginal prices is especially relevant in service areas in which demand is user-led and the volume or quantity of services consumed by a particular patient is the main concern. These conditions apply to, for example, general practitioner consultations and, in some cases, to pharmaceutical prescriptions. In both of these areas, marginal prices may be an important determinant of demand.

Moving on from the classification of different types of cost-sharing arrangement, determining the criteria to use in evaluating the performance of a cost-sharing scheme is important. Kutzin (1998) reviewed the main economic criteria, namely, efficiency and equity. In this context, efficiency has several connotations. If the aim of cost-sharing is to discourage 'unnecessary' demand, its effect on the utilization of services is the key measure. Beyond this, however, disaggregating changes (reductions) in utilization is important to examine whether these have involved appropriate (effective) or inappropriate (ineffective) services, if these can be distinguished. This, in turn, addresses the effects of cost-sharing on health status. Establishing the effects of cost-sharing on the level and pattern of demand allows performance to be assessed in terms of allocative efficiency.

In some countries, however, the aim of cost-sharing is not so much to reduce demand but to generate revenue for funding health care when alternative funding (such as tax revenue) is not available. This objective is sometimes discussed under macro-efficiency – because it focuses on reducing public expenditure on health – but it really has little to do with the concept of efficiency as developed by economists. Rather, it is a policy for public-sector cost containment. As such, cost-sharing can be judged in terms of its success in meeting this objective, although the underlying desirability of the objective is less well established than that of allocative efficiency.

The criterion of equity in health care is complex and is often only loosely defined in discussions of cost-sharing. For practical purposes, however, it is probably sufficient to investigate whether imposing cost-sharing arrangements disproportionately affects lower-income groups as observed through changes in their utilization of services. A slightly wider definition may wish to observe effects on especially vulnerable groups, such as elderly people and people with chronic diseases, independently of their income. Equity in financing as well as equity in utilization may have to be considered; that is, the financial burden of user charges as a proportion of income among different socioeconomic groups.

Economists mainly use efficiency and equity to assess the performance of most health policy instruments. However, other considerations also apply to general health policy. The cost and feasibility of administering cost-sharing arrangements is an important consideration. Although these are often identified separately, these are really an aspect of efficiency and are dealt with as such here. Finally, there is the question of the public acceptability of cost-sharing. In many countries, cost-sharing is a hotly debated political issue. As such, public attitudes can constitute an important constraint on implementing cost-sharing arrangements.

To summarize the discussion on evaluative criteria, any cost-sharing scheme should be assessed in terms of its effects on efficiency, equity (including on health status) and public acceptability.

An overview of cost-sharing in Europe

Two studies have reviewed cost-sharing arrangements in western Europe (Mossialos and Le Grand 1999) and in CEE and FSU countries (Kutzin 1998). Tables 7.1 and 7.2 summarize some of the main findings from these studies. Although obtaining data that are completely standardized across countries is difficult, the tables provide a broad indication of the cost-sharing arrangements found in each country in the main service areas to which they are applied: primary care consultations and ambulatory care, specialist consultations, inpatient care, pharmaceuticals and dental care. Table 7.1 also shows the relative importance of cost-sharing in each country as indicated by the share of total health expenditure financed from out-of-pocket payments (both direct and indirect cost-sharing).

This international comparative analysis produced the following findings.

Pharmaceuticals are a major area of cost-sharing. All 15 European Union countries apply cost-sharing in relation to this sector. In most cases, this takes the form of co-insurance, with the rate varying between different classes of products. Drugs used to treat life-threatening diseases or which have major therapeutic effects are typically subject to lower rates of cost-sharing than those offering more marginal improvements in the quality of life. But not all countries employ co-insurance. In the United Kingdom, and for some drugs in Belgium and Italy, cost-sharing takes the form of a flat rate co-payment. Germany also has a set of flat-rate co-payments but, in this case, they vary according to pack size. Ireland has a maximum quarterly expenditure that acts as a deductible. Germany, the Netherlands and Sweden use reference pricing, and consumers pay the costs exceeding the reference price.

Policies on cost-sharing in relation to general practitioner consultations and ambulatory care vary between countries. Nine countries apply cost-sharing systems in this sector. These include co-payments (such as Ireland and Sweden), co-insurance (such as Austria, Belgium and France) and balance billing (such as Denmark[2] and Greece). Set against these practices, however, Germany, Italy, the Netherlands, Spain and the United Kingdom do not levy user payments for general practitioner consultations.

Most countries (11 of 15) use some form of cost-sharing in relation to specialist consultations. These are often applied in similar ways to the relevant cost-sharing arrangement for general practitioner services. Thus, France and Luxembourg apply the same rates of co-insurance – 30 per cent and 35 per cent, respectively – to both general practitioner and specialist consultations. In most countries, balance billing is not allowed. It is, however, used in Belgium, Denmark[3] and France for specialist consultations.

Table 7.1 Cost-sharing in health care in the 15 European Union countries

Country	General practitioner	Specialist	Inpatient	Pharmaceutical	Dental	Out-of-pocket payments as a percentage of total expenditure on health
Austria	No payment for 80% of the population; the remainder pay about 20% of the cost	Same arrangements as general practitioner services	€3.6–4.4 per day for up to 28 days	€3.1 per prescription	Co-insurance of about 20% for most of the population, with payments of up to 50% for special services, such as fitting crowns	18.3% (1998)
Belgium[a]	8% of fee (for low-income and disabled people, pensioners, widows and orphans) to 30% for others	Charges ranging from 8% (for low-income groups) to 40%	Charges ranging from €33.9 per day (days 1–8) to €12.1 per day for stays over 90 days. Lower charges for low-income groups	Co-insurance rates of 0%, 25%, 50% and 60% of cost depending on drug categories. Price ceilings apply. Reduced rates for low-income groups	Large co-payments or full-cost pricing for most groups. Limited free services for children (under 18 years)	17% (1994)
Denmark	None for most people, although balance billing applies to about 2% of the population who choose to have direct access to general practitioners and specialists	Same as general practitioner services	None	Co-insurance rates vary depending on the individual annual out-of-pocket expenditure: 100% up to DKr500 per year, 50% for DKr501–1200, 25% for DKr1201–2800 and 15% for over DKr2800. For chronically ill patients who spend over DKr3600 on drugs per year, the co-insurance rate is 0%	Co-insurance rates ranging from 35% to 100%. Cost-sharing accounted for about 75% of total cost in 1994	16.5% (1999)

Table 7.1 (cont'd)

Country	General practitioner	Specialist	Inpatient	Pharmaceutical	Dental	Out-of-pocket payments as a percentage of total expenditure on health
Finland	Municipalities set payments for services they provide – either an annual payment of €16.8 or charges of €16.8 per consultation. For services covered by the national insurance scheme, co-insurance of up to 40% plus balance billing	Same as general practitioner services	Co-payment of €21.0 for short stays; charges linked to patient's income for longer stays	A flat-rate co-payment of €8.4 per prescription plus co-insurance of 50% of the remainder of the price	10% for dental examinations and preventive treatment; 40% for other treatments. No charges for children (under 18 years)	19.8% (1998)
France	Co-insurance rate of 30% plus some balance billing. Direct payments represent about 23% of the total costs of ambulatory care	Co-insurance rate of 30% (25% in public hospitals)	Co-insurance rate of 20% (up to 31 days in acute care) plus small co-payment for hotel expenses	Co-insurance rates of 0%, 35% and 65% depending on category of drugs. No reimbursement for products not included on national list. Direct payments represent about 20% of the total cost of pharmaceuticals	Co-insurance of 30% for preventive care and treatments. Co-insurance of up to 80% for dentures and orthodontics	10% (1999)

Country							
Germany	None	None	None	€8.7 per day up to a maximum of 14 days per year. Supplements for private rooms. Full or partial exemptions for children (under 18 years), unemployed people, those on income support and students receiving grants	Charges of €4.1, €4.6 and €5.1 depending on pack size plus 100% of cost above the reference price. Cost-sharing accounted for 12% of total costs in 1996	Basic and preventive care free of charge. Co-insurance rates of between 35% and 50% for operative treatments (such as fitting crowns and dentures). Exemptions for children (under 18 years)	11.9% (1997)
Greece	None for National Health Service services, but balance billing among private physicians	No payments for office-based physicians. Co-payment of €2.9 for outpatient visits to public hospitals	None		A general co-insurance rate of 25% together with lower rates (10%) and higher rates (100%) for specified categories of drugs. User charges represented about 10% of total pharmaceutical expenditure in 1994	None for children (under 18 years). Co-insurance rate of 25% for dental prostheses. Balance billing commonplace among private dentists, who comprise over 95% of the total	40.4% (1992)

Table 7.1 (cont'd)

Country	General practitioner	Specialist	Inpatient	Pharmaceutical	Dental	Out-of-pocket payments as a percentage of total expenditure on health
Ireland[b]	No charges for less affluent people (about one-third of the population); co-payments of €19.0–25.4 for people with an income above a defined ceiling (Category 2 patients)	No charges for either category for specialist services. Co-payments of €15.2 for hospital outpatient consultations	Co-payment for Category 2 patients in public wards of €25.4 per day up to a maximum of €254 in any 12-month period	None for Category 1 patients. Category 2 liable to a deductible of up to €114 per quarter. Exemptions for certain long-term illnesses and disabilities	No charges for Category 1 patients and schoolchildren. Other people covered by social insurance receive dental examinations and diagnosis without charge and subsidized treatments. People outside the social insurance scheme pay the full cost. Private expenditure accounts for an estimated two-thirds of overall dental expenditure	12.3% (1995)
Italy	None	Deductible of €36.2 for outpatient consultations	None	Three categories of drugs. Co-payment of €1.5 for class A products. Co-payment of €1.5 plus 50% co-insurance for class B. Full cost for class C	Most dentistry is private and subject to full-cost pricing. Low-income groups may receive free treatment at National Health Service health centres	23.5% (1999)

Luxembourg	Co-payment of €1.5. Extra for home visits	Co-insurance rate of 35%	Co-insurance rate of 35%	Co-payment of €5.3 per day for 'second-class' hospital beds. Additional charges for 'first-class' beds and additional physician's fees in 'first-class' beds	Three categories of drugs subject to 0%, 20% and 60% rates of co-insurance	Dental services covered by health insurance are subject to a deductible of €29.7 plus co-insurance of 20%. Different cost-sharing arrangements for other dental services	7.4% (1997)
Netherlands	None for people insured by the statutory health insurance because their income is below the defined ceiling	None for people insured by the statutory health insurance because their income is below the defined ceiling		Co-payment of €3.6 per day	Reference pricing and co-payments for some drugs	No charges for children under 17 or for preventive and specialist dental care. All other care subject to full-cost pricing	5.9% (1998)
Portugal		Co-payment of €2.0 for specialists in district hospitals and €3.0 for specialists in tertiary hospitals		None	Three categories based on therapeutic value: 0% for category A, 30% for category B and 60% for category C. Cost-sharing accounted for 33% of the drug bill in 1995	Mostly private with full-cost prices	44.6% (1995)

Table 7.1 (cont'd)

Country	General practitioner	Specialist	Inpatient	Pharmaceutical	Dental	Out-of-pocket payments as a percentage of total expenditure on health
Spain	None	None	None	Co-insurance of 40% with a reduced rate (10%) for chronically ill people	Free check-ups for children (under 18 years). Free tooth extractions in the public sector. Full-cost pricing for other services	16.9% (1998)
Sweden	Co-payments of SKr60–140. Rates determined by municipalities	Co-payments of SKr120–260 for outpatient visits to hospital specialists	Co-payment of SKr80 per day	Deductible of SKr900 and thereafter tapered co-insurance of 50% (SKr900–1700), 25% (SKr1700–3300) and 10% (SKr3300–4300). Maximum liability of SKr1800 in any 12 month period	Preventive care provided free to everyone under 20 years. Co-insurance for rest of the population. User charges represented about 50% of total expenditure in 1995	16.9% (1993)
United Kingdom	None	None	None but co-payments for superior National Health Service (amenity) beds	Co-payment of £6 per item (2000)	Co-insurance of 80% up to £325	10.8% (1998)

[a] Data on out-of-pocket payments includes expenditure on private health insurance
[b] Category 1 patients are those eligible for a medical card and whose income is below a defined level. Category 2 patients are those with limited eligibility due to their level of income.

Source: Mossialos and Le Grand (1999), updated using *Health Care Systems in Transition* country profiles from the European Observatory on Health Care Systems and OECD (2000)

Table 7.2 Cost-sharing in health care in selected CEE and FSU countries

Country	Health insurance and user charges	Services with user charges
Albania	Health Insurance Institute created in 1995, covering primary health care and basic essential drugs. User charges had fallen to very low levels before 1995	Small co-payments on some services covered by insurance, such as outpatient services and drugs
Belarus	No formal cost-sharing arrangements and few user charges	Charges for outpatient drugs, a small group of services and medical aids, etc. Hospitals can charge for non-essential services such as cosmetic surgery, but few do so. Vulnerable groups, those with chronic illness or 'socially important' communicable diseases are exempt from drug costs
Bulgaria	Cost-sharing legalized in 1997; the 1998 Health Insurance Law allows for co-payments for certain services covered by insurance	Visits to physicians, dentists and other inpatient and outpatient care if not referred by the family physician. Patients pay for ambulatory drug costs
Croatia	Some co-payments within health insurance system introduced by Health Insurance Act of 1993. Co-payments accounted for 10% of direct service costs in 1999	Every primary care consultation, home visits by health professionals, ambulance transport, some specialist care, 'hotel' charges for inpatient care, some medical aids and prescription drugs. People on low income, unemployed people, war veterans, children up to 15 years and those with certain illnesses are exempt
Czech Republic	Cost-sharing on a minor scale; out-of-pocket payments represented 5% of total health care expenditure in 1995	Selected drugs, dental services and some medical aids, and small co-payments for ambulatory care
Estonia	Cost-sharing introduced for various services and products in April 1995; exemptions introduced a few months later	Public ambulatory care subject to a small user fee. In hospital care, co-payments only apply to extras such as a single room. For most prescription drugs, co-payments are about 25%. Retired people, disabled people and children are exempt from user fees
Hungary	Act of 1975 set up health insurance and wide scope of services covered. Initially co-payment maintained only for prescribed medicines, medical aids and spa treatments	Since 1975, co-payments also for ambulance transport, dentistry, sanatorium treatments and long-term care, hotel aspects of hospital care and specialist services obtained without referral. 'Socially indigent' people are exempt from co-payment based on a local government means test

Table 7.2 *(cont'd)*

Country	Health insurance and user charges	Services with user charges
Kazakhstan	User charges legalized in 1995	Most oblasts (regional authorities) charge fully for non-essential services, such as cosmetic surgery and some dentistry. Substantial co-payments for outpatient drugs, aids, etc., and often for inpatient food and drugs too. Socially vulnerable groups and certain diagnostic groups such as cancer patients are exempt from outpatient drug charges. In theory, all patients are exempt from inpatient drug charges, although often not in practice
Kyrgyzstan	Official user fees permitted since 1991. Policy on user fees, basic health care packages and exemptions still being developed	User fees charged for a defined list of 17 health services, drugs, laboratory tests, extra amenities in hospital such as single rooms, etc. Semi-official charges made by hospitals for drugs and other supplies. Children, students and disabled people have free health services. However, they will soon be included in the health insurance system and may no longer be exempt from charges
Russian Federation	Health insurance scheme does not include cost-sharing co-payments. There are user charges for some services dating from the Soviet era	Official user charges for dental care, optical services, most medical aids and prostheses, drugs for outpatients and other services excluded from insurance. Veterans, tuberculosis patients, diabetics and another 28 categories of patient are exempt from charges for essential drugs. Unemployed people exempt from insurance contributions
Slovakia	Patient co-payments on some products according to the legislation on the financing of health insurance (1993) and amendments (1995 and 1997)	Rising number of co-payments for drugs (those outside the 'essential' category covered by insurance) and some prostheses, dental products, spectacle frames, etc. Exemptions (such as for unemployed people and employers of disabled people) apply more to insurance contributions than to co-payments

Country		
Slovenia	Services covered by compulsory insurance system vary in extent (defined in law in 1992 and after), with many services subject to co-payment	Several services within compulsory insurance subject to co-payments. Full payment for services outside this basic package, for which they can take out voluntary insurance. Socially disadvantaged groups (such as unemployed people) are fully covered by compulsory health insurance (contributions paid by the state) and do not pay user charges
Tajikistan	User charges officially account for about 1% of health care expenditure (probably more)	Health care facilities allowed to charge approved prices for services such as dentistry, some diagnostic procedures, abortions, etc. People often buy their own drugs because of shortages in hospitals. Patients must pay for optical services, orthopaedics, resort treatment and cosmetic treatment. Veterans, children under 3 years of age, disabled people, tuberculosis patients, etc., are exempt
The former Yugoslavian Republic of Macedonia	Co-payments (usually 10% or 20%) on many services, since the Health Care Law of 1991 and subsequent amendments	Health services and drugs for outpatient treatment (20%) and inpatient treatment (10%); treatment received abroad (20%); hearing aids and dentures (20%); orthopaedic braces, etc. (50%). People over 65 years pay reduced co-payments for drugs. Cash payments are required for services outside the basic health care covered by insurance and from non-insured patients
Turkmenistan	Fees for services introduced alongside the voluntary health insurance system in 1996	Drugs for outpatients, services for self-referred patients, some diagnostic procedures, cosmetic surgery, dental care and physiotherapy. Veterans, some disabled people, people affected by the Chernobyl nuclear accident, pregnant women, children under 1 year of age and people with diabetes, asthma, cancer, mental illness, kidney transplants, tuberculosis, syphilis, AIDS and leprosy have no user charges
Uzbekistan		Hospital inpatients pay own food costs; co-payments for drugs and some services. Official out-of-pocket payments or co-payments for products and services comprised 5.8% of health care spending in 1995

Source: Kutzin (1998), updated using *Health Care Systems in Transition* country profiles from the European Observatory on Health Care Systems

Nine countries apply charges to inpatient care, usually a flat-rate co-payment per day with a ceiling placed on the number of paid days for which the patient is liable (such as Austria, Germany and the Netherlands). Sometimes the rate of co-payment declines as the length of stay increases (such as Belgium and Ireland). In France, a small additional co-payment is levied for 'hotel' services. In Luxembourg, differential co-payments are payable on 'first- and second-class' hospital beds.

All the European Union countries charge for dental services. In several countries, dentistry is mainly private (such as Belgium, Italy and Portugal) and patients pay the full costs of care. Elsewhere, basic preventive services are frequently provided free of charge, but a variety of co-payments and co-insurance arrangements apply to other services (such as Germany, Ireland, Spain and the United Kingdom). In many countries, dental services are seen as marginal to the public health system and, for this reason, cost-sharing usually constitutes a larger proportion of dental costs than of the costs of other areas listed in Table 7.1.

Despite the widespread use of cost-sharing, especially for pharmaceuticals and dental care, all countries offer some exemptions, such as for people under the age of 18 years, people on low incomes, elderly people and people suffering from long-term illness and disability.

The contribution of cost-sharing to the overall funding of health care varies substantially between countries. Table 7.1 shows the proportion of total health care costs met by cost-sharing (user charges) in each country. These data should, however, be treated with caution. Charging arrangements and accounting conventions vary substantially between countries. Moreover, in most cases, the figures cited in Table 7.1 include total out-of-pocket payments; that is, both direct (co-payments, co-insurance and deductibles) and indirect (such as full cost charging on items totally excluded from public reimbursement) cost-sharing. Nevertheless, the data broadly indicate the extent to which individuals in different countries are protected from the costs of health care at the point of use, through some form of social protection, and the extent to which they are expected to draw on their private resources. Thus, except for Greece, Italy and Portugal, all countries raise 20 per cent or less of total health care funding through cost-sharing. Within this context, some countries depend very little on cost-sharing (such as Germany, the Netherlands and the United Kingdom) and some moderately so (such as Denmark and Sweden).

Systematic data on cost-sharing in CEE and FSU countries is less easy to obtain. Moreover, as Chapter 8 shows, informal payments are widespread in practically all these countries. In many cases, these represent the most important form of user payment but are generally illegal and unrecorded. Given these measurement difficulties, Table 7.2 could not be constructed on the same basis as Table 7.1. Instead, it has been constructed to indicate how recent policy has encompassed formal cost-sharing and the areas to which it is applied.

Several countries introduced cost-sharing arrangements during the 1990s as part of their newly established health insurance schemes, such as Albania, Bulgaria, Croatia and Slovakia (Table 7.2). As in western Europe, practically all these countries apply cost-sharing to pharmaceutical prescriptions. These charges often represent a sizeable proportion of pharmaceutical expenditure (such as 25 per cent in Estonia and 35 per cent in Hungary in 1997). Faced with a financial crisis in the pharmaceutical sector, Slovakia has recently introduced a reference pricing system that is leading to substantial growth in cost-sharing. Small charges for primary or ambulatory care and for home visits are also common. Charges for specialist services and inpatient care are less common, although Croatia levies charges for hospital hotel services, Estonia charges for single rooms and Hungary imposes charges for specialist services obtained without referral. Most countries have exemptions from charges for vulnerable groups such as people with chronic illness, elderly people, young people and people on low incomes.

Evidence on the potential substitution of formal cost-sharing for informal, under-the-table payments is mixed. In Croatia, it is claimed that under-the-table payments have become less widespread since social insurance was introduced in 1993. In the Russian Federation, replacing informal payments with official charges is a specific policy objective. Lithuania has had a long history of informal payments. However, a survey conducted by the State Patient Fund in 1998 suggests that their incidence is falling as a result of competition and greater control over providers. In contrast, under-the-table payments in Albania appear to remain widespread despite the growth of formal out-of-pocket payments, which financed an estimated 16 per cent of total health care in 1996. Similarly, although formal payments are growing, there is little sign of a reduction in informal payments in Poland. Between 1992 and 1995, the proportion of the population reporting informal payments rose from 16 per cent to 29 per cent.

The impact of user charges

The analytical framework set out previously suggests that policies on cost-sharing can be evaluated using three main criteria: efficiency, equity and public acceptability. In this section, I assemble evidence to assess the performance of different cost-sharing arrangements in terms of these criteria. This evidence has been drawn from the research literature, from intelligence derived from the work of the European Observatory on Health Care Systems and from three case studies carried out for this project based on the national experiences of Germany, Sweden and the United Kingdom.

Cost-sharing and efficiency

Given that theory predicts that the absence of user charges may lead to moral hazard and excessive demand for health care services, most empirical research has focused on how cost-sharing affects health service utilization. The RAND Corporation carried out the most exhaustive study in this area in the United States during the 1970s. The RAND Health Experiment was a randomized trial of 7708 individuals designed to examine the effects of cost-sharing on both the demand for health services and health status. The experiment was long term; participants were recruited from 1974 to 1977 and followed for 3–5 years. Each participant was offered one of 15 different health insurance plans. The plans varied in terms of the form and extent of cost-sharing.

The RAND findings indicate that health service utilization (measured in terms of the probability of using medical services, inpatient care, admissions and outpatient visits) decreased as cost-sharing increased. However, the pattern of reduced utilization in a wide range of service areas (such as hospital admissions, antibiotic prescriptions and medical care) suggested that cost-sharing reduced utilization of both effective and ineffective – or inappropriate – procedures. Moreover, cost-sharing was also linked to poorer health outcomes on several different indicators. These findings raise serious doubts about the effects of cost-sharing on micro-efficiency as opposed to micro-cost containment.

The RAND study has several limitations that restrict its ability to be generalized, especially in Europe. For example, some critics have challenged its findings because it could not measure the effect of cost-sharing on overall health expenditure (Evans *et al.* 1995). In other words, although the RAND results showed that cost-sharing reduced third-party payer expenditure on the services subject to these charges, providers could, over time, expand activity on alternative services and thereby increase overall expenditure. The study has also been criticized for failing to take account of the fact that physicians rather than patients make many decisions on utilization. Fahs (1992) showed how physicians in the United States responded to the reduction in demand following the introduction of cost-sharing for members of a union insurance programme by inducing greater utilization among non-cost-sharing patients. Finally, the RAND study focused on younger (people over 62 years of age were excluded) and healthy populations.

Nevertheless, several less rigorous studies have confirmed the main thrust of the RAND findings – that cost-sharing reduces utilization. Rubin and Mendelson (1995) reviewed 19 studies that examined the effect of different types of cost-sharing on health service utilization. These studies focused on physician visits, hospital admissions and lengths of stay, and pharmaceutical prescriptions. All but three of the studies examined the effect of cost-sharing in the United States. The overwhelming picture was that cost-sharing was associated with reduced utilization in all the areas studied.

For example, physician visits often declined by 20–30 per cent in response to co-payments of different levels. Nolan (1993) reports similar findings for visits to general practitioners in Ireland for cost-sharing and non-cost-sharing patients. Similarly, hospital admission rates fell by up to 30 per cent in response to deductibles and co-insurance. Nine studies examined how cost-sharing affects pharmaceutical prescriptions. These showed dramatic reductions of up to 30 per cent in the United States and more modest reductions in the United Kingdom.

Rubin and Mendelson (1995) also examined how cost-sharing affected patterns of demand. They identified eight studies covering physician services and pharmaceuticals, all related to United States populations. Their findings supported the RAND conclusions that cost-sharing tended to reduce both appropriate and inappropriate demand. In the case of pharmaceuticals, for example, co-payments and co-insurance tended to reduce the demand for both essential drugs (defined as having important effects on morbidity and mortality) and discretionary drugs, although demand tended to decline more for discretionary or symptomatic drugs, or drugs of limited efficacy, than for essential drugs.

Although most research in North America and western Europe has concentrated on how cost-sharing affects utilization, interest in several CEE and FSU countries – as in many developing countries – has focused on using cost-sharing to raise revenue. Scheiber and Maeda (1997) argue that the evidence on user charges in developing countries is extensive. Certain findings are relevant to CEE and FSU countries.

- Although user charges can supplement public revenue, total revenue from official user charges has not met expectations. It has rarely exceeded 5 per cent of total revenue. Nevertheless, total private spending and informal payments remain high.
- There is some evidence of adverse effects on health outcomes.
- User charges have strongly reduced utilization, with disproportionate effects upon poor people (see the next section on 'equity'), both as a direct response and indirectly, as charges for public services have led to higher prices for private services.
- User charges need to be considered in the context of the managerial and administrative capacity necessary to implement them and the time costs they impose.

The final point raises administrative cost and feasibility. Evidence on cost-sharing schemes in the European Union suggests that they can be complex and expensive to implement and administer (Mossialos and Le Grand 1999). This is likely to be true especially if efforts are made to preserve equity and social solidarity through exemptions from payment for vulnerable groups. This suggests that cost-sharing as a means of reducing demand or raising revenue may not be as cost-effective as alternative policy instruments. Nevertheless, for CEE and FSU countries, the absence of plausible alternative methods of raising revenue may make this direct method the only feasible option.

Cost-sharing and equity

The RAND Health Insurance experiment showed that cost-sharing tended to be associated with especially marked reductions in the probability of medical use and outpatient visits among lower-income groups. These effects were strongest in relation to services for poor children. Moreover, although the probability that a low-income person would use the health service was significantly lower, the average cost per service they incurred tended to be higher.

Rubin and Mendelson (1995) raised similar concerns about the effects of cost-sharing on equity. They examined the links between cost-sharing and health status and found evidence that cost-sharing adversely affected the health of unemployed and homeless people. As reported above, evidence from developing countries also suggests that reductions in utilization are disproportionately concentrated on poor people.

Case study evidence provided for this project confirms this pattern. For example, surveys conducted in Stockholm County in 1993, 1995 and 1996 indicate that between 20 and 25 per cent of the population refrained from seeking care at least once during a given 12 month period because of financial reasons (Anders Anell, unpublished data). Moreover, the same studies showed that individuals on low incomes (such as unemployed people, students and immigrants) tended to be affected more strongly than other groups. These findings have been interpreted as being consistent with the need to use cost-sharing to restrict unnecessary demand but inconsistent with overall equity objectives.

To counteract the adverse impact of cost-sharing on vulnerable groups, most countries offer full or partial exemptions to young and elderly people, people with certain chronic diseases and low-income households. These policies can protect vulnerable groups from the full costs of illness and disability (in the United Kingdom, for example, 84 per cent of pharmaceutical prescriptions were dispensed to people claiming exemptions during the mid-1990s (Eversley 1997), but inevitably add to the complexity of managing a cost-sharing scheme and tend to raise administrative costs.

Public acceptability

Cost-sharing has often been the subject of heated public debate. Attitudes towards its acceptability have been sharply polarized. Recent experiences in relation to this policy instrument in the United Kingdom, Germany, Sweden and Bulgaria illustrate a range of contrasting public attitudes.

The United Kingdom makes very limited use of user charges. The provision of universal service free at the point of use was a fundamental feature of the National Health Service as it was established in 1948. Early decisions to introduce user charges for spectacles in the 1950s caused considerable political turmoil and ministerial resignations. Since then, however, politicians and the public have generally accepted the limited application of charges in pharmaceutical, dental and ophthalmic services. The widespread exemption from charges for pharmaceutical prescriptions has undoubtedly reduced resistance to charging. From time to time, user charges have been suggested in primary and secondary care – both to deter, for example, inappropriate general practitioner consultations and to raise extra revenue for health care. Such suggestions have, however, generally met widespread and strong resistance. None of the main political parties supports the extension of user charging, and this is unlikely to be a part of National Health Service policy in the foreseeable future.

Germany's policies on user charging have shifted according to the political climate. The first explicit cost-containment law establishing user charges was introduced in 1977 by a Social Democratic–Liberal coalition government. However, the government had difficulty in reconciling the introduction of user charges with its prevailing views on social justice and equity. Moreover, the policy was extremely unpopular with the government's traditional blue-collar supporters. Nevertheless, user charges comprised a far more consistent component of the programmes pursued by successive Conservative–Liberal coalition governments from 1982 onwards. For them, individual responsibilities and social solidarity were imbalanced. Their view was that, only if individuals were unable to care for themselves – or if their families and other networks could not do so – should the state intervene to offer a safety net.

Despite this general stance, however, even governments of the centre-right were aware of the sensitivity of user charges, and so there were few major increases during the 1980s. The situation changed dramatically in the 1990s following reunification, when there was an unprecedented debate on the roll-back of social health insurance expenditure and privatization of health care costs (Matthias Wismar, unpublished data). At the same time, on the supply side, the health sector was seen as a growth industry and a potential source of future employment. For this reason, there was reluctance to strangle it through excessive cost containment. The policy that reconciled these conflicting object-ives was a dramatic expansion in user charges (Busse and Wismar 1997).

In the federal election campaign of 1998, the subject of user charges – espe-cially in relation to dental treatment – was an important area of debate. Support for this policy probably contributed to the defeat of the Conservative–Liberal coalition. The newly elected Social Democratic–Green coalition immediately set about reducing user charges and lowering the threshold for exemptions. For the immediate future, expanding user charging has been ruled out politically.

Sweden is politically to the left of centre but has extensive user charges. In fact, the argument that public health services should be provided free at the point of use – for reasons of equity – does not command wide support among health decision-makers. For example, several politicians and medical leaders have complained that the recent introduction of health services free of charge to children (under 18 years of age) will lead to a reallocation of resources away from patients with greater needs. Some county councils have reinstated user charges for children's outpatient services following changes in political major-ities at the 1998 elections.

In Sweden, the general approach to user charging in health care is to levy uniform charges irrespective of incomes and to protect individuals from unac-ceptably high expenditure through the high-cost protection scheme. For many elderly and chronically ill people, this means that many services are free of charge because they have paid the maximum amount (that is, the marginal price is zero). Many decision-makers consider the absence of incentives to economize on use beyond the maximum payment to be a problem. The intro-duction of an administrative fee for prescription medicines for patients who have reached the payment ceiling was discussed as part of the changes intro-duced in June 1999. It was not, however, implemented.

For the future, there is debate in Sweden about reconciling patient choice with societal decision-making. It has been suggested that lower subsidies and less full-cost charging should be introduced for new medical innovations, such as newly available pharmaceuticals, that do not meet the cost-effectiveness criteria for public funding.

Public attitudes towards cost-sharing appear to be different in the CEE and FSU countries. Given the widespread existence of informal payments, their replacement by transparent charging mechanisms that embody clear equity principles has undoubted appeal. Recent developments in Bulgaria exemplify this phenomenon.

Informal payments for health care were common in Bulgaria during the 1980s and 1990s. In a survey carried out in 1994, 43 per cent of 1000 respondents reported having paid cash for services that were formally provided free of charge at state medical facilities in the preceding 2 years. A survey carried out in Sofia in 1999 found that 54 per cent of respondents had made informal payments for state-provided services. Under-the-table payments were common in obtaining drugs, outpatient services and elective surgery. Faced with these circumstances, nearly two-thirds of respondents favoured the introduction of official user charges.

Recognizing the burgeoning problem associated with informal payments and the climate of public opinion favouring a more open and equitable formal system, the government legalized cost-sharing in 1997. The Ministry of Health prepared a unified tariff of co-payments in 1999 covering a range of health care services, including inpatient and outpatient services (Hinkov *et al.* 1999).

These case studies illustrate different patterns of interplay between public attitudes and policy-making on cost-sharing. In the United Kingdom, long-standing bipartisan opposition to cost-sharing in core areas of health care is well established, and policy changes are restricted largely to increasing the charges for pharmaceuticals and dental services. There is little public debate as long as charges are confined to these areas, although increased charging for long-term care has attracted quite strong public criticism. In contrast, in Germany, different stances on cost-sharing by the major political parties have contributed to changes in government. In Sweden, the high level of user charges has generated extensive public debate on the implications of their use, which may lead to changes in policy. In Bulgaria, the transitional phase of development following the abandonment of communism has led to new arrangements for financing health care. Among these, public preferences for formal cost-sharing have been mirrored in official adoption of this policy.

Discussion

Most health policy analysts consider that cost-sharing is a weak instrument for achieving the objectives of efficiency and equity in the allocation of health care resources. This view is based on evidence from several sources.

The most exhaustive study of cost-sharing was carried out by the RAND Corporation. This suggested that cost-sharing can reduce utilization and, therefore, discourage excessive use of services, contributing to enhanced efficiency. Nevertheless, cost-sharing tended to reduce the demand for both effective and ineffective services and, as such, failed to improve allocative efficiency. Other studies confirm this picture. Most report that cost-sharing is associated with reduced utilization but that it tends to reduce both appropriate and inappropriate care. There are also doubts about the ability of cost-sharing to control aggregate health-sector costs given supplier responses leading to increased activity in areas not subject to cost-sharing.

Research on the equity consequences of cost-sharing also raises concerns. The RAND experiment and other studies suggest that cost-sharing is likely to affect low-income and vulnerable groups disproportionately. Offering full or partial exemptions counteracts some adverse consequences but is often complex and expensive to administer.

Recognizing these limitations, Dawson (1999) argues that, if the purpose of cost-sharing is to deter unnecessary utilization of services resulting from moral hazard, this objective could be achieved more effectively by countering the moral hazard of physicians who recommend excessive treatment for patients with insurance coverage. Excessive utilization is thus a supply-side rather than a demand-side problem. If this is the case, it would be counteracted more effectively through the greater use of supply-side financial incentives and micro-techniques for managing clinical activity, such as clinical guidelines and protocols.

Despite all these objections, however, cost-sharing is very widely used as a policy instrument. Why are policy-makers drawn to this policy despite the well-documented evidence regarding its shortcomings? One reason would appear to be the powerful appeal of user charges to parties on the right of the political spectrum. To them, user charging is often seen as a component of a market-based approach, on economic grounds, and as a symbol of individual responsibility, on political grounds. The recent experience in Germany demonstrates quite clearly how support for user charges has ebbed and flowed with changes in the political complexion of government. On this level, theoretical (or ideological) arguments may carry more force than empirical ones, especially when there is a lack of definitive empirical evidence.

Robert Evans (personal communication) has a different 'political' explanation for the persistence of user charges. He argues that examining how cost-sharing affects income distribution may be required to understand its persistence. In particular, which groups gain from such a policy and which ones lose? Viewed in these terms, user charges may prove popular among elite provider groups because it offers a means for sustaining expenditure on health care (and supplementing their incomes) during times of restrained public expenditure. It is likely to be less popular among user groups, but they usually have less political influence.

Yet another reason why policy-makers often resort to user charges relates to the feasibility of different policies. It may well be accepted that full social insurance or tax-based financing is preferable on grounds of efficiency and equity but that increases in contributions or taxation may not be an option for political reasons. These arguments have been heard in several western European countries as governments have sought election on platforms of reducing taxation. But the same arguments are even more strongly expressed in CEE and FSU countries. Difficulties in securing tax payments in times of low (or sometimes negative) economic growth and a wariness about government-based schemes in the post-communist world have contributed to the appeal of cost-sharing as a direct means of raising much-needed revenue for health care. Moreover, the widespread existence of informal payments has meant that policies to replace them with formal user charges are seen as a way of increasing transparency, thereby basing policy on more equitable criteria and reducing corruption.

These arguments suggest that cost-sharing is likely to play a role in the future in both western Europe and in CEE and FSU countries. In most cases, however, it is likely to be used as an adjunct to more important demand-side and supply-side policies rather than as a substitute for them. It may be used to generate additional revenue or to discourage utilization at the margins, but it is unlikely to become a major policy instrument in its own right.

Nevertheless, even within this more limited guise, current experience with user charges suggests several aspects of the policy that decision-makers would be well advised to consider in designing specific cost-sharing schemes, if the objectives of efficiency and equity are to be better achieved in the future. For example, there is reason to believe – and evidence to show – that responses to cost-sharing differ depending on whether the patient or physician initiates the service. Differential responses can also be expected in relation to preventive services versus curative treatments. Careful attention needs to be paid to exemption criteria to avoid adverse effects on equity. In line with policy initiatives designed to discourage ineffective interventions, cost-sharing based on the relative effectiveness of treatments merits further consideration. In all cases, however, better policy-making would be assisted by more thorough evaluation of specific cost-sharing schemes.

Notes

1 I thank Anders Anell and Matthias Wismar for providing background material on cost-sharing in Sweden and Germany. I also thank Robert Evans and Joe Kutzin for comments on an earlier draft of this chapter.
2 In Denmark, extra billing only applies to 2% of the population who opt for free choice of general practitioner and direct access to all specialists (group 2). Most people choose a general practitioner, who then acts as a gatekeeper, and do not have direct access to (most) specialists (group 1).
3 See Note 2.

References

Busse, R. and Wismar, M. (1997) Health care reform in Germany: the end of cost containment?, *Eurohealth*, 3(2): 32–3.

Chalkley, M. and Robinson, R. (1997) *Theory and Evidence on Cost Sharing in Health Care: An Economic Perspective*. London: Office of Health Economics.

Dawson, D. (1999) Why charge patients if there are better ways to contain costs, encourage efficiency and reach for equity?, *Eurohealth*, 5(3): 29–31.

Evans, R., Barer, M. and Stoddart, G. (1995) User fees for health care: why bad ideas keep coming back (or what's health got to do with it?), *Canadian Journal of Aging*, 14(2): 360–90.

Eversley, J. and Webster, C. (1997) Light on the charge brigade, *The Health Service Journal*, 107(5562): 26–8.

Fahs, M. (1992) Physician response to the United Mine Workers' cost sharing program: the other side of the coin, *Health Services Research*, 27(1): 25–45.

Hinkov, H., Koulaksuzov, S., Semerdjiev, I. and Healy, J. (1999) *Health Care Systems in Transition: Bulgaria*. Copenhagen: European Observatory on Health Care Systems.

Kutzin, J. (1998) The appropriate role for patient cost sharing, in R. Saltman, J. Figueras and C. Sakellarides (eds) *Critical Challenges for Health Care Reform in Europe*. Buckingham: Open University Press.

Mossialos, E. and Le Grand, J. (eds) (1999) *Health Care and Cost Containment in the European Union.* Aldershot: Ashgate.

Nolan, B. (1993) Economic incentives, health status and health services utilisation, *Journal of Health Economics*, 12(2): 151–69.

OECD (2000) OECD *Health Data 2000: A Comparative Analysis of 29 Countries.* Paris: Organisation for Economic Co-operation and Development.

Rubin, R. and Mendelson, D. (1995) A framework for cost sharing policy analysis, in N. Mattison (ed.) *Sharing the Costs of Health: A Multi-country Perspective.* Basle: Pharmaceutical Partners for Better Health.

Schieber, G. and Maeda, A. (1997) A curmudgeon's guide to financing health care in developing countries, in G. Schieber (ed.) *Innovations in Health Care Financing.* Washington, DC: World Bank.

chapter eight

Informal health payments in central and eastern Europe and the former Soviet Union: issues, trends and policy implications

Maureen Lewis[1]

Introduction

Informal payments in the health sector in the countries of central and eastern Europe (CEE) and of the former Soviet Union (FSU) are growing and are becoming an important source of health care financing. They can also be a major impediment to health care reform. Informal payments can be defined as payments to individual and institutional providers in kind or in cash that are outside official payment channels or for purchases meant to be covered by the health care system. This encompasses 'envelope' payments to physicians and 'contributions' to hospitals as well as the value of medical supplies purchased by patients and drugs obtained from private pharmacies but intended to be part of government-financed health care services. Voluntary purchases from private providers are not considered informal payments but a market transaction at the discretion of the consumer.

Direct private payments to physicians, nurses and other health personnel are essentially an informal market for health care occurring within public health care service networks. This expenditure is also outside the financial controls, policy rubric and audits of countries' health care systems. Like the informal sector more generally, it is often illegal and unreported.

Informal health payments have been reported and often documented in virtually all CEE and FSU countries with the possible exception of the Czech Republic (World Bank 1999a, 2000a). This issue has raised considerable concern in some CEE and FSU countries (Gaal 1998, 1999), but its relative importance is only beginning to be understood. Part of the difficulty has been measuring its extent, the nature of the process and the burden on households. Given its uncertain status – in some countries it is clearly illegal, whereas in others its legality has remained ambiguous – such evaluation is often difficult. These circumstances have also impeded the development of solutions to the problem.

In this chapter, I outline the key policy issues, summarize available data on the scope and nature of informal payments across CEE and FSU countries and outline the policy implications and possible strategies to address the problem.

Background and historical context

The health sectors of CEE and FSU countries are characterized by an excess supply of both buildings and human resources, including physicians and nurses. The numbers of hospital beds, physicians and lengths of stay in hospital are two to three times those in countries in the Organisation for Economic Co-operation and Development (OECD) (World Bank 1998, 2000b). As revenue has declined in many CEE and FSU countries since the early 1990s, health expenditure has also fallen but with little change in the number of staff or beds. The result has been a large health system with underpaid and sometimes unpaid staff. Some countries, notably the FSU countries, have shortages of medical equipment, drugs and supplies. Some efforts have been made to require patients to officially pay part of the cost, especially for pharmaceuticals, but this has been inadequate to meet the shortfall in resources.

World Bank studies in the early 1990s estimated that 25 per cent of expenditure for health services in Romania and 20 per cent in Hungary were out-of-pocket payments and gratuities (World Bank 1993). Thus, private payments to gain access to care were documented early on in the process of transition.

The tradition of grateful patients rewarding or thanking physicians for services provided is long-standing in central Asia. In CEE and FSU countries, the publicly controlled health services under communism and the introduction of under-the-table payments are more closely linked, as has been documented in Hungary (Gaal 1998). Lack of accountability and endemic corruption among public officials may also play a role. Government-dominated systems without adequate accountability lend themselves to informal payments for services that are faster (such as jumping the queue) or perceived to be better. Underfunding exacerbates the problem. Indeed, declining government budgets and excessive capacity have forced governments to lower the salaries of medical staff. Combined with the lack of accountability, this has contributed to incentives to require informal payments from patients (World Bank 2000b).

Why informal payments?

One reason informal payments increased during the transition was the desire of public servants to ensure or maximize income, evade taxes and, effectively, 'beat the system'. Many CEE and FSU countries, especially those in central Asia, have delayed introducing formal charges despite declining resources. Constitutionally enshrined health services free of charge have translated into 'free' services regardless of wage arrears and limited discretionary resources (World Bank 2000b). Informal payments have resulted. Unlike formal charges, these payments go directly to individual providers, thereby compensating individuals rather than the system. Second, these payments lead to public-sector corruption, undermining the credibility of government. Third, the system of waivers for indigent people is randomly, if ever, assigned. Despite uneven application of waivers in formal fee systems, the process and eligibility are defined and enforcement is possible. With informal arrangements, all exchanges are outside the public domain and enforcement is irrelevant.

Unresponsive government

When health care revenue collapsed after 1990, governments in most CEE and FSU countries did not make commensurate cutbacks in health care services (see Chapter 4) (World Bank 2000b). The numbers of hospitals, beds and physicians have become unaffordable, leading providers to charge fees to maintain their incomes.

Preker *et al.* (1999) have examined the limitations of government health care systems within an institutional economics framework, and empirical work by La Forgia *et al.* (1999) and Lewis *et al.* (1999) has documented some of the egregious shortcomings under government-controlled and -operated systems in developing countries. In most countries, public system problems are manifested in the absence of key health personnel in hospitals, especially physicians, and the need for patients to supply their own consumables, drugs and sometimes completed diagnostic tests (Lewis *et al.* 1992, 1996; Chawla 1995). These practices reflect government inability to establish, monitor and enforce regulations. The practices can also be seen as breeding corruption.

Unlike the countries in transition, most developing countries, especially those classified as middle-income countries, have a parallel private market that serves private patients, and public physicians commonly refer public patients to their private practice. Evidence on informal payments within public systems has been documented in India and several African countries. Inadequate funding and limited public accountability also serve to fuel the practice in these countries. Informal payments do not exist in most OECD countries. The lack of a developed private infrastructure impedes a similar private market in CEE and FSU countries, especially for inpatient and diagnostic services.[2] Hence, physicians, nurses and other health workers and managers use the vehicle of public facilities to supplement their incomes.[3]

Informal fees make providers responsive to patients. This is an improvement over the common situation in which providers are not held accountable to anyone. But provider services are extended for personal gain, contrary to the intent of public service. The result of this is that greater attention is given to those able and willing to pay for services.[4]

Wage bills are generally met in most developing countries. In CEE and FSU countries, conversely, resources are simply insufficient to keep the oversized health care systems operating, leading to a range of measures that undermine the basic operation of health care. In some countries, physicians' salaries have declined precipitously in both absolute and relative terms (such as Georgia, the Russian Federation and Ukraine) and arrears in meeting payrolls are common. Improvement is not likely without serious restructuring of the organization of care and a reduction of personnel.

Where physician wages have kept pace, as in the Czech Republic and Slovenia, the average earnings of physicians are at or above average national earnings, and informal payments are rare (World Bank 1999b, 2000a). But in many FSU countries, wages are low and often unpaid, which necessarily leads to either an absence of service or an implicit, illegal fee-for-service system. In addition, high personal taxation makes informal payment attractive to providers.

Inadequate government oversight

The lack of government oversight of the system combined with the absence of benchmarks and alternatives for a private health sector make the growth of informal payments almost inevitable. With no alternatives or effective government enforcement of standards and performance, the consumer's only recourse is direct payment to ensure alternatives and more responsive treatment, and hopefully better quality. Patients cannot vote with their feet by shifting to an alternative system, but they can circumvent the oligopolistic public system. Even where there has been choice of physician, it has had no apparent impact on informal payments. Moreover, with the private sector in its infancy, governments retain a monopoly on infrastructure, equipment and, therefore, service provision, especially for inpatient services.

One of the most disturbing implications of informal payments is that it fuels growth of the grey economy, undermining governments' efforts to improve accountability and public-sector management. Moreover, they are part of the larger growth in corruption that plagues many CEE and FSU countries. The importance in Ukraine was highlighted by a survey among consumers, on governance, which found that respondents listed health care second to automobile inspection as the most corrupt public services (Ukraine Legal Foundation 1998). In Slovakia, a nationwide survey identified health as the most corrupt of government institutions (Anderson 2000).

Lack of accountability is reinforced by the low likelihood of getting caught and the minimal sanctions if the practice is discovered, as punishment for such behaviour is virtually non-existent. Governments in CEE and FSU countries are largely unwilling or unable to monitor the system in general, much less identify and address informal payments. Indeed, management information systems, quality assurance or other systematic tools for management and oversight generally do not exist or are unevenly applied or not at all.

Discretion of health providers is extensive, especially for physicians, who make all medical decisions with minimal supervision. Similarly, hospital directors are often audited on public expenditure but are not evaluated on performance or quality of services. Either would provide a basis for monitoring and oversight. Accountability requires this kind of information. The lack of true accountability to a higher authority – to the ministry of health, director of the hospital, the general public or patients – is limited, as performance is rarely, if ever, the basis for reward or sanction. This fundamental lack of public oversight and enforcement allows informal payments to be perpetuated outside the purview of government but within the public system.

Despite the nurturing environment for informal payments, their nature and structure remain vague. Who is paid, how much and by whom is only beginning to be understood, but this is important in understanding how to address and cope with the abuses. The source of the practice has been outlined; the importance and the magnitude of the issues are the topics of the next sections.

Why informal payments matter

By definition, informal payments are unaudited and unreported. As such, they have implications for governance, government priorities, the incentives faced by both health providers and managers, access and equity.

Governance and government priorities

The informal nature of payments reduces the role of public policy and of resource allocation decisions in the public interest. Since payments are set with virtually no involvement of the sponsors of the system – that is, the government – the random prices and willingness to pay of patients determine where resources flow into the system. Thus, priority expenditure (such as in maternity) cannot be realized, as the market makes these decisions, driven largely by decisions of providers as to who should benefit from care. In short, public policy objectives become marginalized.

The inefficiency and poor quality of the health systems in many CEE and FSU countries will persist under the current organizational, financial and regulatory arrangements, since funds often go to individuals rather than to facilities or the overall system. Upgrading of medical equipment, improved efficiency of heating systems, cost-effective medical protocols, raising nursing standards and other elements of a functioning health care system do not receive adequate financing, undermining the quality, efficiency and effectiveness of the system. This, however, could be addressed by both systematically reducing staff and facilities and allocating formal fee revenue to raising the quality of infrastructure and equipment and to subsidizing poor people. Such an arrangement would also improve transparency and encourage financial oversight.

Reform requires that those who run the health systems – both medical and administrative leaders – become convinced of the benefit of shifts in incentives, behaviour and practices that define reform. If the individual losses are too great, resistance can undermine efforts for change. Indeed, management theory hinges corporate restructuring on change agents who lead and convince key players in the system to move towards new and better ways to work. Leaders in the health care sector, both in ministries of health and in major health centres, are the agents of change for the sector. If there is systematic resistance, reforms will be difficult to establish and will not take root. Indeed, where the existing system is lucrative for these major players and the future uncertain, engendering reform will be difficult and resisted. Given the upheavals since the early 1990s in CEE and FSU countries, change is unlikely to be embraced with alacrity.

Hence, the more entrenched informal payment arrangements become, the more difficult reforming the system will be. Reform always produces winners and losers. If the powerful, who are currently benefiting from informal payments, are the losers, reform will be difficult, both because the powerful do not buy in and because the levers of the system cannot be reached to promote change.

Access and equity

Requiring payments from patients restricts access to those who can pay, makes the payment levels and terms arbitrary and can render essential services unaffordable. One of the primary reasons for government involvement in financing health care is to ensure equity, especially for those who cannot afford health care. The present arrangement often undermines that objective, leaving effectively a private system operating within a public shell. The system is largely unregulated as well. In private systems, government regulation is meant to maintain both fairness and fiscal responsibility. Neither exist with informal payments. Both quantitative and qualitative studies suggest that poor people may be disadvantaged and discouraged from using the system as they are unable to pay, although, as discussed later, the objective in some settings is convenience or speed of care (Feeley *et al.* 1999; Gaal 1999; GUS 1999; Lewis 2000; Narayan 2000). In some countries, there is anecdotal evidence of exemptions for low-income households, especially in rural areas, but these are unsystematic and *ad hoc*, which provides no guarantee of access for poor people. Moreover, qualitative evidence in Armenia suggests the opposite: refusal to care for people unable to pay informal fees (Kurkchiyan 1999).

Measuring informal payments

Informal health payments are difficult to measure for the same reasons that the underground economy is only a best guess: there are no records of transactions or of pricing, and much is accomplished in secret and rarely discussed openly. By definition, payments pass between payer and payee informally and without records or audits and, if such payments are illegal, they are even more difficult to trace and estimate. These same characteristics impede the collection of information and data on the subject.

Generalizations about such payments are also inappropriate. Since they are illegal in many CEE and FSU countries, providers have been reluctant to admit or discuss informal payments. In the FSU countries, such payments are not always illegal, partly because the tradition of gifts blurs the line between gratitude and required payment. Similarly, the patterns of requesting, pricing, collecting and distributing proceeds also differ by country. For example, in Poland, administrators reportedly share the proceeds from physicians; in other countries they do not. Individual payment to every service provider is demanded in some countries but uncommon in others. The difficulty of obtaining data combined with inconsistencies across settings and countries make generalization unreliable.

The vague definition and the differing interpretation of questions makes the process of collecting and analysing data difficult. For example, is a gift given after services are provided considered an informal payment? Can a gift in-kind be seen as a bribe? Are purchases of drugs formal or informal expenditure? Differing perceptions of these kinds of questions can lead to uncertain answers and ambiguous results.

Despite the difficulties, there is a growing body of relevant and interrelated information and evidence on the practices and importance of informal payments in allowing health systems to operate. Table 8.1 summarizes the types of surveys of informal health payments. They include small qualitative efforts, series of in-depth interviews with users and providers, major surveys of multiple rounds and dedicated household surveys that focus exclusively on informal payments. Such efforts have been ongoing since the first half of the 1990s.

General household surveys are the most common source of measurement. The World Bank's Living Standard Measurement Surveys and variants of them are the best source for comparisons given the standard questionnaire, representative samples and the application of special health modules that allow more detailed information. To date, informal payment information is available for Albania, Armenia, Azerbaijan, Bulgaria, Georgia, Kazakhstan, Kyrgyzstan, Romania, the Russian Federation and Tajikistan.

General household surveys by government also contribute to data on the phenomenon. The Central Statistical Offices in Poland (GUS) and Hungary collect informal payment data as part of general surveys, and in future these promise to be the main source of such data. However, quality is uneven based on just two countries. Poland's data correspond well with other surveys (Chawla *et al.* 1999; GUS 1999), but those in Hungary report an incidence of informal payments one-third to one-tenth of those reported by other surveys (various sources reported in Gaal 1999; Hungarian Central Statistical Office 1993, 1994, 1995, 1996, 1998). The source of discrepancy will be important as such data collection is mainstreamed and confidence in existing data is undermined by the sharp divergence.

Dedicated household surveys, such as those of Feeley *et al.* (1999) for the Russian Federation, Abel-Smith and Falkingham (1996) for Kyrgyzstan, the Polish Statistical Office (GUS 1999) and World Bank (2000c) for Armenia, are

Table 8.1 Summary of studies and surveys of informal health payments in CEE and FSU countries

Country (survey year)	Sources (year)	Type of survey	Sample size (number of individuals)	Types of informal payment measures
Albania (1996)	World Bank (1997a)	Living Standard Measurement Survey household survey	523	Survey covered three cities. Survey not totally representative
Armenia (1999)	World Bank (2000a)	National Institutional Review Survey of households	100 households	Detailed survey of official and unofficial payments
Armenia (1999)	Kurkchiyan (1999)	Interviews with managers, medical staff and others	99 interviews, 17 focus groups	Costing of informal payments for related diagnoses. Interviews conducted at 10 hospitals and four polyclinics
Azerbaijan (1995)	World Bank (1997b)	Azerbaijan Survey of Living Conditions	2000	
Bulgaria (1994)	Delcheva et al. (1997)	Survey of State Health Services	700	Average cost of treatment and per-capita income
Bulgaria (1997)	Balabanova (1999)	Survey and focus groups	1547	Informal payments by gender, in kind/cash, payments by quartile, timing of payments
Bulgaria (1997)	Gallup Organization (1997)	Bulgaria Integrated Household Survey	9750	Little health expenditure data
Georgia (1997)	World Bank (1999b)	Household survey (Living Standard Measurement Survey)	14,486	

Table 8.1 (cont'd)

Country (survey year)	Sources (year)	Type of survey	Sample size (number of individuals)	Types of informal payment measures
Georgia (1999)	Georgian Opinion Research Business International (1999)	Focus groups	50 focus groups	Only includes providers; six different focus groups
Georgia (1997)	Mays and Schaefer (1998)	Government accounts	NA	Health expenditure (government accounts)
Hungary	Hungarian Central Statistical Office (1993–1998) (reported in Gaal, 1999a,b)	Household budget survey	NA	Household expenditure survey
Kazakhstan (1996)	Sari et al. (2000)	Living Standard Measurement Survey household survey	7223	Per-capita income by location, poor/non-poor, national spending
Kyrgyzstan (1994)	Abel-Smith and Falkingham (1996)	Kyrgyz Health Financing Survey, survey of household informal payments	8509	Detailed information on formal and informal cost to households, how they cover costs and deterrents to consumption
Poland (1994)	Chawla et al. (1998)	Household survey (GUS)	12,359	First household survey of medical care use and expenditure, with details on informal payments
Poland (1997)	Chawla et al. (1999)	Household survey of outpatient services in Krakow	12,359	Cost of treatment. Details on payments to different kinds of providers. Distinguishes formal and informal payments

Country (year)	Source	Survey	Sample size	Description
Poland (1998)	GUS (Central Statistics Office Warsaw) (1999)	Household survey	11,983	Gratitude payments to physicians and medical staff; payment for drugs and supplies; other inpatient services
Republic of Moldova (1999)	Ruzica et al. (1999)	Survey of physicians, nurses and patients	390	130 physicians, 130 nurses and 130 patients interviewed in Chisinau (75 per cent) and two administrative districts. Group interviews also conducted
Romania (1997)	World Bank (1997c)	Integrated Household Survey (Living Standard Measurement Survey)	76,852	
Russian Federation (1997–98)	Feeley et al. (1999), Boikov and Feeley (1999)	Household informal payments survey	3000	Detailed survey of formal and informal payments, use of private sector and equity effects of policies and practices
Russian Federation (1997)	World Bank (1997d)	Russian Longitudinal Monitoring Survey (RLMS)	8701	Health module
Tajikistan (1999)	World Bank (2000e)	Living Standard Measurement Survey household survey	14,142	First national household survey
Ukraine (1998)	Kiev International Institute of Sociology (1999)	Exit and household quantitative surveys and qualitative methods: interviews, focus groups, patient diaries	100/200	In-depth discussions with providers as well as patients. Focus on perceptions
Ukraine (1999)	Way (1999)	Qualitative surveys in three cities	200	Interviewed patients and providers

best suited to understanding the extent and nature of the practices, as questions probe to understand the details of the process, but they are often unique, applying country-specific questionnaires. The drawbacks of the general household surveys are their breadth and the correspondingly limited attention to the health sector. For example, they often simply ask whether informal payments were required. In countries accustomed to gratitude payments or where in-kind gifts are not perceived as payment, the resulting informal health care market may be underestimated, and the dedicated surveys can avoid these limitations. However, as noted above, the lack of comparability impedes generalizations from the dedicated informal payment surveys. Both types of surveys focus exclusively on users, ignoring the equally important providers who define and operate the informal payment system.

Another promising and possibly less costly survey approach is canvassing patients. As data collection is systematized in health insurance bodies, patient-based surveys will be viable. This can also be accomplished through exit surveys, as was done in Vietnam (World Bank 1993) and on a more limited basis in Ukraine (Kiev International Institute of Sociology 1999), or by telephone (Chawla *et al.* 1999). However, recent experience in Poland suggests that such approaches in CEE and FSU countries may not be feasible. In the latter circumstance, a random sample of inpatients and outpatients was surveyed after discharge or completed outpatient treatment to elicit feedback on informal and formal payments, satisfaction of patients and other factors. Efforts to apply the exit surveys were predominantly met with non-compliance. The history of informants may explain reluctance to discuss such practices on the premises of health services, and the illegal nature of the practice in some countries makes acknowledgement, much less discussion of the practice, undesirable for patients. The selected alternative, which should be increasingly feasible in tracing patients, is identifying users through insurance rolls.

Qualitative methods in, among others, Armenia (Kurchiyan 1999), Bulgaria (Delcheva *et al.* 1997; Balabanova 1999), Georgia (Georgian Opinion Research Business International 1999), the Republic of Moldova (Ruzica *et al.* 1999) and Ukraine (Kiev International Institute of Sociology 1999; Way 1999) target patients and providers and shed light on the motivation and process of informal payments from both the provider and patient perspectives. Qualitative data can explain quantitative findings and make sense of them. In many instances, surveys are clumsy tools for capturing the perceptions and beliefs that underpin the practices of informal payments, and the results suggest that these are not uniform. Given the sensitivity of the issue, providers are often reluctant to participate but can be willing to anonymously join focus groups. The same can be said of patients who may avoid identification but have information and views that can be captured through discussion. Like all qualitative results, these results are not necessarily representative and generalization needs to be evaluated accordingly.

The comparative analysis below draws on all these sources, attempting to use the disparate data to shape a view of the practice of informal payments and its attendant issues. They reflect the creativity and breadth of efforts over the past few years to understand and measure the phenomena of informal payments.

Extent of informal payments for health care

In this section, I provide an overview of the average payment for inpatient care, outpatient services and drugs, drawing on available data, and explore some additional patterns in less depth, drawing on the quantitative and qualitative results of existing research. Distinguishing between formal and informal payments proves difficult, as the definition is blurred both in the posing of the questions and in the understanding and perceptions of respondents. Moreover, the status of out-of-pocket payments for things like drugs is ambiguous, since they are only informal if the government is meant to cover such costs. The same holds true for health resources. If it is a stated policy that government does not finance drugs, then these purchases are expected and technically do not constitute informal payments. The reverse follows that, when health services are meant to be free, all out-of-pocket expenditure is informal. The intent here is to capture the informal payments and, where possible, to distinguish them from formal payment. The mentioned confusion, however, results in uneven capture, since the two may well be mixed.

Formal fee policies vary across the countries in the sample. At the time of the surveys, free services were guaranteed in Albania, Azerbaijan, Kazakhstan, Kyrgyzstan, the Republic of Moldova and Tajikistan; in Poland, inpatient care was free, but the patients were responsible for outpatient medication (and all dentistry). Romania required co-payments only for prescriptions. To the extent possible these differences are taken into account and, as mentioned above, some of the surveys specifically distinguish between what is formally and informally paid.

Some countries, however, including Armenia, Bulgaria, Georgia and the Russian Federation, formally charge something, and patients pay twice. In general, informal fees are higher than formal charges (Lewis 2000). In Armenia, one of the few countries for which such data are available, the introduction of formal charges has reduced the level and frequency of informal revenue and the total number of patients (Kurkchiyan 1999).

Figure 8.1 summarizes the average informal health expenditure per capita by country using reported totals or, if these are not available, aggregating inpatient, outpatient, drugs and other categories of informal payments.[5] The other categories encompass fees for diagnostic tests, specialist consultations, direct physician contributions and consumables if these data are available. Thus, the average levels for each country provide a snapshot of the total expenditure, without the benefit of detailing the distribution of that expenditure across categories of payment.

Figure 8.2 presents the average out-of-pocket payment in US dollars by expenditure type: outpatient, inpatient and drugs.[6] In some cases, these are not strictly comparable across countries, but existing data have been adjusted to conform as closely as possible to definitions of average expenditure in each type of service. Not surprisingly, inpatient care is significantly more costly than outpatient services, and average drug expenditure often exceeds the cost of ambulatory care. Since drug expenditure can capture more than a single episode (and possibly other family members as well), the average expenditure can be quite high. Drug costs also vary according to the pharmaceutical

Figure 8.1 Average informal payments (in 1995 US dollars adjusted for purchasing power parity) per capita for people who sought care in five CEE and FSU countries, 1996 or 1997

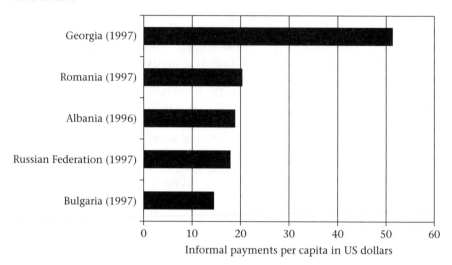

Sources: per-capita income from World Bank (2000d) and informal payments data from World Bank (1996, 1997c, 1999b), Balabanova (1999), Boikov and Feeley (1999) and Feeley *et al.* (1999)

Figure 8.2 Average informal payments (in 1995 US dollars adjusted for purchasing power parity) per visit for outpatient care, inpatient care and drugs for seven CEE and FSU countries, 1996, 1997 or 1998

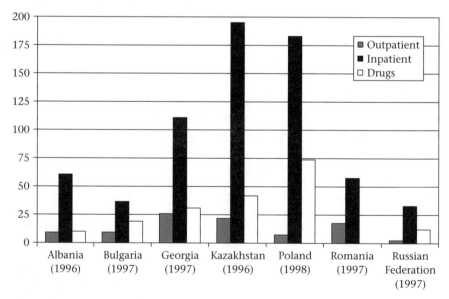

Sources: World Bank (1996, 1997c, 1999b), Balabanova (1999), Boikov and Feeley (1999), Feeley *et al.* (1999), GUS (1999) and Sari *et al.* (2000)

Table 8.2 Percentage of people seeking health care reporting informal payments by category of health service in selected CEE and FSU countries

Country	Year of survey	General hospital	Physicians	Nurses or other health care personnel	Drugs	Tests or supplies	Other	Total
Bulgaria	1997	6	66	12	16	NA	NA	100
Kazakhstan	1996	28	32	NA	6	34[a]	NA	100
Kyrgyzstan	1994	0	18	0	61	14	7	100
Republic of Moldova	1999	10	7	0.5	49	16	18[b]	100
Poland[c]	1998	6	42	9	16	3	25[d]	100
Poland: Krakow[e]	1997	8	NA	92	NA	NA		100
Russian Federation	1997–98	31	21	7	18	NA	23[f]	100

[a] Defined by the author as 'procedures'. [b] Mainly additional food payments and other therapeutic services; general hospitals includes about 5 per cent for food already. [c] This study only includes inpatients. [d] Includes payments for outside assistance, private hospital payments and undetermined expenses. [e] Includes outpatients only. [f] Largely privately financed dental care. NA = not available.

Sources: Balabanova (1999), Chawla *et al.* (1999), Abel-Smith and Falkingham (1996), Feeley *et al.* (1999), GUS (1999), Ruzica *et al.* (1999) and Sari *et al.* (2000)

cost structure in each country, something that is not controlled for in the reported data.

The distribution of patient purchases for health care indicates where patients contribute to health care costs. Table 8.2 shows the circumstances in which payment was made across six categories for a small number of CEE and FSU countries. The results suggest considerable variation – indeed, a lack of any consistent pattern in informal payments. For example, the percentage of payments made for drugs ranged from 6 per cent in Kazakhstan to 49 per cent in the Republic of Moldova. Even physician payments do not converge, although the discrepancy is narrower. These findings suggest the variability of the extent to which informal payment is required across CEE and FSU countries and, if Poland is a guide, across inpatient and outpatient services within countries.

The importance to households of informal payments can be seen by examining the frequency of informal payments and in comparing expenditure per episode as a percentage of per-capita income. Together these measures provide a sense of the relative burden of payments on the average household.

The frequency of informal payments varies considerably between countries; for example, 78 per cent of inpatients in Poland versus 21 per cent in Bulgaria in 1997. The percentage for Bulgaria is below the 1994 proportion of 43 per cent, when urban areas were oversampled. This may explain the apparent decline in reported informal payments, as such payments appear to be more common in urban areas (Balabanova 1999).

The 74 per cent for the Russian Federation relates only to informal hospital payments; only 16 per cent of patients made informal payments to physicians.

Table 8.3 Average monthly income per capita and average percentage of monthly income spent on health care and drugs[a] by people seeking care in seven CEE and FSU countries

Country	Year of survey	Average monthly income per capita in the year of the survey (in US$)	Average expenditure as a percentage of income	Drug expenditure as a percentage of income
Albania	1996	193	9.1	4.8
Bulgaria	1997	334	4.4	5.8
Georgia	1997	164	20.6	12.4
Kazakhstan	1996	290	NA	11.2
Poland	1994	432	NA	10.3
Romania	1997	359	4.1	NA
Russian Federation	1997	355	3.9	2.6

[a] Adjusted for purchasing power parity, from the World Development Indicators (World Bank 2000d). Per-capita income calculated from the World Development Indicators. NA = not available

Sources: see Table 8.1 for a summary of survey sources

This study distinguishes between formal and informal payments. There are considerable formal payments, and pharmaceutical drug purchases account for 55 per cent of all household health expenditure, both formal and informal. If it is assumed that the health system should provide these, then the estimate of informal expenditure would rise accordingly (Feeley *et al.* 1999).

For countries with available data, drug payment exceeds expenditure for health care services. In contrast to low service payments, 90 per cent of patients in Bulgaria and 98 per cent in Poland purchased drugs (Balabanova 1999; GUS 1999). Data for outpatient care in Krakow, Poland showed that drugs constituted 68 per cent of all informal outpatient expenditure (Chawla *et al.* 1999); in Kyrgyzstan, three-quarters of admitted patients were required to purchase drugs that were meant to be free (Abel-Smith and Falkingham 1996). In the Russian Federation, private purchase has become the norm, resulting in a low proportion of the population paying informally for drugs; 16 per cent already purchase pharmaceuticals outright (Feeley *et al.* 1999).

Table 8.3 compares per-capita income with the percentage of income devoted to all health care and the percentage of income spent on drugs. The latter is a subset of the total and may capture discretionary pharmaceutical purchases, but it is very important to households given that such expenditure can be made both with and without benefit of medical advice and, therefore, covers the cost of self-treatment.

The reasons for making informal payments are somewhat complex. In Ukraine, focus groups noted the low wages and arrears in payment to physicians as important, as without patient payment the system could not function. One patient summed up the situation differently, indicating that 'no grease, no motion' (Kiev International Institute of Sociology 1999). Patients in

Bulgaria made similar references but also said that patients sometimes paid to seek higher-quality care or to improve the attitude of staff towards them and their health problems. The data also suggest that higher-income and more urbanized populations are more likely to pay for services, which is not surprising since upper-income households can pay for better services (Balabanova 1999). In Hungary, various studies have reported that gratitude motivates under-the-table payments, although in some circumstances convenience and provider attitudes have also emerged as important (Gaal 1999).

Interestingly, the results of a 1997 opinion survey in the Russian Federation indicated that 25 per cent of respondents were not confident of the professional qualifications of public-sector physicians and sought private care, and another 20 per cent noted the 'lack of sensitivity' of medical personnel in public clinics, both consistent with the perceptions in Bulgaria (Feeley *et al.* 1999). The need to expedite, to ensure responsiveness and quality, to encourage the system to continue working and to compensate underpaid health care workers, all seem to contribute to willingness to pay. The question is whether all patients can pay.

Services financed and provided by the government are intended to ensure access without regard to differences in income. The need to make under-the-table payments can restrict access for people unable to pay for care. Here, I summarize available information on impediments to equity and access to health care services, including drugs.

The income of households appears important in determining the utilization of health services when illness occurs. In the 1998 survey in the Russian Federation (Feeley *et al.* 1999), official payments were found to constitute 27 per cent of the monthly income of the lowest quintile of households in contrast to 9 per cent for the highest quintile; informal payments were reported to have a negligible effect on incomes at all levels. In contrast, the 1997 survey found that 41 per cent said they could not afford drugs and 13 per cent could not pay for health care. Thus, there is some discrepancy, although the more careful distinction between informal and formal payments in more recent work may explain the differences.

How much low-income and high-income groups spend on health care can be seen through the structure of payments across income groups. Richer households tend to spend more in absolute terms but less as a percentage of their total income. In Ukraine, the average expenditure per household varied from 50 hryvna for poor households to four times that for higher-income households. In Kazakhstan, poor families that experienced hospitalization spent 252 per cent of monthly income for care, whereas more affluent people spent 54 per cent of monthly earnings for the same type of service (Sari *et al.* 2000).

Reports of inability to afford care in specific circumstances complement this. In Poland, 11 per cent of the population could not afford prescription drugs and another 26 per cent sometimes found it too costly. The rate of unaffordable prescription drugs rose to 14 per cent for retirees, suggesting that, even in relatively affluent Poland, out-of-pocket costs are high and place some forms of health care out of reach of certain segments of the population (GUS 1999). The results of the 1997 survey in the Russian Federation indicate considerable inability to afford health services and prescription drugs.

A useful indicator for determining affordability is the need to borrow, sell off, produce or otherwise raise funds for health care. In Ukraine, about 15 per cent of users dipped into savings or borrowed from family members (Kiev International Institute of Sociology 1999). Not only does this mean that health care costs can be a significant burden on the economic well-being of some families, it also implies that low-income households get less care than those from more affluent families since durable goods, borrowing and assets tend to be less accessible to poorer households, thus removing a possible safety valve for covering health care costs. In Kyrgyzstan, one in three inpatients borrowed money, and in rural areas 45 per cent sold produce or livestock to cover the costs of hospital care. Thus, an inpatient episode can have a devastating economic effect on a family, especially those from low-income households.

Conclusions and policy implications

The implicit or explicit acceptance of informal payments is most troubling, as it places government in the position of either ignoring or abetting irregular practices. In some countries, anecdotal evidence suggests that governments estimate such payments to determine physicians' wages. Discussions with providers indicate that they need to solicit gratuities or 'envelope' payments to supplement low salaries and arrears in earnings. Permitting informal payments acknowledges the government's inability to meet its costs under the current system.

There are no benefits to, or acceptable rationales for, tolerating informal payments. Doing so places government in the position of condoning random charges by its own employees from citizens who are in the unfortunate position of needing health care. Informal payments are at odds with transparent public policy and trust in government, fundamental premises of democracy and good government. Thus informal payments are damaging to the health sector, the government and society.

Solving the increasingly entrenched practice of informal payments is neither painless nor easy, but without action, access to health services becomes difficult, as does setting and maintaining basic standards of care. The cultural tradition of such payments makes addressing the problem even more difficult. As discussed below, many of the initiatives most likely to address the problem effectively entail major restructuring of the sector. As a result, solutions must address that structure and its effects on provider behaviour. Moreover, any single intervention is unlikely to be adequate on its own; a multi-pronged strategy is therefore required.

First, a clear policy framework that clarifies the government's position regarding informal payments and off-budget financial exchanges between public employees and citizens would be needed to set the parameters for acceptable behaviour. Second, the existing public health care systems are too large and function in many settings as employment services rather than public services. Reduction to a manageable size that is affordable is desirable if reform is to take hold. In many countries, budgets cannot cover the costs of the excessively large workforce, expensive inpatient services, large numbers of hospitals and broad service coverage. There are too many inputs and inadequate funding, leading to solicitation of alternative sources of funding by front-line providers.

A good example is physician numbers and salaries. With little attrition and declining or modestly increasing expenditure, real wages have declined. Reducing the number of physicians should offer the opportunity to downsize hospital capacity, reduce costs and raise the salaries of the remaining physicians. Two examples help to illuminate this. In the Czech Republic, the number of physicians has declined somewhat (although further reduction is needed) and earnings have exceeded or kept pace with growth in overall wages. In the Czech Republic, unlike other CEE countries, informal payments to physicians appear uncommon (World Bank 1999a, 2000a). Poland is a more robust example. Average informal payments paid to different public providers in 1998 ranged from nearly 26 million Zloty for public outpatients to only 164,000 Zloty for public emergency care. Only the capitated primary care physicians did not make an additional charge, as their earnings were highest given the adequacy of the capitated payment and the patterns of demand (Chawla *et al.* 1999). These examples provide some indication that higher earnings may offer a partial solution, at least in some settings. However, this is unlikely to be a solution by itself. Indeed, physician salaries in Greece were raised and informal payments declined temporarily only to rise again thereafter (Elias Mossialos, personal communication), a sobering example of a possible longer-term failure to effectively suppress informal payments and to hold providers accountable to the public.

Third, comprehensive, free services are not affordable in a budget-constrained environment. Governments in many CEE and FSU countries have difficulty affording what is already in place. The scope of financed services may need to be reduced or users will need to formally cover the costs of some aspects of care. Given national income levels, these alternatives deserve serious consideration.

Hospitals and clinics could be scaled back. Incentives could be used to encourage reducing capacity. In many countries, budgets remain driven by input requirements, creating perverse incentives to maintain excess capacity. Policy-makers need to focus on the budgeting process and the over-emphasis on input if they are to be able to downsize and thus have the resources to ensure efficiency and raise quality.

Formally charging users, which would hopefully replace the existing arrangements, could take many forms:

- charging marginal payments for many services, a variant of current practices;
- offering upgraded hotel services and personal attention for a premium, a practice already applied in some systems;
- per-day payment for inpatient care, even if the amounts are nominal;
- payment for private physician services in public hospitals;
- supplementary health insurance to cover the costs of input (such as for drugs and supplies) for which patients are often responsible, a recent formal system that appears to be successful in Kyrgyzstan;

- across-the-board payments that charge everyone something but disproportionately subsidize inpatient care or drugs or other services that are a heavy
burden to patients; and
- full subsidies for poor people and some form of charging of more affluent
patients on a sliding fee scale.

These represent options and any or all can apply in a given setting. Patients
are already paying and there clearly exists a willingness to pay; the issues are
how much should be charged and who should pay. These issues need to be
resolved at the country level, preferably within the context of comprehensive
health system reform.

Numerous options exist and debate and experimentation can help guide
policy. The basic principle of cost-sharing is inevitable either to finance the
range of services desired (especially in CEE countries) or to make only basic
services available (especially in FSU countries). In effect, governments should
decide what and whose health care to give priority and subsidize within its
own fiscal constraints.

Fourth, health systems require basic oversight and accountability for all
providers. Performance is both hard to measure and a new concept in health
care. However, achieving a more affordable, fair and equitable system requires
that relative performance be assessed, performance benchmarks be set and
providers held accountable for the results. Fundamental to this is the use of
acceptable accounting standards and retrospective auditing of hospital accounts
combined with tools to ensure that hospital managers comply with national
policies regarding informal payments.

Finally, private alternatives can be allowed and promoted for those who
choose to use them. The lack of private alternatives for both providers and
patients contributes to a market within the public system. The two would be
more effective if separated and the government is in a position to foster this.
Currently government directly finances much of the 'private care' or physicians use public infrastructure to treat their private patients.

The political economy of phasing out informal payments is serious. It
requires a consistent, broad plan, as the incentives of its beneficiaries are to
maintain the system as it exists. Although complex, the initiatives that do
exist deserve serious consideration either alone or as part of a broader reform.
Establishing priorities has political and social implications, including the
acknowledgement that the government cannot do everything given the income levels and public revenue of most CEE and FSU countries. Without such
commitment, informal payments are likely to continue to define public health
care systems in CEE and FSU countries.

Notes

1 I thank the participants in the European Observatory on Health Care Systems Workshop on Funding Health Care: Options for Europe (held in Venice, Italy in December
1999 and supported by the Veneto Region), especially Peter Gaal and Alexander
Preker for comments on an earlier draft of the manuscript. Dina Balabanova and Peter
Gaal prepared background case studies on informal payments in Bulgaria and Hungary,

respectively. John Voss provided able research assistance and Ian Conachy produced the manuscript. The findings and recommendations do not necessarily reflect the policy or views of the World Bank Group.

2 Dental care, however, is increasingly private and with fees for services in CEE and FSU countries.

3 In some countries, such as Georgia and Ukraine, non-payment of salaries has meant that informal payments are the sole source of income. In others, such as Hungary and Poland, they supplement relatively low salaries.

4 Formal fees are less likely to elicit a similar responsiveness to patients, since the individual provider does not benefit. If provider units (hospitals or clinics) retain these formal fee revenues, they have an incentive to satisfy patients.

5 The data for the tables are drawn largely from statistically representative samples for each country. The data from qualitative sources are not statistically representative. The data sources are described in Table 8.1; if samples are not representative, this is noted.

6 Exchange rates were drawn from the International Monetary Fund tables for the year of the survey and adjusted for purchasing power parity. The purchasing power parity conversion factor is the number of units of a country's currency required to buy the same amount of goods and services in the domestic market as the US dollar would buy in the United States (World Bank 2000d). When available, the exchange rates reported in the studies are used.

References

Abel-Smith, B. and Falkingham, J. (1996) *Financing Health Services in Kyrgyzstan: The Extent of Private Payments*. London: London School of Economics and Political Science, LSE Health and Department of Social Policy.

Anderson, J. (2000) Corruption in Slovakia: results of diagnostic surveys, unpublished. Prepared at the request of the Government of the Slovak Republic by the World Bank and the United States Agency for International Development.

Balabanova, D. (1999) Informal payments for health care in Bulgaria, unpublished. London: Health Services Research Unit, London School of Hygiene & Tropical Medicine.

Boikov, V.E. and Feeley, F.G. (1999) *Russian Household Expenditures on Drugs and Medical Care*, unpublished. Boston, MA: Boston University.

Chawla, M. (1995) *Factors Determining Dual Job-Holdings in the Health Sector: Some Evidence from Egypt*, PhD dissertation. Boston, MA: Boston University.

Chawla, M., Berman, P. and Kawiorska, D. (1998) Financing health services in Poland: new evidence on private expenditures, *Health Economics*, 7: 337–46.

Chawla, M., Berman, P., Windak, A. and Kulis, M. (1999) *Provision of Ambulatory Health Services in Poland: A Case Study from Krakow*, Boston: International Health Systems Group, Harvard School of Public Health. http://www.hsph.harvard.edu/ihsg/publications/pdf/No-73.PDF (accessed 25 February 2001).

Delcheva, E., Balabanova, D. and McKee, M. (1997) Under-the-counter payments for health care, *Health Policy*, 42(2): 89–100.

Feeley, F.G., Sheiman, I.M. and Shiskin, S.V. (1999) *Health Sector Informal Payments in Russia*, unpublished. Boston, MA: Boston University.

Gaal, P. (1998) Under-the-table payment and health care reforms in Hungary, unpublished. Bucharest: Health Service Management Training Centre, Semmelweis University of Medicine.

Gaal, P. (1999) Informal payment in the Hungarian health services, unpublished. Bucharest: Health Service Management Training Centre, Semmelweis University of Medicine.

Gallup Organization (1997) Background paper for the Bulgaria Poverty Assessment Study, unpublished. Washington, DC: World Bank.

Georgian Opinion Research Business International (1999) *Health Care Reform in Georgia: A Focus Group Study*. Tbilisi: Georgian Opinion Research Business International.

GUS (Central Statistics Office Warsaw) (1999) *Health Care in Households in 1998*. Warsaw: GUS.

Hungarian Central Statistical Office (1993) *Household Budget Survey 1992*. Budapest: Hungarian Central Statistical Office.

Hungarian Central Statistical Office (1994) *Household Budget Survey 1993*. Budapest: Hungarian Central Statistical Office.

Hungarian Central Statistical Office (1995) *Household Budget Survey 1994*. Budapest: Hungarian Central Statistical Office.

Hungarian Central Statistical Office (1996) *Household Budget Survey 1995*. Budapest: Hungarian Central Statistical Office.

Hungarian Central Statistical Office (1998) *Household Budget Survey 1996*. Budapest: Hungarian Central Statistical Office.

Kiev International Institute of Sociology (1999) Level of availability and quality of medical care in Ukraine, unpublished. Kiev: Kiev International Institute of Sociology.

Kurkchiyan, M. (1999) The change in health care in post-Soviet countries: a case study of Armenia, unpublished. World Bank Report on Health Care in Armenia. Washington, DC: World Bank.

La Forgia, G., Levine, R., Diaz, A. and Rathe, M. (1999) Fend for yourself: systemic failure in the Dominican health market and prospects for change, paper presented at the IHEA Conference, Rotterdam, the Netherlands, 5–8 June.

Lewis, M. (2000) *Who is Paying for Health Care in Europe and Central Asia?* Washington, DC: World Bank.

Lewis, M.A., La Forgia, G.M. and Sulvetta, M.B. (1992) Productivity and quality of public hospital staff: a Dominican case study, *International Journal of Health Planning and Management*, 6: 287–308.

Lewis, M.A., La Forgia, G.M and Sulvetta, M.B. (1996) Measuring public hospital costs: empirical evidence from the Dominican Republic, *Social Science and Medicine*, 43(2): 221–34.

Lewis, M., Eskeland, G.S. and Traa-Valerezo, X. (1999) *Challenging El Salvador's Rural Health Care Strategy*, Policy Research Working Paper No. 2164. Washington, DC: World Bank.

Mays, J. and Schaefer, M. (1998) Preliminary analysis of risk pooling potential in the health care financing system of Georgia, unpublished. Annandale, VA: Actuarial Research Corporation.

Narayan, D. (2000) *Voices of the Poor: Can Anyone Hear Us?* New York: Oxford University Press.

Preker, A., Harding, A. and Girishankar, N. (1999) The economics of public and private participation in health care: new insights from institutional economics, paper presented at the Economist Forum, Alexandria, VA, 4, May.

Ruzica, M., Lisnic, V., Orlova, N. and Nedera, S. (1999) Moldova health reform: social and institutional assessment (SIA), unpublished. Washington, DC: World Bank.

Sari, A., Langenbrunner, J. and Lewis, M. (2000) Out-of-pocket payments in health care: evidence from Kazakhstan, *EuroHealth*, 6(special issue 2): 37–9.

Ukraine Legal Foundation (1998) *Questions on National Integrity: Analytical Report*. Kiev: Ukraine Legal Foundation.

Way, L. (1999) Decentralization of social services in Ukraine, unpublished. San Francisco: University of California.

World Bank (1993) *World Development Report*. Oxford: Oxford University Press.

World Bank (1996) Data set, Albania, unpublished. Washington, DC: World Bank.

World Bank (1997a) *Albania: Growing Out of Poverty*. Washington, DC: World Bank.

World Bank (1997b) *Azerbaijan: Poverty Assessment*, Vol. I. Washington, DC: World Bank.

World Bank (1997c) World Bank LSMS Household Survey 1997 for Romania, unpublished. Washington, DC: World Bank.

World Bank (1997d) Russian Longitudinal Monitoring Survey (RLMS), unpublished. Washington, DC: World Bank.

World Bank (1998) *Health Strategy Paper for Eastern Europe and Central Asia*. Washington, DC: World Bank.

World Bank (1999a) *Czech Republic Country Economic Memorandum*. Washington, DC: World Bank.

World Bank (1999b) *Georgia: Poverty and Income Distribution*, Vols I and II. Washington, DC: World Bank.

World Bank (2000a) Health, in Czech Republic: public expenditure review, unpublished. Washington, DC: World Bank.

World Bank (2000b) *Making Transition Work for Everyone: Poverty and Inequity in Eastern Europe and Central Asia*. Washington, DC: World Bank.

World Bank (2000c) Armenia institutional and governance review, unpublished. Washington, DC: World Bank.

World Bank (2000d) *World Development Indicators Central Database CD-ROM*. Washington, DC: World Bank.

World Bank (2000e) LSMS Household Survey, Tajikistan, unpublished. Washington, DC, World Bank.

nine

Lessons on the sustainability of health care funding from low- and middle-income countries

Anne Mills and Sara Bennett [1]

Introduction

There are diverse experiences in health care financing outside industrialized countries, arising both from what governments have tried to do and from what individuals and private agencies have done in the absence of government action. Low- and middle-income countries outside Europe have used a wide range of financing options, including social health insurance, community-based insurance, user fees, increased tax financing and various combinations of these. Experiences have been very mixed. Some approaches, such as social health insurance, may have worked well in certain contexts but have been problematic in others. Successes and failures cannot be assessed without examining the context within which changes are designed and implemented.

A key feature of the health financing debate in low- and middle-income countries is the extent to which it is influenced by policy trends in more affluent countries. The multilateral and bilateral systems of development assistance, the influence of education and training programmes in industrialized countries and the general flow of ideas and ideologies across the world all make less affluent countries vulnerable to the inappropriate importation of ideas. Hence, any discussion or evaluation of financing reforms must examine the extent to which they conform to the general characteristics of low- and middle-income countries.

In this chapter, we seek to understand some successes and failures of health financing reform in low- and middle-income countries. Successes and failures are defined with respect to efficiency and equity criteria and the extent to which countries implemented changes effectively. Central to the discussion is the belief that the financing system needs to be congruent with government capacity, interpreted broadly to encompass both internal aspects of capacity and institutional structures and socioeconomic context (Batley 1997). We therefore explain successes and failures by referring to these broader characteristics. We focus on the three main alternatives to financing by government tax revenue that have been explored in low- and middle-income countries: social health insurance, community-based health insurance and user fees. Cutting across each of these sections is the theme of government capacity to design new financing mechanisms, to garner support for implementing them and to implement them. The final section draws lessons for low- and middle-income countries in Europe (Europe being defined here as including countries in western Europe, central and eastern Europe and the former Soviet Union). First, however, we address common characteristics of the health sectors of low- and middle-income countries relevant to the choice of financing option, and present an analytical approach to thinking about capacity to design and implement changes.

Common characteristics of health sectors in low- and middle-income countries

The key characteristics of the health sectors of low- and middle-income countries are:

- low absolute expenditure on health services;
- a large proportion of total health financing is privately generated and flows to private providers, both formal and informal; and
- out-of-pocket payments comprise a large proportion of health expenditure.

For example, total health expenditure per capita in low-income countries was about US$22 (1994 prices), with only 37 per cent spent through the public sector (Bos *et al.* 1998). In middle-income countries, these figures were US$209 and 52 per cent. Influencing all three of these characteristics is the limited participation in the formal labour market characteristic of many low- and middle-income countries, which has several direct implications for health financing.

Tax revenue is very limited, especially from direct taxes. Governments have not generally perceived increased tax revenue for health as feasible; many low- and middle-income countries have therefore sought to complement tax revenue with alternative sources of financing. Reliance on indirect taxes can mean that tax financing is relatively inequitable. For example, in the Philippines, indirect taxes comprise 60 per cent of public funds for health care, and the effective (indirect and direct) tax rates for lower, middle and higher income classes are 27 per cent, 32 per cent and 18 per cent, respectively (World Bank 1993).

Achieving universal coverage with social health insurance is difficult: many long-standing schemes, especially in Latin America, have failed to cover more than a minority of the population and have exacerbated inequity in access to health care between different segments of the population. More recently, several countries in south-east Asia have introduced social health insurance and they, too, are now grappling with issues of how to provide universal coverage when a relatively small proportion of the working population is in formal employment.

Because establishing compulsory insurance for informally employed populations is inherently difficult and because general tax revenue for health care is limited, user fees are greatly relied on as a source of revenue, especially in low-income countries. Consequently, there is much interest in, and experimentation with, community-based health insurance schemes, because these promise to protect against the adverse welfare implications of out-of-pocket payments. In the long term, it is hoped that these schemes can be knit together into a system of universal protection.

Thus, health financing systems in low- and middle-income countries rely on a mix of funding sources. This pattern has emerged as a result of low taxation capacities and the fact that no one source alone can generate enough revenue to provide health services for the whole population.

Concepts of capacity

Capacity-building has traditionally been associated with education and training (Brinkerhoff 1994), but recent writers on capacity have substantially enlarged this concept. The capacity internal to an organization is commonly distinguished from that external to the organization (Batley 1997). The dimensions of internal capacity generally examined include human resources, management and information systems and financing. The broader public-sector institutional context will also affect capacity, in particular the presence of concurrent policies, management practices, rules and regulations, and formal and informal power relationships, which may all influence a particular task (Hildebrand and Grindle 1994). Capacity will also be affected by the even broader environment, which includes economic factors (such as private-sector development and the structure of the labour market), political factors (such as political stability and leadership support) and social factors (such as the development of civil society and human resources). The institutional context, including laws and regulations, may also be important.

In addition, the literature emphasizes the capacity to change. This can be interpreted in two ways. First, the ability of government to change the *status quo* is a highly political question that depends on such factors as the presence of strong leadership and political windows of opportunity. Second is the notion of capacity to adapt or learn from experience, which is important because reform is normally a dynamic process and not a one-off event.

Expansion of coverage of social health insurance

Where compulsory social health insurance schemes exist in less affluent countries, they tend to offer a much higher quality and quantity of care than that available to those not in formal employment, who must rely on often under-funded and poorly distributed services from the ministry of health. A notable feature of health financing policy trends in the last few years has been interest in several countries in achieving universal coverage (Nitayarumphong and Mills 2000). In south-east Asia, this has been fuelled by economic growth and an awareness that improvements in access to health care and protection against income loss from illness can be both the fruits of economic growth and an important contribution to a flourishing economy. In Latin America, institu-tionalized inequality in access to care is finally being tackled in some coun-tries as part of the liberalization of economic and political systems. However, the means of achieving universal coverage are very uncertain. Key issues, exemplified in the case study on Thailand at the end of this section, are how best to bring together the different financing schemes for different segments of the population and whether the internal and external capacity constraints are conducive to making progress towards universal coverage.

Compulsory payroll contributions seem to have greater political acceptance than increased general tax revenue as the central element of the funding mix and are more acceptable to employees. Given this reliance on compulsory social insurance, the key issues facing countries seeking to extend coverage have been how to finance and administer the extension to self-employed people and low-income workers. Several possibilities are apparent from country experiences (Mills 2000).

- The cost of insurance premiums has been kept low by providing highly subsidized public hospital care to poorer groups of the population, such as in Thailand, for those purchasing a voluntary health card and, in Singapore, for those self-selecting into hospital wards with fewer amenities.
- Social insurance funds have been used to cross-subsidize care for low-income populations; this appears most feasible in countries such as Costa Rica, where most of the population is formally employed and covered by social health insurance.
- All compulsory health insurance premiums have been subsidized by public funds (in Thailand, employers, employees and the government pay equal shares) or only the premiums of low-income employed and self-employed people, identified through a means test (such as in the Republic of Korea and Turkey).
- Innovative ways have sometimes been found to incorporate farmers, who usually comprise most self-employed people, including payment at the time of harvest or payment related to assets as well as or in place of income, such as in the Republic of Korea.
- The government can encourage voluntary schemes that may become com-pulsory in time, such as in the Philippines and Thailand.

Sometimes a separate and self-contained insurance arrangement is created for self-employed people, whereas elsewhere government funding is used to bring them under the umbrella of the compulsory insurance scheme. The experience of countries in Asia suggests that the former is the preferred or most feasible option in the first instance; for example, Japan, the Republic of Korea and Taiwan have had historical experience of separate arrangements for different population groups. Over time, the different schemes are standardized and made more compatible and, when it is affordable, the government increases the subsidies for lower-income groups so their benefits match those of formally employed people.

A related issue is how to finance the extension of coverage to those without any steady income: many aged, unemployed and disabled people. Many elderly people as well as children can be covered as the dependants of those employed in the formal sector; this, for example, is being recommended as the next stage in the extension of Thailand's social health insurance scheme (Donaldson *et al.* 1998).

Many social health insurance schemes involve high co-payments, as they may permit the contribution rate to be set at a level that is affordable and acceptable (Republic of Korea and the Philippines) and may also help to constrain demand. Co-payments may also be seen as a symbol of family responsibility for its own health care (Republic of Korea and Singapore). Their main disadvantages are that they are regressive and they will hinder the achievement of the overall aim of insurance schemes by reducing the level of risk protection.

Social health insurance schemes have aroused quite substantial concerns over efficiency, because of how health services have been paid for and the fragmentation of the health care system they frequently encourage. Selecting an appropriate payment method has become one of the key policy questions facing countries seeking to introduce or reform such schemes. Some social health insurance schemes in middle-income countries, such as the Republic of Korea and Taiwan, have purchased care from public and private facilities on a fee-for-service basis. Fee-for-service payment in Taiwan during the period 1980–94 was undoubtedly a major factor behind the annual per-capita increase in health spending of 15.7 per cent compared with an annual GNP increase per capita of 12.1 per cent (Chiang 1997). In the Republic of Korea, health expenditure as a share of gross domestic product increased from 2.8 per cent in 1975 to 4.3 per cent in 1986 and 7.1 per cent in 1991 (Peabody *et al.* 1995). The Ministry of Health and Social Affairs attempted to contain costs by mandating lower fees, but this was countered by volume increases. Such problems have created considerable interest in case-based payment and capitation.

Introducing social health insurance in a context of relatively low formal-sector employment makes fragmentation almost inevitable; this has occurred in many countries, especially in Latin America. Fragmentation adversely affects efficiency by duplicating certain functions (such as provider payment) for populations and providers in the same geographical area. Fragmentation is also a problem for the coherence of health policy. The responsibility of a ministry of health for national policy and regulatory functions is frequently not binding or is difficult to ensure for the social security part of a health care system.

Case study 1: social health insurance in Thailand

Thailand offers an interesting case study of the difficulties of merging different health financing arrangements for different segments of the population into a universal system. The key risk protection arrangements are:

- The Social Security Scheme established in 1990, compulsory for all employees in establishments of 10 or more workers.
- The Civil Servants Medical Benefit Scheme, covering all civil servants.
- The Low Income and Elderly Scheme, covering those below an income threshold and those over 65 years of age: a low income card can be applied for or, alternatively, fee waivers are available from health facilities.
- The Health Card Programme, a voluntary insurance arrangement.

The uncovered part of the population must pay substantial fees at public facilities or use private providers. A very small number have private insurance coverage. The main differences between these arrangements are summarized in Table 9.1. Each of these schemes covers different segments of the population and uses different payment mechanisms and different means of collecting revenue. Merging the schemes would create potential for efficiency gains in administration as well as for equity gains.

Table 9.1 shows the grossly inequitable distribution of government subsidies, which affects levels of utilization and the benefit package offered by different schemes. Some measures to reduce inequity have been introduced, for example increasing the public subsidy to the low-income scheme. In addition, the very rapid cost increases experienced by the Civil Servants Medical Benefit Scheme, plus the financial crisis, have forced some measures to restrict access to private providers (Tangcharoensathien *et al.* 1999). However, the basic differences between the arrangements have yet to be addressed, for reasons that can be explained in terms of the elements of capacity identified earlier (Bennett *et al.* 1998a).

Of the three main dimensions of internal capacity – human resources, management and information, and financing – only the last represents a real constraint to the Thai government. Financing has been a constraint because a relatively small proportion of the population is covered by compulsory social insurance and voluntary insurance, which maintains quite a large role for public funding. However, the Ministry of Finance has been consistently reluctant to envisage a substantial increase in tax funding for health care.

Until the financial crisis, financial and economic conditions looked conducive to the extension of risk protection and, indeed, initial planning for enabling legislation for universal coverage began. However, the financial crisis delayed progress and extended the feasible timetable. Although the crisis provided a window of opportunity to redress inequality and attempts were made to reduce the cost of the Civil Servants Medical Benefit Scheme, attempts have so far failed to restructure the various schemes more fundamentally. The key problems appear to have been political.

First, the most inequitable part of the health financing arrangements, the Civil Servants Medical Benefit Scheme, has behind it the power of the civil service. Efforts have concentrated on reforming the payment arrangements to bring it closer to the Social Security Scheme. However, the capitation payment of the Social Security Scheme has received some poor publicity arising from complaints that private hospitals have excessively restricted the care provided; hence a move away from fee-for-service payment is being resisted. Second, politicians oppose an excessive welfare orientation, espousing free market ideologies, including in the social sectors (Mills *et al.* 2001). Third, less advantaged people

Table 9.1 Risk protection arrangements for social health insurance in Thailand

Scheme characteristics	Social Security Scheme	Civil Servants Medical Benefit Scheme	Low Income and Elderly Scheme	Health Card Programme
Percentage of total Thai population (1997)	7	11	41	9
Definition of beneficiaries	Worker only	Worker plus dependants (children and parents)	Household for low-income card; individual for fee waivers	Choice of household or individual
Benefit package	Comprehensive; tied to chosen contractor hospital (public or private)	Comprehensive; some limitations on access to private providers	Public only; referral channels to be observed	Public only; referral channels to be observed
Payment mechanism	Capitation to contractor hospital	Fee-for-service	Special budget for each facility for low-income card	Partial reimbursement of costs incurred by facilities
Financing sources	Employer, employees, general tax revenue	General tax revenue	General tax revenue for low-income card holders; those with waivers usually pay part	Household; general tax revenue
Per-capita expenditure in 1993 (baht)	805	916	317	141
Per-capita tax subsidy in 1992 (baht)	270	916	164	68

Source: Tangcharoensathien et al. (1999)

are not readily heard in policy circles in Bangkok, and although their cause has been strongly championed by a few senior civil servants in the Ministry of Health, it appears to be a continuous struggle to shift resources in their favour.

Community-based health insurance: an additional route towards universal coverage?

Many governments and other organizations in low- and middle-income countries have looked towards the development of small-scale, not-for-profit health insurance schemes for people outside employment in the formal sector. They may be based around geographically defined areas or may group together people working in a similar trade (such as farmers or market traders). Such schemes exist in low- and middle-income countries; a review found 82 (Bennett *et al.* 1998b). Community-based health insurance is popular for several reasons. First, limited tax funds and the difficulties of social health insurance in the absence of a substantial formal labour market mean that alternative forms of risk-pooling are often thought to be needed. Second, such schemes may be especially needed in many low- and middle-income countries, where out-of-pocket payment for health care is high. Third, many countries have had risk-pooling mechanisms at the community level historically, although often for other types of loss (such as bereavement or disability); community-based health insurance may be viewed as extending these more traditional arrangements.

Few schemes have been successful in providing sustainable financing for health care while promoting both efficiency and equity. Several problems with efficiency are widespread (Bennett *et al.* 1998b):

- Benefit packages are frequently poorly defined, allowing providers to deliver and be reimbursed for a range of services, many of which are not cost-effective.
- Limited monitoring of service provision means that quality standards are not enforced.
- Fee-for-services is the predominant form of payment, predictably giving rise to problems of containing costs, given the absence of cost controls or utilization review.
- Basic aspects of scheme management and administration, such as investment of revenue, have been poorly handled; insurance funds, therefore, quickly decapitalize and schemes collapse.
- Effective mechanisms are lacking to counter problems of adverse selection. Therefore, the schemes frequently attract people at higher risk of illness, leading to the archetypal adverse selection problem of escalating premiums and a dwindling number of enrollees.

Community-based health insurance schemes have frequently been advocated as a means to increase equity, but their actual effects on equity in financing and utilization of health services appear mixed. With respect to financing, very few schemes offer sliding-scale premiums, and the poorest households often cannot afford membership. This inequitable situation may be exacerbated by the substantial external subsidy (from governments or donors) often attracted. The schemes may adversely affect the equity of utilization: enrolment in community-based health insurance schemes is higher among households located close to health facilities, and utilization increases far more among this group than among people who are more remote. Finally, as discussed in the earlier case study, there are substantial concerns about equity between different health insurance schemes. Under the Chinese Cooperative Medical System, the resources available within the community substantially affected the quality of care provided: poorer communities could often afford to cover only primary care and not inpatient services (World Bank 1997).

Despite – or perhaps because of – these negative experiences, the schemes offer several lessons. Context is important to the successful design of the scheme. Different external environments mean that schemes have different objectives and should thus be designed differently. For example, in some cases (such as the former Zaire) government was very weak or had collapsed completely; in such contexts, relatively simple schemes can play a critical role in allowing the population access to health services, and links to the broader health system are less important (or insignificant). Where there is an established and functioning health system, schemes need to play a different role (for example, facilitating financial access to the private sector) and, consequently, may need a more complex design, with more attention being paid to coordinating the scheme with the rest of the health system.

Governments can play a critical role in promoting the good design and implementation of community-based health insurance schemes. The countries that have had most success in increasing coverage (such as China, the Republic of Korea and Thailand) have established clearly defined policy frameworks, have often developed specific operational guidelines and have frequently judiciously used government subsidies to encourage enrolment. Technical support and operational guidelines appear important, as seen in the next case study, as so many community-based health insurance schemes have neglected basic principles of insurance, such as preventing adverse selection and ensuring that payment mechanisms create appropriate incentives. Although the potential of schemes to mobilize extra funds appears limited, there does appear to be considerable potential for improving the efficiency of existing expenditure by developing an effective purchasing role.

Community-based health insurance schemes also have implications for the government's strategy for sector subsidy. Government financing needs to complement the role of community-based health insurance. For example, if community-based health insurance only covers limited risks, then public subsidies may be best targeted at services that lead to relatively catastrophic expenditure.

Case study 2: community-based health insurance in Zambia

From independence until the early 1990s, the Zambian government provided free health care for all its citizens. This policy was officially reversed in 1993 and, between 1992 and 1994, most health facilities in the country introduced some form of fees. During 1993–94, interest in the development of community-based health insurance schemes emerged, stimulated by concern about declining utilization of health facilities resulting from fees. It was thought that community-based health insurance might provide a means to maintain or even increase revenue while not preventing people from seeking health care when it was needed.

The government began to implement community-based health insurance schemes in 1994, focusing on three tertiary hospitals. Some district management teams have since developed similar schemes. However, these schemes have suffered multiple problems in both design and administration. The schemes have been successful in raising revenue, but they have not functioned as proper insurance schemes, pooling risk. Many of the problems faced in Zambia can be traced to capacity constraints. The success of community-based health insurance schemes depends on conveying knowledge about the basic principles and administrative needs of health insurance schemes to people at the local level who manage such schemes and may even be responsible for their design. In Zambia, several capacity constraints, both internal and external, were especially problematic. The internal capacity constraints included the following.

- Although officials at the central level understood the concepts of health insurance, responsibility for designing and implementing schemes was devolved to the facility and district level, where knowledge about health insurance was limited.
- Until recently, no guidelines were available to guide the implementation of health insurance schemes.
- The reform programme has sought to improve financial systems, but improvements at the facility level are only just beginning to materialize. Furthermore, many systems such as patient records are not well adapted to scheme implementation.
- Community-based health insurance was implemented at a time of immense change in the health system. Health staff were struggling to understand and implement not only new ways of financing health care, but also new planning systems, organizational structures and treatment procedures.

The external capacity constraints included the following.

- The history of care without user charges led to a lack of acceptance of charging among the general population.
- Political intervention led to rapid implementation and precluded proper planning.
- Changes in the Minister for Health led to shifts in policy direction and also delays in capacity-building.
- The continued macroeconomic crisis reduced the value of the government budget for health care in real terms, forcing health facilities to raise more funds at a time when the general population was especially short of money.

User fees as a source of revenue

Two broad categories of user fee system have been identified: national user fee systems implemented at the tertiary, secondary and primary levels throughout the country, and community financing initiatives at peripheral levels of the health system, often supported and coordinated at the national level (Jarrett and Ofosu-Amaah 1992; Bennett and Ngalande-Banda 1994; Nolan and Turbat 1995; Gilson 1997). Both systems implicitly aim to tackle problems of sustainability in the health system by generating revenue to improve health services (Gilson 1997). We have chosen to review national systems here.

Analysts and donors have advocated national user fee systems as a means of addressing inefficiency and inequality in the health system (World Bank 1987,

1993; Griffin 1992; Shaw and Griffin 1995). Efficiency can, in theory, be improved by a cascading fee system that promotes better use of the referral system and by using fee revenue to address input shortages and improve the quality and utilization of primary care facilities. The equity benefits of fees, by far the more contentious assertion, can be achieved if revenue is reallocated and targeted to poorer and underserved sections of society and if an effective exemption system is implemented to protect poor people.

Substantial research shows that improving quality, efficiency and equity critically depends on supportive policy contexts and policy measures, and government capacity to implement policy effectively (Gilson *et al.* 1995; Kutzin 1995; Nolan and Turbat 1995; Bennett *et al.* 1996; Gilson 1997). Mills *et al.* (2001) identify the following as being the most critical:

- Decentralized retention of revenue to provide incentives to collect fees and to allow local improvements in quality.
- Information systems for accounting, auditing and financial management that support management at all levels.
- Financial management skills, especially at sub-national levels where revenue is managed.
- Well-motivated staff with balanced financial incentives that encourage adopting new charging and management practices but discourage overzealous or illegal charging.
- A well-designed and appropriate exemption system, with information that permits the target group to be reached.
- Central leadership, training and guidance on implementing exemption policy and using revenue.
- Maintaining government funding levels to ensure that fee revenue is additional and can be used to improve quality and motivate staff.
- Public willingness and ability to pay.

As the following case study on Ghana indicates, these conditions are often not present. This case study is of particular interest, given that this experience is often quoted as a success story.

Case study 3: the experience of user fees in Ghana[2]

In the 1980s, against a background of economic crisis, Ghana significantly increased long-standing but low user fees and introduced full-cost recovery for drugs. The main objective of the policy was to raise revenue for the health sector, with a secondary objective to curtail the frivolous use of services.

From the mid-1980s to the mid-1990s, the legislative framework permitted drug fees to be revised continuously to keep pace with inflation. Other fees, however, remained at the levels specified in the law and could not be revised except by passing a new legislative instrument. Fear of political backlash and a genuine concern for the rural population, who form the core constituency of the ruling party, have blocked subsequent efforts by the Ministry of Health to revise the fees. As a result, inflation steadily eroded the real value of fees and this, together with continued budgetary pressures, resulted in increasingly widespread local charging practices with or without the tacit approval of the Ministry of Health. In part, this was symptomatic of a broader public-sector malaise in which rent-seeking was common, which probably dated from the collapse of public-sector pay and morale in the early 1980s. However, the introduction of much higher fees for health care may have conferred a legitimacy on charging the patient that was not there before.

Revenue

The user fee policy appeared to have been reasonably successful in raising revenue. Expressed as a proportion of government-financed Ministry of Health recurrent expenditure, total revenue from user fees averaged 8.5 per cent between 1985 and 1993 and reached over 10 per cent in 1987 and 1988. In real terms, revenue from user fees grew considerably over the period. The vast majority of user fee revenue came from drug charges, especially for smaller health facilities without inpatient or diagnostic facilities, and from a small number of larger (usually urban) facilities. Because the headquarters or regional level controlled and administered a considerable portion of government financial resources, user fee revenue assumed increasing importance (as a proportion of financial resources under local control) at lower levels of the health system.

Efficiency

Cost recovery for drugs markedly improved drug availability and thus resulted in a better input mix and hence improved technical efficiency. Stock control and procurement were also generally felt to have improved. But user charges also decreased technical efficiency.

- Unit costs increased greatly and staff productivity declined as a result of the drop in utilization following the fee rise (Waddington and Enyimayew 1989, 1990).
- Unclear guidance from the centre on uses for non-drug revenue caused risk-averse managers to leave them in bank accounts, where their value was eroded by inflation. In other cases, local authorization procedures for fund disbursement required health centre managers to obtain authorization from the regional office, with the same result.
- The cost of collecting fees could be as high as 35 per cent of total revenue collected for small facilities with low utilization, and 15 per cent in busier facilities. The practice of charging separately for each service resulted in a large number of revenue points, higher collection costs and a greater waiting time and inconvenience for patients.
- Drugs offered the main opportunity for facilities to raise extra money, through prescribing more items, more profitable items or increasing their margins. This clearly offered an incentive for inappropriate prescribing and pricing.

Equity

The user fee rise resulted in a 50 per cent decline in outpatient attendance in the Volta region, a trend that was reversed over time in urban areas but not in rural ones (Waddington and Enyimayew 1990). There is every reason to believe that poor people, and especially rural poor people, were seriously affected, and there is much qualitative evidence that low-income households were substantially deterred from seeking care by lack of money to pay fees (Norton *et al.* 1995). The problem was probably made worse by uncertainty about the level of charges to be paid because of the widespread informal charging.

Attempts to relate fees to ability to pay were poorly targeted. 'Paupers' were exempt from fees, but exemption based on an inability to pay was very rare (Waddington and Enyimayew 1989, 1990), especially because it represented foregone income and a potential threat to the viability of the drug revolving fund.

Capacity constraints

To what extent can these problems with performance be explained by limits to government capacity? The overriding objective was to raise extra revenue at a time when government finances were in crisis and the government administration was in a state of near collapse. Harmful effects on efficiency and equity were largely attributable to the design of policy and legislation at the outset and the fact that allocative efficiency and equity were not the primary objectives of the policy. The Ministry of Health seized a window of political opportunity to introduce user fees, leaving capacity concerns aside. Many different capacity constraints hindered implementation. The internal capacity constraints included:

- a lack of accounting staff at facility level and central medical stores;
- a lack of operational guidance – where guidance did exist, there was a lack of clarity, especially on spending fee revenue;
- poor compliance with the accounting systems introduced in 1994;
- weaknesses in the drug supply system, which meant stock-outs, expired drugs, etc.; and
- a lack of social welfare officers who were made responsible for assessing whether or not someone should be exempted from fees.

External capacity constraints included:

- low and irregular cash incomes, which created problems in designing the exemption system; and
- a closed political system that excluded user views from the policy arena.

Finally, the introduction of user charges generated new stakeholders. By presenting managers with an opportunity to raise substantial amounts of revenue in contrast to a constrained government budget, the policy won many converts. Managers at the facility level were the principal proponents for raising fees and extending cost recovery. This and the anecdotal reports of widespread unofficial levies illustrate the slippery-slope character of user fees.

Capacity constraints and capacity-building approaches

Implementing change

Several preliminary steps are required to successfully implement reforms: developing a clear policy framework; generating commitment to the policy, both from internal actors such as health staff and external actors such as politicians; and thinking through an implementation strategy (Mills *et al.* 2001). Failure to perform effectively one or more of these tasks in low- and middle-income countries has frequently suspended the implementation of health financing reforms.

Ministries of health frequently lack the ability to elaborate a policy framework. Although consultants can help in translating policies into operational plans, operational details often imbue policies with a very particular flavour, and local ownership cannot be maintained if this task is delegated to external consultants. Once a clear policy framework is in place, the next necessary step is to develop and elaborate an implementation strategy. All too often, this step has been omitted altogether or given only superficial attention.

In many countries, a very small policy elite makes substantial decisions about the scope and direction of health financing reform: senior national technocrats and external policy advisers. This leads to several adverse consequences. First, implementation of reforms may suffer because key stakeholders such as politicians, health workers and health service users do not own the reform programmes. Second, reform proposals may be technically sound but not always politically feasible. The technocratic perspective of many donors and external consultants has probably contributed to this problem. Third, the almost complete exclusion of implementers from policy circles has implications not only for the ownership of reforms but also for how they are designed. This has been especially evident in some countries in sub-Saharan Africa, where a common understanding among the policy elite about the direction of the reform programme can result in relatively sophisticated programmes and plans that mask real difficulties in implementation (Russell *et al.* 1999).

Garnering support for a policy may be critical for implementation. Proper communication campaigns to inform the general public of the nature of reforms are very rare. Information, education and communication capacity should be strengthened within ministries of health, or at least ministries should recognize the importance of information, education and communication in policy reform and should contract for such services.

In low-income countries, financing policy is often made at a time of financial crisis. This often means that unrealistic time frames are set for implementing policies, inhibiting the development of realistic implementation strategies. This was clearly the case for the implementation of user fee policy in Ghana and for community-based health insurance in Zambia, as the case studies show. In addition, economic crisis tends to prevent adequate investment in the necessary changing and developing of systems. Economic crisis may create windows of opportunity for reform, but the crisis may also weaken government capacity to plan for and implement change. Researchers examining the policy process around health financing reform since the first democratic elections in South Africa concluded: 'A time of radical change in national policy goals has enabled health policy change, but the accompanying change in personnel, governance and administrative structures and macro-economic strategies has also made it exceptionally difficult to develop well-designed policy and to implement policy effectively' (Centre for Health Policy, University of Witwatersrand and Health Economics Unit, University of Cape Town 1999).

Finally, reform experience in low- and middle-income countries emphasizes the importance of careful phasing of financing reform programmes to build support and negate opposition, strengthen capacity, generate trust in government and adopt new roles and expectations.

- *Building support and negating opposition.* Careful phasing of reform programmes can introduce first the more popular elements of reform or at least ensure early successes that build support. Some aspects of reform may be especially controversial yet also critical to success. For example, under-the-counter payments, which are prevalent in many low- and middle-income countries, may prevent successful financing reform but are very difficult to eliminate without first improving staffing conditions.
- *Strengthening capacity.* Each country has different forms of capacity, and a well-phased programme of financing reform takes advantage of existing capacities and gradually builds capacities in new areas.
- *Generating trust in government.* In some low- and middle-income countries, people have very little trust in government, perceiving that government exists to serve the interests of certain classes or groups of people (for example, bureaucrats). Even well-intentioned financing reforms may suffer from this and from the unwillingness of the broader community to comply with new laws or rules.
- *Adopting new roles and expectations.* Health financing reforms often envisage a new role for the general population, from a passive role of patient towards a more active role of consumer. Communicating key elements of reform programmes to consumers may help to generate new expectations, which may help reinforce reforms. For example, beneficiaries of social health insurance programmes who are aware of their rights may be more active in monitoring providers and ensuring that they receive adequate services.

Internal capacity-building for health financing reform

Certain types of health financing reform require the establishment of very new functions within ministries of health or even the development of new organizations such as social health insurance offices. Functions that are often only weakly (or not at all) established in traditional ministries of health include regulating and monitoring, providing information, collecting revenue and purchasing services and paying providers.

- *Regulating and monitoring.* Both health care providers and health insurance organizations need to be regulated and monitored.

- *Providing information.* Information is needed both about the reform policies and as a continuing function, including informing people about their rights under new social health insurance laws, or disseminating the results of performance monitoring of providers and insurers such as price and quality data.
- *Collecting revenue.* Ministries of finance have traditionally collected revenue, but all three forms of financing discussed here may increase the involvement of ministries of health in revenue collection.
- *Purchasing services and paying providers.* Traditional forms of government financing for health care in low- and middle-income countries commonly allocate funds according to facility budgets. Health insurance development has led to the adoption of a wider variety of forms of purchasing and payment, such as capitation and case-based payment, which often require more complex information and systems.

Ministries of health generally need to plan and implement a programme of capacity-building encompassing developing new human resource skills and new systems and possibly changing existing organizational structures to perform these new functions properly. The core of capacity-building is frequently training for staff either in formal courses overseas or in less formal workshops (Paul 1995), although on their own these are inadequate. Exchange visits and acting as counterparts to expatriate technical advisers are more informal ways to build skills. The type of knowledge required to implement new financing mechanisms successfully often cannot be acquired through tuition alone but requires hands-on experience. Reform programmes need to build opportunities for individuals to assess experience and learn from their mistakes or those of other people. They may also need to address the more fundamental factors that lead to low standards of performance, such as poor personnel management and a lack of incentives for efficient working practices.

The external environment

Broader capacity constraints, such as organizational culture or bureaucratic constraints outside the ministry of health, are frequently not addressed. Four key types of external constraint are:

- constraints in the broader bureaucratic environment;
- political interference or lack of political commitment to reform;
- macroeconomic crisis; and
- widespread corruption.

The scope for health financing reform may be constrained by broader government regulations issued by the ministry of finance or a civil service commission, which constrain action by the ministry of health. For example, in Zimbabwe, substantial increases in the user fees charged in public facilities initially had little effect on revenue collected, since all revenue had to be returned to the Ministry of Finance and health staff had very little incentive to collect fees (Mills *et al.* 2001).

Health-financing measures can be politically very sensitive, and politicians may therefore try to retain control over key dimensions of policy. This was clearly the case in Ghana, where increases in fee required the approval of parliament. Furthermore, credible and successful financing reform requires strong and evident government commitment to the reform. However, reform policies have often been formulated during periods when economic crisis was rocking the foundations of government. Under such circumstances, it is hardly surprising that there was frequently no true political commitment to reform programmes. In addition, raising extra revenue, whether from health service users or employers, is likely to be most difficult at times of economic recession.

Finally, corruption poses several constraints on the effective implementation of new forms of financing and may damage their credibility to such an extent that they are no longer viable. Although corruption is an issue in pre-reformed systems, reform that decentralizes financial control and the ability to generate revenue may aggravate it.

Addressing such external capacity constraints can be very difficult, especially for ministries of health acting on their own. Either the constraints must be treated as given and ways found of minimizing their effects or they need to be addressed by changing specific rules, such as those on retaining revenue, or through a broader programme of government reform.

Lessons for low- and middle-income countries in Europe

Low- and middle-income countries in Europe share some of the characteristics of such countries elsewhere, but there are also some significant differences. Unlike other countries in Asia, Africa and Latin America, the countries of central and eastern Europe and the countries of the former Soviet Union had extensive health systems providing universal coverage during the communist era. The dismantling of the communist state, accompanying privatization measures and severe economic recession in some of these countries has led to the development of features very similar to those of the countries reviewed here. For example, tax revenue is low, a small proportion of the population is in formal-sector employment, managerial capacity is limited, government is weak and enjoys limited trust, and levels of corruption and informal payment are high. However, the legacy of their form of universal coverage includes a very large number of health facilities and an excess supply of many types of trained staff, especially physicians. Thus, the question of capacity in many low- and middle-income countries in Europe is especially complex: capacity is frequently inadequate in certain dimensions and excessive in others. Health financing reform in low- and middle-income European countries must address both dismantling existing institutions and establishing new ones.

In a widespread economic crisis, there appear to be few alternatives to relying on multiple health financing mechanisms, probably including health insurance, user fees and tax revenue. Fragmented health financing can adversely affect both efficiency and equity, and especially the development of tiering and geographical inequity. Government needs to have a strong role in both providing an overarching policy framework for health financing and directly subsidizing or organizing subsidies for poorer parts of the population to offset these problems. If government plays a strong role in shaping the financing and organizational arrangements in the sector, multiple funding sources should be possible without fragmenting the health system.

Of the specific health financing mechanisms discussed here, social health insurance is clearly very attractive to low- and middle-income countries within Europe and elsewhere. However, it is likely to cover only a limited proportion of the population, and experience suggests that economic growth is probably the only engine that will enable progress towards universal coverage using this mechanism. Community-based health insurance schemes appear to offer some promise as implemented in some countries in south-east Asia as part of a broader strategy to achieve universal coverage. Nevertheless, European countries are likely to suffer from many of the same implementation problems experienced elsewhere, notably limited understanding of the concept of insurance among the community and limited understanding of important design elements of voluntary insurance schemes among implementers. Again, a strong government role in providing operational guidance and a policy framework is needed to offset these problems and prevent fragmentation of the sector.

Many European countries already have some user fees, but the fees are often less significant than parallel informal fees, confirming the slippery-slope nature of fees highlighted in the Ghana case study. Unfortunately, although there is increasing research and understanding of informal fees in low- and middle-income countries outside Europe, there have not been concerted policy efforts to 'formalize' informal charges, and there are thus few clear lessons on how to manage this problem.

Perhaps the most significant lessons for low- and middle-income European countries from outside Europe concern the process of health financing reform. As elsewhere, those in Europe are especially susceptible to 'imported' ideas. Reform plans must not only be technically congruent with existing systems in the country but also capacity must be sufficient to implement these plans properly. The lessons from outside Europe in some respects appear very obvious:

- ensuring an adequately long time frame for implementation;
- focusing on the elements of reform most critical to its overall success;
- carefully phasing reforms to build capacity, develop political support and ensure that technical changes occur in the correct order; and
- paying adequate attention to the skills of people and financial and information systems so the new financing mechanism functions as intended.

All too frequently, however, in the rush to implement within a window of political opportunity or to fit in with a donor project, these critical rules are overlooked.

Notes

1 Anne Mills and Sara Bennett work in the Health Economics and Financing Programme of the London School of Hygiene & Tropical Medicine, which receives a

research programme grant from the United Kingdom Department for International Development.
2 The case study draws extensively from Smithson *et al.* 1997.

References

Batley, R. (1997) *A Research Framework for Analyzing Capacity to Undertake the 'New Roles' of Government*, Role of Government in Adjusting Economies Publication No. 23. Birmingham: Development Administration Group, University of Birmingham.

Bennett, S. and Ngalande-Banda, E. (1994) *Public and Private Roles in Health: A Review and Analysis of Experience in Sub-Saharan Africa*, Current Concerns Series, SHS Paper No. 6. Geneva: World Health Organization.

Bennett, S., Russell, S. and Mills, A. (1996) *Institutional and Economic Perspectives on Government Capacity to Assume New Roles in the Health Sector: A Review of Experience*, Department of Public Health and Policy Publication No. 22. London: London School of Hygiene & Tropical Medicine.

Bennett, S., Mills, A., Russell, S., Supachutikul, A. and Tangcharoensathien, V. (1998a) *The Health Sector in Thailand*, Role of Government in Adjusting Economies Publication No. 31. Birmingham: Development Administration Group, University of Birmingham.

Bennett, S., Creese, A. and Monasch, R. (1998b) *Health Insurance Schemes for People Outside Formal Sector Employment*, Current Concerns Series, ARA Paper No. 16. Geneva: World Health Organization.

Bos, E., Hon, V., Maeda, A., Chelleraj, G. and Preker, A. (1998) *Health, Nutrition, and Population Indicators: A Statistical Handbook*. Washington, DC: World Bank.

Brinkerhoff, D.W. (1994) Institutional development in World Bank projects: analytical approaches and intervention designs, *Public Administration and Development*, 14: 135–51.

Centre for Health Policy, University of Witwatersrand and Health Economics Unit, University of Cape Town (1999) *Analysing the Process of Health Financing Reform: South Africa Country Report*. Johannesburg and Cape Town: Centre for Health Policy, University of Witwatersrand and Health Economics Unit, University of Cape Town.

Chiang, T.L. (1997) Taiwan's 1995 health care reform, *Health Policy*, 39(3): 225–39.

Donaldson, D.S., Pannarunothai, S. and Tangcharoensathien, V. (1998) *Health Financing in Thailand. Technical Report*, ADB # 2997-THA. Boston, MA: Management Sciences for Health.

Gilson, L. (1997) The lessons of user fee experience in Africa, *Health Policy and Planning*, 12(4): 273–85.

Gilson, L., Russell, S. and Buse, K. (1995) The political economy of user fees with targeting: developing equitable health financing policy, *Journal of International Development*, 7(3): 369–401.

Griffin, C. (1992) Welfare gains from user charges for government health services, *Health Policy and Planning*, 7(2): 177–80.

Hildebrand, M.E. and Grindle, M.S. (1994) *Building Sustainable Capacity: Challenges for the Public Sector*. Cambridge, MA: Harvard Institute for International Development.

Jarrett, S. and Ofosu-Amaah, S. (1992) Strengthening health services for MCH in Africa: the first four years of the Bamako Initiative, *Health Policy and Planning*, 7(2): 164–76.

Kutzin, J. (1995) *Experience with Organizational and Financing Reform of the Health Sector*, Current Concerns Series, SHS Paper No. 8. Geneva: World Health Organization.

Mills, A. (2000) The route to universal coverage, in S. Nitayarumphong and A. Mills (eds) *Achieving Universal Coverage of Health Care: Experiences from Middle and Upper*

Income Countries. Nontaburi: Office of Health Care Reform, Ministry of Public Health, Thailand.

Mills, A., Bennett, S. and Russell, S. (2001) *The Challenge of Health Sector Reform: What Must Governments Do?* Hampshire: Palgrave.

Nitayarumphong, S. and Mills, A. (eds) (2000) *Achieving Universal Coverage of Health Care: Experiences from Middle and Upper Income Countries*. Nontaburi: Office of Health Care Reform, Ministry of Public Health, Thailand.

Nolan, B. and Turbat, V. (1995) *Cost Recovery in Public Health Services in Sub-Saharan Africa*. Washington, DC: World Bank.

Norton, A., Arytee, E.B-D., Korboe, D. and Dogbe, D.K.T. (1995) *Poverty Assessment in Ghana Using Qualitative and Participatory Research Methods*, Poverty and Social Policy Department Discussion Paper No. 83. Washington, DC: World Bank.

Paul, S. (1995) *Capacity Building for Health Sector Reform*, Forum on Health Sector Reform Discussion Paper No. 5. Geneva: World Health Organization.

Peabody, J.W., Lee, S.W. and Bickel, S.R. (1995) Health for All in the Republic of Korea: one country's experience with implementing universal health care, *Health Policy*, 31(1): 29–42.

Russell, S., Bennett, S. and Mills, A. (1999) Reforming the health sector: towards a healthy new public management, *Journal of International Development*, 11: 767–75.

Shaw, P. and Griffin, C. (1995) *Financing Health Care in Sub-Saharan Africa through User Fees and Insurance*. Washington, DC: World Bank.

Smithson, P., Aamoa-Baah, A. and Mills, A. (1997) *The Case of the Health Sector in Ghana, Role of Government in Adjusting Economies* Publication No. 26. Birmingham: Development Administration Group, University of Birmingham.

Tangcharoensathien, V., Supachutikul, A. and Lertendumrong, J. (1999) The social security scheme in Thailand: what lessons can be drawn?, *Social Science and Medicine*, 48(7): 913–24.

Waddington, C.J. and Enyimayew, K.A. (1989) A price to pay: the impact of user charges in Ashanti-Akim District, Ghana, *International Journal of Health Planning and Management*, 4: 17–47.

Waddington, C.J. and Enyimayew, K.A. (1990) A price to pay, part 2: the impact of user charges in the Volta Region of Ghana, *International Journal of Health Planning and Management*, 5: 287–312.

World Bank (1987) *Financing Health Services in Developing Countries: An Agenda for Reform*. Washington, DC: World Bank.

World Bank (1993) *World Development Report 1993: Investing in Health*. New York: Oxford University Press.

World Bank (1997) *Financing Health Care: Issues and Options for China*. Washington, DC: World Bank.

chapter ten

Funding long-term care: the public and private options

Raphael Wittenberg, Becky Sandhu and Martin Knapp[1]

Introduction

> The late twentieth century brought to many the ultimate gift: the luxury of ageing. But like any luxury, ageing is expensive. Governments are fretting about the cost already; but they also know that far worse is to come. Over the next 30 or 40 years, the demographic changes of longer lives and fewer births will force most countries to rethink in fundamental ways their arrangements for paying for and looking after older people.
>
> (Beck 1996: 3)

The need for long-term care arises from a combination of many factors, usually dominated by ageing-related deterioration in health and the ability to care for oneself. The tremendous achievements of previous decades in reducing morbidity and mortality have created unprecedented levels of need for long-term care across the world, posing major challenges for economies, societies and governments. These needs will grow hugely in the next few decades.

In this chapter, we describe models for funding long-term care in Europe and examine their consequences. We first discuss the broad architecture of long-term care and models of provision within broader systems of care and treatment. The debate on how best to fund long-term care has understandably generated many demands for accurate projections of levels of future need and demand, and we thus examine projections of the scale of funding likely to be required over the next 20–30 years. We then outline some possible systems for financing long-term care, discussing approaches in the private and public sectors (separately and jointly) and examining how far the approaches meet criteria of efficiency and equity. We conclude by looking at attitudes to long-term care funding and the main policy issues in this field.

Providing long-term care

Long-term care services are delivered to older people either in their own homes or in substitute care settings, especially residential homes, nursing homes and hospitals. They include assistance with the tasks of everyday living – dressing, bathing, shopping, preparing meals and cleaning – as well as skilled therapy and carefully tailored care services to reduce, lessen the consequences of or compensate for disability, cognitive impairment and loneliness. Ageing is often accompanied by an impoverished quality of life that originates partly in ill health but is more likely to stem from wider demographic, economic and social trends for both individuals and the wider community.

Across Europe, a variety of agencies deliver long-term care services financed by numerous sources. The balances of responsibility between the public (government) and private (non-governmental) sectors and between formal and informal arrangements (that is, organizational and familial roles) lie at the heart of any description of long-term care. Indeed, service provision across Europe produces common policy and practice themes:

- the boundary between health care and social care, with potential consequences for the nature of both types of service and their funding;
- the role of the family and questions of how and when care responsibilities move from the family to the state or some other (formal) organization;
- the balance between residential and home-based care, and how decision-making and funding arrangements facilitate or hinder movements from one setting to another as individual needs change;
- the respective provider roles of the state and non-state bodies and shifts in market shares; and
- the form that public subsidies of care might take, especially the balance between support in kind and support in cash.

Each of these features is relevant to the financing of long-term care, either through their effects on costs or cost-effectiveness or because they influence the balance of funding between stakeholders.

Health and social care

Many of the needs of older people clearly stem from a deterioration in health and can be met by health care services. Equally, social needs can be met by social services providers. In between lie needs that are variously met by health or social care agencies depending on national culture, the structure of the care system, the availability of appropriate professional inputs and, quite often, the caprices of day-to-day working. Who provides care may also depend on the funding system in place, since a social care system that charges users for the services they receive might find itself in less demand if the parallel health care system offers services free at the point of delivery.

In the Netherlands and France, long-term institutional care is provided in hospitals and nursing homes as part of the health insurance system. The Netherlands added an 'exceptional costs' element to the health insurance system in 1980 to cover nursing homes and other services. France's health insurance system covers the nursing component of care in some communal establishments. Long-term care was not covered under the old health insurance system in Germany, leaving the responsibility for funding to individuals, except for means-tested social assistance arrangements. Recent reforms have introduced changes. For example, in Finland and Sweden, the boundaries of responsibility between the health and social care sectors have shifted, and the 1990 National Health Service and Community Care Act in the United Kingdom introduced much-needed clarification. Sweden transferred responsibility for long-term care for elderly and disabled people to the municipalities in 1992. The municipalities are now responsible for funding hospital care when it is no longer required for health reasons and discharge is delayed by a lack of adequate community services. A similar change was introduced in Denmark, also in 1992.

The distinction between health and social ('long-term') care has potentially important implications both for the level of cost (for example, needs may be excessively medicalized or specialist treatment underprovided) and for the balance of funding (if different eligibility criteria influence threshold levels of dependence, for instance). In turn, these could create (perverse) incentives for the type of care chosen by stakeholders. This distinction also has implications for the interpretation of international comparisons of 'health' spending.

Formal and informal care

The largest provider in the care of older people is the informal sector – the families, neighbours and community groups that offer support without funding, without charging and often without recognition. The availability of informal care heavily influences the level and type of need for formal care for which, by definition, resources must be found. But therein lie many challenges: 'Just as some demographic change is increasing the numbers of very elderly people in need of some care, other demographic and social changes may be reducing the potential of the younger (female) population to provide care for their older relatives' (Royal Commission on Long-term Care 1999b: 159). This is an international phenomenon. Middle-aged female relatives comprise most informal care-givers (Kendig et al. 1992). Changing demographic patterns, family composition, labour force participation and geographical mobility are all reducing the (potential) pool of family care-givers. Projections of the future costs of long-term care are clearly sensitive to assumptions made about the future supply of informal care (see later), which is one reason governments introduce support arrangements for care-givers.

Residential and home-based care

There has been long-term debate about the appropriate balance between institutional and home-based care. A study by the Organisation for Economic Co-operation and Development (OECD 1996) found movement towards convergence at a level of about 5 per cent of older people supported in institutional settings, ranging from below 1 per cent in Greece and Turkey to above 6.5 per cent in Canada, Finland, Luxembourg, the Netherlands, New Zealand and Norway. The countries with a level of bed provision above the average are trying to reduce it and those below it are trying to increase it. Although no level is 'right', demography and health status have substantially influenced the level of institutional provision in OECD countries (Royal Commission on Long-term Care 1999b: 160).

Discussions on the appropriate balance of care have included arguments about relative effectiveness (for whom is residential care more effective, and when?), relative cost (both in total and to various agencies, especially health and social care) and user and family preferences (themselves conditioned or influenced by many factors, including perceptions of quality, availability of informal care, the broader family-centred culture in certain societies and personal cost). This last consideration – or its wider equivalent – is often pivotal, because many care systems have perverse incentives.

Countries vary much more in the provision of home-based care (home help, meals, day care, community nursing, and so on). For example, no more than 5 per cent of older people in Austria, Germany, Ireland, Italy, Portugal and Spain receive home help versus more than 10 per cent in Denmark, Finland, Norway and Sweden (OECD 1996). The extent and nature of development of intermediate-care arrangements (housing with various levels of care support) also vary considerably.

In contrast, long-stay hospital services have been nearly universally reduced and replaced by residential and nursing home care. However, arrangements for funding replacement services vary between countries: some are financed from health care budgets, some from social services budgets and some by users themselves. Many countries provide wider public funding for some services than for others. The National Health Service in the United Kingdom covers hospital and community health services but not residential or domiciliary social care. France's health insurance covers care costs in long-stay hospital and nursing home care and nursing at home but not home care services. The Netherlands' special national fund for long-term care covers nursing home care and community health services but not residential care and home care. Germany's social insurance scheme for long-term care, however, covers both residential and home care.

Public and private provision

Provider pluralism is a long-standing feature of long-term care systems in most European countries. The public sector has often been the largest provider of formal services, but not-for-profit (voluntary) and for-profit (private) organizations have also been high-volume and high-profile contributors in the mixed economy of care (Kramer 1981; Evers and Svetlik 1994; Knapp *et al.* 2000). Policy debates in some countries have kept services and financing quite distinct when discussing the future of long-term care, such as in the United Kingdom (Knapp and Wistow 1996), although the two are often closely connected in practice. For example, in 1993 much public funding for residential and nursing home care in the United Kingdom was re-routed from the Department of Social Security to local authorities (and from payments controlled by the user to ones controlled by the state purchaser) on the condition that 85 per cent of the transferred money was spent on independent services. The sectoral balance of provision affects funding balance and responsibility; for example, charitable donations can be and often are used to subsidize state or individual funding of some care services. It may also affect the overall cost of care if one sector is demonstrably and consistently less expensive or more cost-effective than another.

Support in cash or kind

Economic theory suggests that, under various conditions, providing cash is more efficient than providing care (Culyer 1980). Cash payments allow the recipients to choose the package of services that, in their view, provides them the greatest benefit, whereas care arranged by a third party might fit the older person's perceived needs less well. However, some older people may not have the ability or the information to make informed choices, especially users of long-term care services with some cognitive impairment, and they may not be able to call on a family member, care professional or independent advocate to arrange their care. The move in many countries to allow older people more informed choice has thus been accompanied by growth in care management and brokerage arrangements.

The cash versus care argument also depends on whether or not taxpayers or insurance fund contributors, who directly or indirectly fund the services used by many older people, are concerned about how the resources are spent. Taxpayers might, for example, prefer to know that their contributions have been spent on care and not on other goods and services. This difficulty could be alleviated in principle by offering cash dedicated to purchase long-term care services only (voucher schemes). In practice, this might not be clearly distinguishable from a care-managed system under which social care professionals arrange long-term care in close consultation with the older person and the family. The Netherlands has introduced 'personal care budgets' under which a minority of elderly service recipients are given cash benefits with which to purchase services.

The care versus cash debate could affect overall expenditure in various ways. Limiting the former may be easier. For instance, the United Kingdom government sets cash limits for health and social services but not for disability benefits or other social security payments. Reforms in 1990 transferred a voucher scheme run by the social security ministry to a services arrangement through local authorities, partly to control the growth in expenditure. In Germany, expenditure is greatly affected by the choice of cash or care, as cash payments are lower (see later).

Funding projections

Key drivers of future expenditure

Future long-term care needs and costs have now been projected for several countries. Several factors affect expenditure on long-term care services:

- the number of older people, and especially very old people, since the latter are the main users of long-term care;
- age-specific dependence rates;
- the availability of informal care, especially personal care provided by spouses, children and other relatives; and
- the real unit costs of care, which seem certain to rise, since long-term care is highly labour-intensive and average earnings are expected to rise.

These four factors are largely exogenous to long-term care policy. Two further factors – arguably endogenous – may be just as important:

- the expectations of future cohorts of older people as to the quality of care – higher retirement incomes and experiences with improving health care in younger years may raise expectations among future users; and
- future patterns of care, which may differ from current patterns depending on the policies and preferences of older people and their care-givers.

Projections for the United States: the Brookings model

The Brookings Institution and Lewin-VHI, Inc. in the United States developed the first long-term care financing projection model using microsimulation techniques in 1986–87 (updated and refined in 1988–89). Their model projected the numbers, financial position, disability status, nursing home and home care use and expenditure of older people to 2020 and (on a broader basis) to 2050. The model has been used to simulate the effects of changes in the system for financing long-term care in the United States (Wiener *et al.* 1994). It started with a sample of 28,000 people that are nationally representative of the adult population – with information on each person's age, gender, income, assets and other characteristics – and simulated individual changes from 1986 to 2020 in onset and recovery from disability and when they would start and stop receiving long-term care services. Based on this, the Brookings Institution projected that the total number of older people in the United States using nursing homes would increase from 2.2 to 3.6 million between 1993 and 2018 and the number of home care users from 5.2 to 7.4 million. Total long-term care expenditure was projected to rise from US$75 billion (1.21 per cent of gross domestic product, GDP) to US$166.2 billion (2.14 per cent of GDP, if real GDP grows by 2.5 per cent per year) in constant 1993 dollars over the same 25 years. Medicaid's share of total expenditure, about one-third of the total, was expected to fall only slightly.

Projections for the United Kingdom

In the 1990s, three studies sought to project the demand for long-term care in the United Kingdom. Nuttall *et al.* (1994) projected the numbers of disabled people in the United Kingdom (expected to grow from 6.4 to 8.5 million between 1991 and 2031) and the costs of caring for them (rising from £42 to £62 billion, or 7.3 per cent to 10.8 per cent of gross national product (GNP)), assuming certain changes in age-specific morbidity rates and that the unit costs of care rise proportionally to growth in GNP. These figures include estimates of the costs of informal care. Richards *et al.* (1996) updated these estimates of the numbers of disabled people and re-examined the supply of informal care, the division between informal and formal care and the public–private division of expenditure. The Department of Health projected public expenditure on long-term care services on a range of assumptions, especially in relation to future levels of dependence and the real unit costs of care (House of Commons Health Committee 1996). The Department projected that, on plausible assumptions, the proportion of GDP devoted to long-term care would remain broadly constant.

More recently, the Personal Social Services Research Unit at the London School of Economics and Political Science projected long-term care demand and financing for England to 2030 under different scenarios (Wittenberg *et al.* 1998). The Royal Commission on Long-term Care (1999b) used this model extended to the whole of the United Kingdom. The Government Actuary's Department projects that the numbers of older people in England (aged 65 years and over) will rise by 57 per cent between 1995 and 2031, and the numbers of very elderly people (aged 85 years and over) will rise by 79 per cent. Long-term care services would need to expand by about 61 per cent between 1995 and 2031 to keep pace if no account is taken of other factors. Such estimates are, however, sensitive to assumed growth rates in the numbers of very elderly people: if the numbers of people aged 85 and over grew by 1 per cent per year more than expected, long-term care would need to expand by 92 per cent rather than 61 per cent.

Expenditure projections are also sensitive to assumptions about dependence rates. If, pessimistically, age-specific dependence rates rose annually by 1 per cent, long-term care would need to expand by 121 per cent rather than 61 per cent, whereas if these rates fell annually by 1 per cent, long-term care would need to expand by only 18 per cent between 1995 and 2031. Another source of sensitivity is the assumption made about changes in the real unit costs of services, which will be affected by such factors as real wages in the care sector, technical efficiency changes in service provision and changes in service quality and expected outcomes. It is assumed as a base case assumption that the real unit costs of social care will rise by 1 per cent per year and those of health care by 1.5 per cent per year. Based on this, total expenditure is projected to grow by 153 per cent in real terms between 1995 and 2031 (from

1.6 per cent to 1.8 per cent of GDP, if GDP grows by 2.25 per cent per year in real terms).

The Personal Social Services Research Unit study also examined the funding balance. Under current funding arrangements, total health service long-term care expenditure would rise by 174 per cent between 1995 and 2031, social services expenditure (net of user charges) by 123 per cent and private expenditure by 173 per cent. These illustrative projections are sensitive to a wide range of assumptions, especially the rate of growth of the very elderly population, trends in age-specific dependence rates, real rises in unit costs and the likely rise in the proportion of care home residents who do not qualify for public funding support because of their housing assets. For example, if unit costs grew by 1 per cent more than in the base case (assuming current patterns of care), total expenditure would rise by 260 per cent, or if age-specific dependence rates fell by 1 per cent per year, total expenditure would rise by only 85 per cent.

Projections for Germany

Schmahl and Rothgang (1996) projected the long-term costs of Germany's new public long-term care insurance scheme. Based on unchanged age-specific rates of disability and service utilization, they projected that the number of frail elderly people covered by public long-term care insurance would rise by 31 per cent between 1995 and 2030. Expenditure on home care was expected to rise by almost 25 per cent over this period (from about DM12 billion to DM15 billion), and expenditure on nursing home care by 44 per cent (from DM12.8 billion to DM18.4 billion) on the basis that 80 per cent of recipients choose cash and 20 per cent choose services and that monthly payments for nursing home care average DM2500. Demographic pressures were thus expected to increase total expenditure under the insurance scheme by one-third between 1995 and 2030. These projections are as sensitive as any model to the assumptions on which they are constructed, in this case with the added element of assuming the proportion of older people choosing cash.

This model linked contribution rates, numbers of contributors, benefit rates and numbers of beneficiaries and assumed that aggregate contributions and benefit payments would balance. Four scenarios were modelled: constant contribution rates, contribution rates rising proportionally to demographic pressures, benefit rates constant in volume terms (care cost inflation) and benefit rates constant in real terms (general inflation). Care costs were assumed to rise proportionally to wages. Average income was assumed to rise by 1.61 per cent annually in 1992–2000, by 2.25 per cent in 2000–2010, by 1.67 per cent in 2010–2020 and by 1.15 per cent in 2020–2030. Under the first scenario, contribution rates would remain constant at 1.7 per cent and real expenditure would rise by 77 per cent between 1995 and 2030. Contribution rates rise under the second scenario proportionally to demographic pressures, to 2.27 per cent, and expenditure rises by 136.7 per cent to DM69.1 billion. Under the third scenario, contribution rates also rise, this time to 2.56 per cent, and expenditure rises by 166 per cent to DM89 billion; this enables a constant level of care to be provided per capita. Under the fourth scenario, contribution rates fall to 1.28 per cent and expenditure rises by 34 per cent to DM39 billion; this enables a constant cash sum to be provided per capita.

Conclusions from the projections

Many factors affect total expenditure on services. Over time, the share of the total that is public expenditure will be affected by public expectations, by future policies on financing long-term care and by the rising housing wealth and real incomes of elderly people. The appropriate division of costs between the state and the individual lies at the core of the policy debates across Europe.

Examination of the affordability of long-term care needs to consider not only future demand pressures on expenditure but also future economic growth. In the United Kingdom, for example, if the economy continues to grow at its long-term trend rate of 2.0–2.5 per cent per year, demand pressures of the magnitude suggested by some of the projections discussed above would not render the system unsustainable. It was on this basis that the Department of Health, the House of Commons Health Committee (1996) and the Royal Commission on Long-term Care (1999a) argued that, based on plausible assumptions about demand factors, a crisis of affordability is not likely. The Rowntree Inquiry, however, was more sceptical (Joseph Rowntree Foundation 1996).

The key conclusion to draw is that there is clearly a wide 'funnel of doubt' about future demand for long-term care and its expenditure consequences. Although there is no 'demographic time-bomb', there may be considerable resource pressures from a combination of factors, including rising numbers of older people, rising real costs of care and possibly rising expectations. Another uncertainty is whether the supply of informal care will rise proportionally with demand. Any system for funding long-term care must therefore be flexible enough to allow for these and other uncertainties.

Models of financing long-term care

There are at least five broad approaches to funding long-term care, differing in the balance between private and public funding and in the nature and extent of risk-pooling:

- private savings, possibly through special savings accounts or the use of housing equity;
- private insurance or, more precisely, the voluntary purchase of private insurance, which could be free-standing long-term care insurance or linked with pensions or life insurance;
- private insurance with public-sector support, such as subsidy, tax concession or partnership arrangements;
- public-sector tax-based support, funded from general tax revenue with services or cash provided based on need and possibly also on income and assets; and

- social insurance, funded through a hypothecated contribution with services or cash provided based on needs and contributions.

The key question is, who carries the risk? These approaches have been listed broadly in order of increasing risk to the public sector. Under the first approach – funding from private savings – the individual and her or his family bears the full risk, the family being involved because of the important role of informal family care and because of the impact of significant long-term care expenditure on inheritance. Under the private insurance option, groups of individuals carry the risk: enrollees in the insurance scheme. This is also the case for the third approach – private insurance with public-sector support – although now part of the risk might be transferred to the public sector. Under the fourth approach, taxpayers will carry the risk, whereas under the fifth approach, contribution payers will; for example, all workers if contributions are based on a payroll tax. Nevertheless, some costs may be passed on; for example, the costs of a payroll tax may be partly passed on to consumers.

Looking across these funding options, the public sector can wield five types of policy instrument: providing information and advice, regulating, subsidizing or taxing, making transfer payments and directly providing services. These instruments can be applied directly to the various funding approaches. Under the first two approaches, for example, the public-sector role would be limited to regulating private-sector financial products and perhaps providing information. Under the third funding approach, the public-sector role would be a form of subsidy (in addition to regulation and information provision) and, under the last two approaches, the role would amount to directly providing insurance.

In practice, many countries operate a mix of approaches (Box 10.1). The public sector usually provides at least a safety net to protect the poorest group of older people needing long-term care. Wealthier people are usually expected to rely on their savings or to purchase private insurance, although the degree of progressivity varies markedly from country to country.

Before these five funding approaches (or mixtures of them) are considered, it is helpful to be clear about the broader objectives of welfare states and about the criteria commonly advocated for comparing funding and provision arrangements within them.

Welfare state objectives

Welfare states pursue numerous objectives in helping individuals by providing services and cash benefits, especially (Hills *et al.* 1997):

- insurance of all against risks such as illness or unemployment;
- redistribution towards those with greater needs, such as for health care, disability or family circumstances;
- smoothing out the level of income over the life cycle; and
- stepping in where the family 'fails'.

Each of these is relevant to long-term care. The concept of insurance against risks is clearly very relevant: many people require little or no long-term

Box 10.1 Approach of five western European countries to funding long-term care

Denmark
Denmark funds health and social services through general taxation. Local taxation finances most long-term care. All community nursing and home care services are provided free of user charges. Institutional care is subject to user charges for rent and basic care. The charge is related to pension levels. The system was reformed during the 1970s to concentrate responsibility for hospital care on the regions and for community health services and social care on municipalities, the most local level of government. About 6 per cent of elderly people are in institutional care and more than 20 per cent receive home care. The public sector provides most services.

France
France's health insurance system covers the nursing component of care in long-stay sections of hospitals and in retirement homes that have a medical section. Social insurance contributions fund the scheme. Hotel costs in hospitals and care homes are subject to user charges. Nursing services at home that are medically prescribed are not subject to user charges. Home care services are subject to user charges based on income. About 5 per cent of elderly people are in institutional care and 10 per cent receive home care.

Germany
Germany introduced a new statutory insurance scheme for long-term care. Home care benefits commenced in April 1995 and institutional care benefits in July 1996. Social security contributions fund the scheme. Until the new scheme was introduced, the social security system did not cover long-term care. Individuals paid the cost subject to a means-tested social assistance safety net. The new scheme provides for three levels of benefit depending on an assessment of care needs. People eligible for benefits can choose cash or services. About 5 per cent of elderly people are in institutional care and less than 5 per cent receive home care. The voluntary sector provides most services.

The Netherlands
Social health insurance funds health services for most of the population and private health insurance for the wealthier part of the population. Contributions by employers and employees supplemented by deficit funding from the central government funds social insurance. A special national care fund set up in 1968 funds long-term care. The fund is based on tax-related contributions supplemented by central government financing. The special fund finances nursing home care and community health services but with co-payments. Local authorities finance residential care and home care and apply a means test. A minority of elderly recipients of long-term care are given cash benefits in the form of a 'personal budget' with which to purchase services. Personal budgets account for less than 5 per cent of total long-term care expenditure for older people. About 6.5 per cent of elderly people are in institutional care and between 5 and 10 per cent receive home care. The private sector provides many services.

United Kingdom
General taxation funds most health services, which are mainly free from user charges. Central and local taxation fund social services, which are mostly subject to user charges. A national means test for residential care considers most income and assets above a prescribed capital limit. Local authorities set charges for home care. The system of funding long-term care was reformed in 1993 to give local authorities responsibility for assessing care needs and arranging care. Services are mixed, involving public, voluntary and private services. About 5 per cent of elderly people in the United Kingdom are in institutional care and more than 10 per cent receive home care and/or community nursing services.

care, but some need substantial support over an extended period. For example, based on current patterns of utilization, the lifetime risk of entering residential or nursing home care in England is about one-sixth for a man and about one-third for a woman (Bebbington *et al.* 1997). About half of all women and one-third of all men who turn 65 years need intensive long-term care for periods that average 2 or more years before they die (Glennerster 1996).

Long-term care services may step in where family care is not available. In the United Kingdom, someone living with her or his spouse or another adult is less likely to receive home care and less likely to enter residential care than someone living alone, after controlling for dependence (Wittenberg *et al.* 1998). To some extent, public funding thus targets those without access to family care. The risk involved in long-term care can be seen as the risk of requiring help with personal or domestic care tasks family members cannot provide.

Systems for financing long-term care also redistribute towards people with greater needs and lower incomes. Redistribution from low- to high-need individuals is integral to insurance, whether private or public, and redistribution from high- to low-income groups arises when needs, and thus benefits, are inversely correlated with income, and also when the resources to fund the scheme are raised progressively in relation to income.

Funding long-term care inevitably involves redistribution across the life cycle. Sums set aside during the working years – personal savings in housing equity or other forms of wealth, premiums for private insurance or contributions to fund a public-sector scheme – are used to cover care needs in old age. Comparisons, therefore, are sometimes drawn between long-term care for older people and pensions. Pensions, although involving an element of insurance, are mainly concerned with saving during working years to provide income for retirement years (Dilnot *et al.* 1994). The financing of long-term care, in contrast, involves redistribution across the life cycle but raises substantial issues of risk-pooling through insurance. The balance between insurance and smoothing out income over the life cycle differs for pensions and long-term care, and the two should probably be considered separately (House of Commons Health Committee 1996). Comparing the funding of long-term care with that of acute health care is more appropriate than comparing it with pensions. In both cases, the welfare state combines insurance and redistribution towards those with greater needs and fewer resources. Consequently, some of the issues discussed elsewhere in this book are relevant to the financing of long-term care.

Criteria for evaluating these approaches

Several criteria have been suggested to assess the success of long-term care arrangements, especially funding routes and mechanisms. One is clearly efficiency: maximizing the quantity and quality of output for a given level of expenditure or minimizing the cost of achieving a specified level of output or effectiveness. In providing and funding long-term care, it is not ultimately service output – the quantity or quality of care delivered – that is valued as much as the outcomes for users and care-givers that flow from them. Outcomes for community care are notoriously difficult to define and measure, but this increases rather than diminishes the need to estimate the probable effects on service users of any funding system.

The achievement of efficiency may be impeded in practice by unsatisfactory (unclear, contradictory or perverse) incentives. The financing of long-term care has arguably long been dogged by this problem, for the division of budgets – and the administrative structure more widely – generates the potential for cost-shifting between agencies. Moreover, if more than one agency bears the costs of care, the agency responsible for assessing care needs may not appreciate the true or full resource costs of different care options. If, for example, users contribute more to residential care than to domiciliary care, public-sector agencies may prefer or encourage reliance on residential care even if domiciliary care would be more cost-effective in the wider context and also more acceptable to the user. The issue of inappropriate incentives should be a key concern of public policy.

The equity criterion is also relevant, provided one considers not only services or benefits but also funding contributions. The issue of what constitutes equity in contributions is clearly normative: perceived fairness may be as important as any particular measure of equity, and this criterion has been influential in discussions of different funding options (see later).

Independence, self-respect, dignity and choice have each been highlighted as general objectives of community care policy. For instance, the *Caring for People* White Paper in England stressed that independence and choice should be central considerations (Department of Health and Department of Social Security 1989). The Labour government's Green Paper, *New Ambitions for Our Country*, included among its principles that disabled people should get the support they need to lead fulfilling lives with dignity (Department of Social Security 1998). The Royal Commission's terms of reference referred to independence, dignity and choice, and the White Paper, *Modernising Social Services*, stressed the importance of promoting independence (Department of Health 1998). Clearly, therefore, when approaches to funding are evaluated, a key concern should be to ensure that the funding arrangements do not unduly limit older people's choice of care, distort their preferences through unsatisfactory incentives or create stigma.

A further criterion often suggested is the promotion of social solidarity (Le Grand *et al.* 1992). One interpretation would be to avoid disincentives to providing informal care by family and friends. Another would be to promote a sense of fairness between generations. It is not fairness between age groups but fairness between generations – that is, successive cohorts – that is important. Finally, affordability and sustainability are important, since resources are always limited. Given the uncertainty about future demand for long-term care and about the associated future expenditure, numerous issues arise as to the flexibility of the funding system and its capacity to control expenditure.

Private savings

Individuals may save for long-term care in many different ways, but in particular through shares, deposit accounts, housing equity and pensions. Under the housing equity approach, older people could fund their care by moving to a less expensive property, taking out a home equity plan or selling the property on entering residential care. None of these savings approaches appears very efficient as a general policy. Since not everyone needs long-term care, everyone does not have to save enough to meet the average cost of care let alone the maximum likely lifetime cost. Individuals with substantial housing assets who are not concerned about leaving a substantial inheritance may prefer to carry the risk themselves without insurance. This is a different scenario from individuals saving specifically to meet potential long-term care costs. In practice, most people do not save enough to meet the maximum likely lifetime costs, and those needing care for a long time tend to be reduced to low levels of wealth. People who do not need significant long-term care may still have saved for care needs and will, therefore, have foregone the benefit of using those resources for other purposes. Many older people may worry about the possibility of needing costly long-term care and the financial effects on them and their relatives. They may feel concern that their inheritance could be used up. Consequently, a policy of risk-pooling through insurance seems more efficient than a policy of individuals saving for long-term care needs.

In addition to these inefficiencies, private savings approaches are not likely to provide equal resources for equal needs. They redistribute resources across the life cycle but do not redistribute from those with lesser needs for long-term care to those with greater needs. They are relatively unfavourable to women; as women face a higher risk of needing care, they need more savings than men. Savings approaches would also not be widely affordable and they would not especially promote social solidarity.

In countries where individuals are left to manage their own risk with limited state pensions and limited universal health coverage, they will have to rely on their savings or purchase insurance privately. There may, however, be competing priorities for these resources. In countries with generous pensions, individuals may be considered to be able to cover long-term care costs out of income, as in Germany before social insurance was implemented. Other countries may have both limited state pensions and universal health care, but for historical reasons only a safety net for long-term care, as in the United Kingdom.

Private insurance

Insurance may be purchased from private companies voluntarily by individuals or may be publicly mandated. Alternatively, it could be purchased through a social insurance scheme. According to Barr (1998), five conditions need to be met for (voluntary purchase of) private insurance to be efficient:

- the probability of one person suffering the adverse event must be independent of the probability of anyone else suffering that event;
- the probability must be less than one, that is, not certainty;
- the probability must be known or estimable – if not, private insurers will be unable to calculate an actuarial premium;
- potential insurance enrollees must not have better information about their own personal probability of suffering the adverse event than insurers (adverse selection); and
- enrollees must not have scope to increase their probability of suffering the adverse event or the extent of their loss (moral hazard).

The voluntary purchase of private long-term care insurance would generally be more efficient than private savings for the reasons discussed previously. It would also redistribute from those with lesser care needs to those with greater care needs, and it could promote choice, independence and dignity. However, private long-term care insurance is likely to face difficulties with all except the second of Barr's conditions. For example, long-term, cohort-specific reductions in morbidity mean some interdependence of risks, potentially upsetting the first condition. If insurance is purchased around retirement age, as is typical for private insurance, this is some 15–20 years away from the time when any claim on the policy would be likely. Uncertainty about future rates of morbidity and about inflation in care costs means that insurers have difficulty in estimating the risk that long-term care will be required or the costs involved, making it difficult to calculate premiums (contrary to the third condition). Difficulties also arise with the fourth and fifth conditions, covering adverse selection and moral hazard, because of the long-term nature of care insurance (Wiener *et al.* 1994; Glennerster 1997).

Pricing is thus problematic, partly because many countries have neither past experience of claims nor quality data with which to estimate the lifetime risks involved, and partly because insurers need to allow for the possibility that enrollees represent above-average risks and that some insurance-induced claims may occur. Although insurers can take steps to counteract these problems – for example, through exclusions, limitations and co-payments, as well as through higher premiums – these actions reduce the affordability and attractiveness of private insurance policies. The corollary is that only a minority of the population could reasonably afford long-term care insurance unless it is purchased early in life (or possibly by releasing home equity). Nevertheless, people have other priorities early in life and may not be well informed about the risks of needing long-term care or the arrangements for public funding. Long-term care insurance thus seems unlikely to achieve widespread take-up in most countries unless it is compulsory.

Since women are more likely to require care, premiums for private insurance are often higher for women than men even though women have lower average incomes. Generally speaking, premiums constitute a higher proportion of the incomes of poor people, since they relate to actuarial risk rather than ability to pay. People who do not end up needing care receive no direct benefits in return for their insurance, although they are assured that potentially catastrophic long-term care costs would be covered. It also releases the use of some savings to be devoted to other purposes.

The Brookings Institution has undertaken substantial studies of ways of funding long-term care in the United States. Although about 5 per cent of the elderly population in the United States already had private long-term care insurance, the Institution projected that only a very small proportion of long-term care costs could be met from insurance benefits in the period to 2020. The authors of the study did not foresee private insurance replacing any significant proportion of projected public-sector expenditure on long-term care (Wiener *et al.* 1994). This finding is almost certainly applicable to European countries (Royal Commission on Long-term Care 1999b).

Public-sector support for private insurance

The rationale for public-sector support for private insurance would be to address some of the problems just mentioned. Subsidies for insurance premiums and partnership arrangements would reduce costs to enrollees. Requiring people to purchase insurance from early in adult life could reduce adverse selection and other informational problems and simultaneously improve affordability. The effects on distribution would be different from social insurance (Burchardt 1997). Compared with social insurance, private insurance benefits wealthier people relatively more than poorer people and benefits men more than women.

Under this approach, the state could take several steps to promote demand for long-term care insurance. One way would be to offer tax relief on premiums, by analogy with contributions to occupational and personal pensions. However, recent experience with private medical insurance for older people in the United Kingdom suggests that tax relief might not affect uptake much and that the tax expenditure might prove to be mainly 'deadweight' loss. Another way to promote demand for private insurance would be to offer a subsidy on the basis that those purchasing long-term care insurance were 'contracting out' of the long-term care part of the welfare state. However, as social care is currently subject to means testing in many countries, the savings to public funds from wider uptake of private long-term care insurance might be very modest.

The public sector could reduce the cost of private long-term care insurance by effectively taking part of the risk. The partnership schemes introduced by some states in the United States and proposed by the previous United Kingdom (Conservative) government have this effect. Those who purchase private insurance offering benefits of a specified minimum amount are treated more favourably under the assets test should they later exhaust their insurance benefits and seek public funding for their care. Partnership policies could have lower premiums than policies with unlimited coverage, because the public sector effectively takes part of the risk. Nevertheless, the uptake of partnership policies has proved disappointing. The reason in the United States, for example, is thought to be the perceived stigma of dependence on Medicaid (the safety net for poor people in the United States), even in the last resort.

The public sector could intervene to make long-term care insurance compulsory. Compulsion is not inherently inconsistent with an important role for private-sector provision. In the United Kingdom, for instance, employees (with earnings above a lower limit) are effectively covered by second-tier pensions, in that they are either contracted into the state earnings-related pension scheme or contracted out into occupational or personal pension schemes. Making private long-term care insurance compulsory for individuals and compelling private insurers to accept all applicants on standard terms would eliminate problems of adverse selection and exclusion of those with higher risks. Insurers might also be able to offer the same premium for men and women: premiums for women are currently markedly higher in the United Kingdom.

A compulsory system raises the issue of how premiums are paid for people unable to afford them. The public sector could pay premiums in such cases or, more realistically, could pay benefits for those who had been unable to afford sufficient insurance. One important question, therefore, is whether a funded private-sector insurance system with a substantial continuing public-sector role is preferable to a public-sector, potentially unfunded, social insurance system.

Public-sector funding schemes

The primary rationale for a public-sector scheme is that it would allow both insurance and redistribution objectives to be achieved, given that insurance appears efficient but private insurance suffers from various forms of market failure and inequity. A public-sector scheme could range from a safety net for poor people with a strict means test to a universal arrangement for the whole population without any means test. The scheme could be funded through general taxation, with no contribution conditions or hypothecated resources, or through a social insurance approach, with hypothecated resources and probably contribution conditions.

A safety-net public-sector scheme involves targeting public resources on poor people with care needs or non-poor people needing very expensive services who would thus become poor if they had to rely on their own resources. This is achieved by combining assessment of care needs and assessment of financial resources. The latter can take account of most or all sources of income and assets. Housing assets may be included, as in the case of most single people in the United Kingdom, or may be ignored, as in the United States and many European countries.

A scheme along these lines can be regarded as a combination of a public-sector tax-funded scheme for poorer people and a private savings or insurance approach for wealthier people. Most countries have safety net coverage for the services for which they do not provide universal coverage. If there is universal coverage for some interrelated services and a safety net for others, there is a risk of perverse incentives and scope for cost-shifting between agencies funding different services and also between public agencies and individuals. There is also the danger that schemes for poorer people are themselves 'poor' because few advocates have political influence.

A means-tested system tends to work best when income is more unevenly distributed – that is, when services can be targeted on a small number of poor people. Everyone contributes but only the poorest receive benefits, and they contribute less because of their low incomes. Those who have paid taxes and who are above the means-test threshold will have to pay their own costs if need arises. The presence of a means test has implications for incentives both to save and to make lifetime gifts of assets. There is a disincentive to save above the means-test capital limit for those able to do so, and there is an incentive to give assets to children or other relatives to circumvent the effect of the means test. The means test may be seen as penalizing the care-givers of the older people who fail the means test but need expensive formal care.

A universal tax-based scheme would pool risks across the entire population. Some countries have universal coverage but only for certain types of care, such as nursing care, as in France. This is likely to cause perverse incentives at the boundary between universal and means-tested forms of care. Few countries universally cover all long-term care services.

A universal system is more likely to apply if the income distribution is more equal and most people have similar incomes. It is likely to involve redistribution from men to women, although it may not be seen as such, since taxes tend to be related to income. It is likely to be progressive, since poorer groups tend to pay less because of their lower incomes. People who do not end up needing care still receive the assurance that potentially catastrophic long-term care costs would be covered if needed. A universal system may be perceived as benefiting care-givers, in particular with regard to protection of inheritance.

An important aspect of any funding arrangement should be to ensure that the mode of care is chosen based on effectiveness, overall cost and client choice and not through considerations of cost-shunting caused by perverse funding arrangements. The more that budgets and responsibilities are brought together and the more forms of care that are covered by these budgets, the less likely are perverse incentives. This suggests that it would be helpful if any universal scheme covered as wide a range of long-term care services and benefits as possible. This is not merely an issue for social insurance schemes but applies more widely: the scope for cost-shifting needs to be reduced.

Social insurance is a different way to provide a universal public-sector scheme. The difference between a tax-funded scheme such as the current arrangement in the United Kingdom and a social insurance scheme such as that in Germany does not lie in insurance, since a tax-funded scheme also involves risk-pooling across the population. The difference lies in the following.

- hypothecation of revenue is central to social insurance;
- insurance implies a link between contributions and benefits, but this may be weak where there are credits for spells of unemployment, etc.;
- national, enforceable eligibility criteria are also implied;
- the last two points imply the absence of a means test, although social insurance, like a tax-funded scheme, can incorporate co-payments and deductibles; the long-term care insurance scheme in Israel has an affluence test for benefits.

Hypothecation has been advocated as a means of guaranteeing a specified level of resources for a specified purpose. Hypothecated funds for long-term care would mean that social care funding would no longer compete directly with funding of other services. Ultimately, however, resources are limited and the need to prioritize is clearly not circumvented. Hypothecation has also been advanced as more acceptable to the public than an increase in general taxation, but this is debatable. It could even be suggested that the revenue raised would not be regarded as taxation. It would, however, be a public-sector scheme, and the scheme's liabilities would clearly be public-sector liabilities.

Hypothecation is not without drawbacks. One problem is that the revenue raised through contributions based on earnings in any year would be affected by the economic cycle. Supplementation from general tax revenue or borrowing might be needed in some years. Another problem is that hypothecation for one purpose raises the issue of the reason that service is getting preferential treatment; a special social insurance contribution for health, education or social services for children and younger adults might also be advocated.

National eligibility criteria have been advocated in the United Kingdom to promote equity (Laing 1993; Joseph Rowntree Foundation 1996). The criteria should be flexible to match services closely with needs and to promote cost-effectiveness.

A possible reason for preferring a social insurance scheme to an arrangement funded from general taxation would be the option of a funded scheme. A funded scheme would mean that contributions were invested so that each generation's long-term care costs could be met from their own past contributions rather than from the current contributions of the following generation. Whereas public funding for long-term care in European countries is currently pay-as-you-go, a social insurance scheme could be funded or pay-as-you-go. Barr (1998) discusses the economic issues that arise in the debate about funded social insurance.

The Rowntree Inquiry (Joseph Rowntree Foundation 1996) recommended a funded scheme for the United Kingdom partly in the belief that this would transfer long-term care resources into the future. A funded scheme could be easier to present than an unfunded scheme, if the public had more confidence in an arrangement under which individuals' contributions were potentially identifiable. It would not, however, provide an absolute guarantee of a higher level of funding for long-term care. Moreover, it seems to require one generation of working age to contribute twice. This could be avoided if either individuals passed the burden on by reducing their level of bequests or the government negated the funding element by increasing public-sector borrowing.

A funded social insurance scheme for long-term care would not necessarily present advantages over an unfunded, pay-as-you-go scheme. The issue of whether it would result in faster economic growth over the longer term is the subject of differing views. The accumulated fund would, in any event, be small in relation to that in second-tier pensions in the United Kingdom, although perhaps not in European countries with less funded pensions. It is doubtful that a funded scheme would have a large effect on the economy.

Mixed private- and public-sector approaches

Several approaches combine social insurance with private funding (Wiener *et al.* 1994). One possibility would be to make public funding available for home care without a means test and for residential care with a means test, since most elderly people have little spare income or capital when living at home, but capital from the home is released when they move to residential care. A problem is that the biggest risk for the individual is that of needing residential care over an extended period, and much of the controversy about the means test relates to how housing assets are treated when applying a means test for residential care.

Another approach would be for the state to fund home care and the first few months of residential care without a means test but to retain a means test for longer periods of residential care. This would facilitate returning home after a short period of rehabilitation in residential care, but once the stay is permanent, capital might be released to pay for care, although this could be seen to be at odds with the purpose of insurance and the aims of alleviating poverty. Conversely, public funding without a means test could be provided for home care and for residential care stays exceeding a few years, with the means test retained for the initial few years of residential care. This would limit the risk of an individual or a private insurance scheme. Long stays in residential care would be publicly funded, and savings or private insurance need cover only a limited period of residential care. A consequence is that, since fewer long-stay residents than short-stay residents are discharged into home care, the main effect would be to benefit the heirs of those needing residential care over an extended period.

In general, countries have tended to choose solutions that fit their existing method of financing health and social services. None of the 'national health service' countries has gone down the social insurance route when financing long-term care, preferring to proceed through setting user charges for services, especially the social care component (Royal Commission on Long-term Care 1999b: 171).

Austria and Germany, two countries with social insurance systems for health, have recently introduced new long-term care entitlements, and France and the Netherlands already do so. In the United Kingdom, with a national health service, a means-tested system for nursing homes has developed to replace the long-term care that has been withdrawn from the health service. Covering most health care by one (universal) system while covering long-term nursing care in institutions by another (means-tested) system is bound to create tensions both in public reaction and allocation of services, regardless of the mechanisms that might be promoted to help with later costs. Shifting any service outside a universal system is never going to be popular.

Attitudes and policy issues

A study by the OECD (1996) considered the implications of an ageing population in industrialized countries for a range of economic and social policies, including long-term care. The study observed that the costs of long-term care are rather modest – less that 2 per cent of GDP in most countries. Although need or demand may increase drastically by, say, 50 per cent because of demographic change, this would only increase expenditure by 1 per cent of

Table 10.1 Percentage of respondents in 12 European Union countries in 1992 agreeing with the statement: 'Those in employment have a duty to ensure, through contributions or taxes, that older people have a decent standard of living'

Country	Agree strongly	Agree slightly	Disagree	Don't know
Belgium	32.5	42.7	17.9	6.9
Denmark	60.1	29.8	8.3	1.8
France	25.9	51.2	17.6	5.3
Germany	30.4	48.4	15.0	6.2
Greece	39.4	35.0	12.5	13.1
Ireland	40.7	40.9	7.5	10.9
Italy	38.4	40.1	9.6	11.1
Luxembourg	34.2	44.8	14.0	7.0
Netherlands	42.4	38.2	13.8	5.6
Portugal	41.2	32.3	17.8	8.7
Spain	45.7	38.1	7.2	9.1
United Kingdom	45.9	37.2	9.3	7.5

Source: adapted from Walker (1996)

GDP. The OECD study concluded that, 'with careful planning and adaptation, such an increase should be reasonably met by most care systems, provided that the resulting burden is spread among workers and older people'. This appears to be in line with the view expressed by the Royal Commission on Long-term Care (1999a) in the United Kingdom that a crisis of affordability is unlikely. But is achieving such a spread politically feasible? Based on the criteria outlined earlier in this chapter, what is the best means by which to turn the principle into practice?

The Eurobarometer surveys of public attitudes to ageing and older people were devised to provide baseline information on attitudes towards older people and some of the related topical policy issues (Walker 1993). These usefully describe the general public's views on whether older people have a decent standard of living and on the preferred methods of financing long-term care. A sample of the general public in each European Union country was asked in 1992 to what extent they agreed or disagreed with the statement that those in employment have a duty to ensure, through the contributions or taxes they pay, that older people have a decent standard of living. The results, summarized in Table 10.1, show a remarkably high level of solidarity across the European Union countries and suggest that 'the social contract is in good shape' (Walker 1993: 3).

The social contract is interpreted as being a social policy contract based on inter-generational transfer of resources through taxation and social expenditure. The 'late twentieth century phenomenon of population aging has raised questions about the main elements of this contract: public pension provision and, to a lesser extent, the provision of health and social care' (Walker 1993: 10). Arguments have been propounded for inter-generational equity – equalizing the contribution and benefits received by cohorts. Kotlikoff and Leibfritz

Table 10.2 Views of respondents in 12 European Union countries in 1992 on the best way of providing long-term care

Country	Compulsory public insurance	Compulsory private insurance	Optional public insurance	Optional private insurance	Public provision of care financed through taxes	Don't know
Belgium	45.7	10.4	8.2	8.2	17.7	9.9
Denmark	17.9	6.0	4.9	5.1	60.3	5.2
France	41.3	7.9	7.1	2.6	32.1	9.0
Germany	48.3	6.6	10.4	5.4	20.6	8.7
Greece	32.2	4.0	8.4	3.6	31.1	20.6
Ireland	19.3	5.7	4.9	4.0	44.0	22.0
Italy	34.9	7.2	5.1	3.0	34.7	15.2
Luxembourg	50.1	7.3	8.4	3.0	18.1	13.2
Netherlands	40.1	9.9	7.9	5.2	27.2	9.7
Portugal	31.3	6.4	7.1	5.0	48.0	2.0
Spain	38.2	2.6	5.7	2.2	29.6	21.7
United Kingdom	17.7	3.8	8.0	5.0	56.7	9.0

Source: Walker (1993)

(1999) argued that, if policies were unchanged in the OECD countries, this 'will sentence their [older generations'] children to sky-high rates of net taxation' or require cuts in social security for both current and future pensioners and reductions in rights of access to health and social care. Table 10.1 shows a high level of consensus that 'Those in employment have a duty to ensure, through contributions or taxes, that older people have a decent standard of living'.

A second issue the Eurobarometer surveys addressed was the best way of providing long-term care (Table 10.2). The general public were asked to choose from a series of possible methods the way they thought was best for financing long-term care. The results revealed:

> surprisingly widespread opposition to the use of the private sector in this field. More than seven out of ten favoured either a compulsory public insurance scheme or public services financed through taxation and, if the 'don't knows' are excluded this rises to just under eight out of ten. The citizens of Europe have spoken with clear voices on this issue: either the public sector should organize the financing of long-term care or it should both finance and provide it.
>
> (Walker 1993: 31)

These public attitudes are consistent with the analysis offered earlier in this chapter. Risk-pooling through insurance is a more efficient way of funding long-term care than relying on savings. It also effectively redistributes resources towards people with greater care needs. But because there are likely to be problems with the voluntary purchase of private insurance – especially some degree of market failure, affordability and perhaps also equity – an important role for the public sector is inevitable. This could range from assisting the spread of private insurance and providing a safety net for those unable to afford private insurance to a comprehensive public-sector arrangement financed from general taxation or financed through hypothecated contributions to a social care insurance scheme.

Note

1 The views of the authors in this chapter are personal and do not necessarily represent the views of the United Kingdom Department of Health.

References

Barr, N. (1998) *Economics of the Welfare State*, 3rd edn. Oxford and Palo Alto, CA: Oxford University Press and Stanford University Press.

Bebbington, A., Brown, P., Darton, R. and Netten, A. (1997) *The Lifetime Risk of Entering Residential or Nursing Home Care for Elderly People*, Discussion Paper 1230/2. Canterbury: Personal Social Services Research Unit, University of Kent.

Beck, B. (1996) The economics of ageing, *The Economist*, 27 January, pp. 3–16.

Burchardt, T. (1997) *What Price Security? Assessing Private Insurance for Long-term Care, Income Replacement during Incapacity, and Unemployment for Mortgagors*, Welfare State Discussion Paper WSP/129. London: London School of Economics and Political Science.

Culyer, A.J. (1980) *The Political Economy of Social Policy*. Oxford: Martin Robertson.

Department of Health (1998) *Modernising Social Services*, Cm 4169. London: The Stationery Office.

Department of Health and Department of Social Security (1989) *Caring for People: Community Care in the Next Decade and Beyond*, Cm 849. London: HMSO.

Department of Social Security (1998) *New Ambitions for Our Country: A New Contract for Welfare*, Cm 3805. London: The Stationery Office.

Dilnot, A., Disney, R., Johnson, P. and Whitehouse, E. (1994) *Pensions Policy in the UK: An Economic Analysis*. London: Institute for Fiscal Studies.

Evers, A. and Svetlik, I. (eds) (1994) *Balancing Pluralism: New Welfare Mixes in Care for the Elderly*. Aldershot: Avebury.

Glennerster, H. (1996) *Caring for the Very Old: Public and Private Solutions*, Welfare State Discussion Paper WSP/126. London: London School of Economics and Political Science.

Glennerster, H. (1997) *Paying for Welfare: Toward 2000*. Hemel Hempstead: Prentice-Hall.

Hills, J., Gardiner, K. and the LSE Welfare State Programme (1997) *The Future of Welfare: A Guide to the Debate*, revised edn. York: Joseph Rowntree Foundation.

House of Commons Health Committee (1996) *Long-Term Care: Future Provision and Funding*, session 1995–96, third report. London: House of Commons.

Joseph Rowntree Foundation (1996) *Meeting the Costs of Continuing Care: Report and Recommendations*. York: Joseph Rowntree Foundation.

Kendig, H., Hashimoto, A. and Coppard, L. (1992) *Family Support for the Elderly: The International Experience*. Oxford: Oxford University Press.

Knapp, M.R.J. and Wistow, G. (1996) Social care markets in England: early post-reform experiences, *Social Service Review*, 70: 355–77.

Knapp, M.R.J., Forder, J.E. and Kendall, J. (2000) The growth of independent sector provision in the UK, in S. Harper (ed.) *The Family in an Ageing Society*. Oxford: Oxford University Press.

Kotlikoff, L.J. and Leibfritz, W. (1999) An international comparison of generational accounts, in A.J. Auerbach, L.J. Kotlikoff and W. Leibfritz (eds) *Generational Accounting around the World*. Chicago, IL: University of Chicago Press.

Kramer, R. (1981) *Voluntary Agencies in the Welfare State*. Berkeley, CA: University of California Press.

Laing, W. (1993) *Financing Long-Term Care: The Crucial Debate*. London: Age Concern England.

Le Grand, J., Propper, C. and Robinson, R. (1992) *The Economics of Social Problems*. Basingstoke: Macmillan.

Nuttall, S.R., Blackwood, R.J.L., Bussell, B.M.H. *et al.* (1994) Financing long-term care in Great Britain, *Journal of the Institute of Actuaries*, 121(part 1): 1–68.

OECD (1996) *Caring for Frail Elderly People: Policies in Evolution*. Paris: Organisation for Economic Co-operation and Development.

Richards, E., Wilsdon, T. and Lyons, S. (1996) *Paying for Long Term Care*. London: Institute for Public Policy Research.

Royal Commission on Long-term Care (1999a) *With Respect to Old Age*, Cm 4192. London: The Stationery Office.

Royal Commission on Long-term Care (1999b) Lessons from international experience, *The Context of Long-term Care Policy*, Research Vol. 1, Cm 4192-II/1. London: The Stationery Office.

Schmahl, W. and Rothgang, H. (1996) The long-term costs of public long-term care insurance in Germany: some guesstimates, in R. Eisen and F.A. Sloan (eds) *Long-Term Care: Economic Issues and Policy Solutions*. Dordrecht: Kluwer Academic.

Walker, A. (1993) *Age and Attitudes: The Main Results from a Eurobarometer Survey*, Eurobarometer Surveys on Opinions and Attitudes of Europeans No. 69. Brussels: European Commission.

Walker, A. (1996) *The New Generational Contract – Intergenerational Relations, Old Age and Welfare*. London: University College London Press.

Wiener, J.M., Illston, L.H. and Hanley, R.J. (1994) *Sharing the Burden: Strategies for Public and Private Long-Term Care Insurance*. Washington, DC: Brookings Institution.

Wittenberg, R., Pickard, L., Comas-Herrera, A., Davies, B. and Darton, R. (1998) *Demand for Long-term Care: Projections of Long-term Care Finance for Elderly People*. Canterbury: Personal Social Services Research Unit, University of Kent.

chapter eleven

Strategic resource allocation and funding decisions

Nigel Rice and Peter C. Smith[1]

Introduction

In this chapter, we examine the methods used to distribute national health care funds to the insurers responsible for organizing health care on behalf of their members, a process we call 'strategic resource allocation'. We first define the concept and describe different contexts within which resource allocation might take place. A discussion follows of capitation and risk adjustment, which have become the favoured instruments for resource allocation in many industrialized countries. We then discuss the explicit and implicit objectives attached to schemes for strategic resource allocation. Next, existing methods of setting health care budgets are summarized. We then describe the needs factors currently used to determine capitation and, finally, we discuss the variation in current methods. The discussion is based predominantly on a survey of the relatively mature resource allocation systems in western European countries. However, we believe the results have important implications for other countries seeking to reform their systems of health care.

What is strategic resource allocation in health care financing?

Despite the enormous diversity in methods of financing health care within Europe, a fundamental challenge confronts almost all systems of health care (Hoffmeyer and McCarthy 1994). Society, often in the form of the national government, seeks to devolve responsibility for arranging health care to a health care 'plan'. This plan might be a local government (as in Scandinavia), a local administrative board (as in the United Kingdom) or a sickness fund (as found in Belgium, Germany, the Netherlands and Switzerland). Whatever their precise constitution, these plans – often referred to as 'purchasers' – are charged with organizing specified types of health care for a designated population, whether defined by geography, employment type or voluntary enrolment, over a given period of time.

Although there are a few examples of self-funding social insurance plans (for example, in Austria), few European health care systems operate an integrated (self-contained) model of financing and delivery for plans. Instead, many of the functions of financing operate effectively at the national level. Even when local plans in the form of local governments or sickness funds retain responsibility for collecting premiums, the plan does not usually have direct access to the funds. Instead, they are effectively pooled at the national level. There is then a formidable task in distributing the national-level health care funds to the plans in accordance with society's equity and efficiency objectives. We call this form of devolved budgeting 'strategic resource allocation'.

Three methods can be envisaged for funding the devolved plans:

- full retrospective reimbursement for all expenditure incurred;
- reimbursement for all activity based on a fixed schedule of fees using, for example, a system of diagnosis-related groups; and
- prospective funding based on expected future expenditure, using fixed budgets.

These three forms of resource allocation imply a progressive shift of risk from the national funder towards the health care plan. Under the first method, the plan assumes no financial risk; under the second method, the plan assumes risk for treatment costs but not patient numbers; and under the third method, the national funder shifts all financial risk to the plan. These methods are points on a spectrum of funding mechanisms, and many intermediate solutions can be envisaged. The first and second methods entail an uncertain total funding commitment, whereas the third method is consistent with a fixed total budget constraint.

European health care systems have increasingly been seeking to move away from the first method and towards the third method along the spectrum of resource allocation mechanisms. In particular, the devolved plans have been an important focus for securing expenditure control (Mossialos and Le Grand 1999). To this end, most health care systems in western Europe have required a global budget for health care expenditure to be set prospectively for each devolved plan. The intention is that the plan should then deliver (or purchase) the required health care to the population at risk within the specified budget, thereby securing the required expenditure control.

Given that a fixed-budget resource allocation mechanism has been chosen, four methods of distributing funds prospectively between plans might be envisaged:

- according to the size of bids from the plans;
- based on political negotiation;
- according to historical precedent; and
- based on some independent measure of health care needs.

The first three options have come under increasing criticism within most health care systems. The first option – based on the size of bids – would generally offer plans the incentive to overstate their needs and, with no countervailing incentive to moderation, would inevitably lead to inflation of bids. The second option – based on political negotiation – can offer a comfortable short-term solution to the resource allocation problem but is vulnerable to accusations of political favouritism and has often proved to be unsustainable in the longer term. The third option – based on historical precedent – has been in widespread use, for example in the form of statistical extrapolation of previous expenditure or using budgets based on services available. It is, however, arbitrary and does not encourage efficiency. All three methods contain the potential for gross inequity, which is often a central concern in European health care systems.

More scientific approaches towards setting budgets based on health care needs have increasingly been used, most notably in the form of capitation, whereby an explicit contribution to the budget is attached to each member of a plan (Newhouse 1998). Most of the health care systems surveyed here use capitation to a greater or lesser extent to allocate resources; we therefore discuss this instrument in some detail in the next section. Nevertheless, most capitation-based budgeting systems are somewhat (and some very greatly) tempered by considerations such as historical precedent and political negotiation. In Portugal, for example, a recently introduced capitation scheme is heavily moderated by the use of historical expenditure (Ministério da Sáude 1998).

Furthermore, explicit mechanisms for resource allocation, in the form of budgets, may be supplemented by implicit systems of resource allocation, such as provision of capital infrastructure or other hidden subsidies, which may favour certain plans relative to others. These implicit instruments are by definition difficult to catalogue and vary in importance between systems. They may nevertheless be important in certain contexts.

The prospective allocation of budgets is only the first stage in allocating resources. It is almost invariably accompanied by a final stage in which prospective allocations are altered retrospectively based on actual expenditure experience. Several arrangements exist for handling retrospective variation in actual expenditure from the prospective budget:

- renegotiating the budget retrospectively with the central payer, as has effectively occurred in Italy and Spain;
- running down or contributing to the plan's reserves, as in many systems of competitive insurance funds;
- varying the premiums or local taxes paid by the plan members, as in Scandinavia and some competitive insurance systems;
- varying the user charges (co-payments) paid by the patients, as in Finland;
- varying the package of benefits available to patients; and
- delaying or rationing health care to the population at risk, as occurs to differing extents in Norway, Sweden and the United Kingdom.

These arrangements might exist in any budgetary system and are especially important when the plans are small and therefore vulnerable to random fluctuation in demand. They imply important differences in the strictness of the budget constraint confronting plans, and suggest that – to differing extents – the apparently scientific methods (such as capitation) used in prospective budgetary schemes might be tempered by many other methods of resource allocation, both prospective and retrospective. As a consequence, the extent to which the financial resources ultimately available to health care plans have been determined by some objective assessment of needs varies considerably between systems.

What is capitation?

Capitation can be defined as the health service funds associated with a plan member for the service in question and for the time period in question, subject to any overall budget constraint. A capitation system puts a 'price' on the head of every member. People's health care needs vary considerably, depending on personal characteristics such as age, morbidity and social circumstances. Considerable effort, therefore, has been expended on the process known as risk adjustment, which seeks an unbiased estimate of the expected costs of the member to the health care plan relative to all other plan members, given the member's personal characteristics. If the overall budget is set at unrealistically low levels, then the capitation sum will be less than expected expenditure. However, in these circumstances, the intention is that the risk-adjusted capitation should continue to reflect people's relative health care expenditure needs.

In this chapter, we focus on capitation for the purpose of strategic resource allocation. We therefore assume that this is required to compensate plans for the expected health care expenditure of their members. Capitation might also be used for other purposes not directly related to health care expenditure needs, such as determining the reimbursement of primary care physicians for the population for which they are responsible. These purposes are not considered further here.

Although a given capitation sum might be notionally assigned to an individual, as a measure of expected expenditure, the health plan is not generally expected to spend precisely that amount on the individual. For example, although a national capitation of, say, £550 per annum may be assigned to a person aged 45–64 years in England, it would be absurd to expect every such individual to incur that expenditure in a particular year. The capitation sum offers an expected level of expenditure that might vary substantially. Under these circumstances, the plan is expected to manage at least some of the risk inherent in the demand for the services for which it is responsible. Furthermore, the plan may not necessarily be required to spend at the assumed level of funding. For example, local governments delivering health care may vary funding levels somewhat from those assumed by the central government by changing local taxes (Rattso 1998), and competitive sickness funds might fund variations in expenditure by varying the insurance premiums they charge from the assumed level (McCarthy *et al.* 1995).

Capitation can be very rudimentary – at its simplest (as in Spain) assigning an equal amount of funding for every citizen, regardless of circumstances

(Consejo de Política Fiscal y Financiera 1998). Successive degrees of refinement using risk adjustment can then be envisaged. For example, in many of the risk-adjustment schemes used in systems of social insurance (such as Germany and Switzerland), capitation is based on simple demographic data, thereby introducing several different categories of individual based on age and sex. Age and sex may be important determinants of expenditure variation, but there are many other potential risk adjusters. In incorporating further factors into the risk-adjustment mechanism, most capitation schemes have been constrained by data availability (see pp. 258–9).

Capitation should relate only to the services for which the health care plan is responsible. In most western European countries, this embraces a comprehensive range of services. However, capitation can in some circumstances be constrained (or 'carved out') for specific sectors, such as mental health services (Ettner *et al.* 2000). In the United Kingdom, which has a significant private health care sector, capitation for the National Health Service (NHS) should in principle reflect the expected use of NHS services only and exclude the use of private services. In circumstances such as these, a useful indicator for risk-adjustment purposes would be whether or not the citizen has private insurance.

A few surveys offer international perspectives on capitation methods (McCarthy *et al.* 1995; Hutchison *et al.* 1999; Oliver 1999; van de Ven and Ellis 2000). This chapter is based on a survey of documentary evidence and personal contacts. Substantial policy changes were proposed or being implemented in several countries at the time of writing, and we have tried to signal these where they are known. The detailed findings for some of the individual countries can be found elsewhere (Rice and Smith 1999). Recent international experience is reported in special issues of the journals *Inquiry* (Swartz 1998) and *Health Care Management Science* (Rice and Smith 2000).

What is the purpose of resource allocation methods?

Here, we look at the resource allocation methods in use in western Europe. Table 11.1 summarizes the 20 countries surveyed and indicates four types of

Table 11.1 The 20 resource allocation schemes surveyed in western Europe according to category

Competitive insurance plans	Employer-based insurance plans	Public sector: devolved	Public sector: centralized
Belgium	Austria	Denmark	Ireland
Germany	France	Finland	Portugal
Netherlands	Greece	Italy	Spain
Switzerland	Luxembourg	Norway	United Kingdom (England,
		Sweden	Northern Ireland, Scotland
			and Wales)

system of health care financing within which the resource allocation scheme is embedded: competitive insurance markets, captive employment-based insurance, devolved public sector and centralized public sector. The public-sector schemes imply a geographical basis for health care plans. The categories are somewhat flexible. For example, Belgium's system is in many respects far from competitive, Germany's system retains many echoes of its precursor, which was employment-based, and Spain's system has elements of both devolution and centralization. However, they indicate the wide range of contexts within which a policy of capitation has been adopted. Hoffmeyer and McCarthy (1994) give fuller details of institutional financial arrangements. The four constituent countries of the United Kingdom use somewhat different systems and are therefore considered separately.

The imperative driving most resource allocation systems is controlling expenditure. If the level of health care expenditure were considered unproblematic, then the interest in setting prospective budgets would largely disappear. Under such circumstances, there is little incentive to move far from the relatively straightforward (albeit highly inefficient) fee-for-service approach to funding, possibly with added incentives to treat underserved sections of the population. However, given that controlling expenditure is of universal concern and that prospective budgets must therefore be set, the question arises: Why are capitation methods increasingly preferred to the other methods of setting budgets noted above? There are two main reasons, relating to equity and efficiency.

The equity arguments for adopting capitation and risk adjustment tend to reflect a requirement to secure equal access to health care (for equal health needs) and equal payments in the form of premiums or taxes (for equal income or wealth). The pursuit of equity plays a central role in securing widespread support for health services funded from tax revenue, and explicit equity objectives underlying resource allocation methods are therefore most frequent in centrally controlled public-sector health care systems. For example, the objective of Italy's mechanism for regional resource allocation is 'to overcome territorial inequalities in social and health conditions' (Mapelli 1998), and the resource allocation formula used in England is intended 'to secure equal opportunity of access to those at equal risk' (NHS Executive 1997).

This type of objective reflects two broad types of concern: securing equity of health and securing equity of access to health care. The former objective is largely rhetorical, and few practical attempts have been made to adjust capitation to address inequality in health. Nevertheless, in England a radically new equity criterion is being contemplated of 'contributing to the reduction of health inequalities'. It remains to be seen whether this can be made operational. In practice, the objective of seeking to offer equal access to health care to those in equal need has been the equity objective – either explicit or implicit – underlying almost all schemes.

A slightly different approach to equity underlies devolved public-sector systems of the type in Scandinavia in which local governments are responsible for organizing most health care. Here, the central government supports health care expenditure with grants in aid, the principal objective of such grants being to enable local communities to deliver some 'standard' level of health care while levying some standard rate of local taxation (Rattso 1998). The equity objective relating to access then remains similar to that found in the centrally controlled state schemes. For example, the Finnish State Subsidy System seeks to secure 'equality of opportunity of access for equal need' (Ministry of Social Affairs and Health 1996). However, local communities might then enjoy certain freedom in determining the level of health care they choose to offer, the associated local taxes they levy and the user co-payments they levy. Thus, such schemes implicitly seek to secure equity based on equality of opportunity, both in access to health care and in levels of payment (in the form of local taxes and charges).

Implicit equity objectives on the payment side also underlie some of the schemes of social insurance in northern Europe. For example, the main objective of the risk-adjustment scheme used in Germany is to reduce variation in health insurance premiums between plans (Files and Murray 1995). The less explicit adjustment scheme used in France, where a citizen's choice of insurance plan is limited, appears to have a similar objective (Hoffmeyer and McCarthy 1994).

Efficiency objectives are implicit in most prospective budgetary schemes, in the sense that all such schemes are embedded within a budgeting system that seeks to make purchasers and providers more responsive to issues of the costs and benefits of their actions. However, efficiency considerations tend to be most conspicuous in the resource allocation methods used for health care systems with competitive insurers, such as those found in Belgium, Germany, the Netherlands and Switzerland (van de Ven and Ellis 2000). Such systems usually legally require plans to set premiums independent of a member's health status or the number of dependants covered. Furthermore, if premiums are related to income, such as in Germany and the Netherlands, plans would – if unconstrained by regulation – wish to recruit members with a high income instead of a low income and members with few instead of many dependants.

If left uncorrected, this situation would give competitive health plans a strong incentive to 'cream-skim' healthy, young, rich citizens with few dependants. They would have an incentive to scrutinize potential members to assess whether or not their expected annual costs exceed the associated income to the scheme and to reject applications if this applies. Even if 'open enrolment' were stipulated (under which a plan must in principle accept all applicants), Newhouse (1994) shows how plans can effectively deter high-risk applicants or encourage high-risk members to leave the plan. Such cream-skimming would lead to increasing inequality in premium rates and profit levels between plans that practised cream-skimming and those that did not. In the extreme, some people might be unable to find insurance.

Many of the systems of 'managed competition' between health plans are highly regulated and, in practice, offer the plans little scope to improve the efficiency of providers, who continue to be reimbursed based on activity (Brown and Amelung 1999; Schokkaert and van de Voorde 2000). This lack of leverage in pursuing provider efficiency increases the incentive for plans to target their energies either towards the socially wasteful activity of cream-skimming or towards the inefficient practice of quality-skimping; for example, delivering less than the socially desirable level of care to patients with high needs. In these circumstances, the purpose of capitation and risk adjustment is to seek to reduce the manifest inefficiency that emerges. Here, however, we do not focus directly on the incentives that emerge in a competitive health care insurance market and, therefore, we ignore the many interesting efficiency issues that emerge when seeking to implement such a market (Giacomini *et al.* 1995; McCarthy *et al.* 1995; Newhouse 1996; van Barneveld *et al.* 1996; Emery *et al.* 1997; Hutchison *et al.* 1999; Oliver 1999; van de Ven and Ellis 2000).

Both the equity and efficiency arguments sketched above generate a policy prescription of risk-adjusted capitation. Essentially, capitation seeks to address how, given that health care expenditure is to be constrained, the limited resources available should be distributed between health care plans in accordance with society's equity and efficiency objectives. The purpose of risk-adjusted capitation is to ensure that plans receive the same level of funding for people with equal 'need' for health care, regardless of extraneous circumstances such as area of residence and level of income.

How can resources be allocated prospectively?

Once the principle of allocating funds based on prospective budgets has been established, the question arises as to how the budgets are to be derived. The first fundamental choice is how much public money is to be allocated to the service. This is principally a political decision and beyond the scope of this chapter. Of the budgetary methods noted above, capitation has become the dominant method of setting budgets for individual plans. Historical precedent and, to a lesser extent, political negotiation are important in determining a proportion of the budget in many systems, but – with a few exceptions – their role is to temper the swings in allocation implied by a pure capitation system, which forms the core of the resource allocation method. We therefore concentrate on the use of capitation methods to determine budgets.

The capitation sum for a given individual can be considered as that person's relative expenditure needs, and the characteristics to be taken into account in calculating the needs as needs factors. The general principles that should be applied when choosing needs factors are that, all other things being equal, they represent demonstrably material influences on the propensity to utilize the health care service under consideration. This raises the important question as to who should decide what constitutes 'need' for a particular health care service. Such decisions could be mainly judgemental. However, the main yardstick for deciding whether a putative 'needs factor' should be used as a basis for risk adjustment has in practice become whether it explains actual spending patterns among plans in a statistically significant manner. That is, the actual spending behaviour of the health care sector is used to infer appropriate needs factors.

Modelling existing determinants of health care utilization may not accommodate some aspects of 'unmet' need within the capitation method. This arises when groups within the population – such as ethnic minorities, those living in rural areas or patients with particular conditions – are not receiving the services to which they are entitled compared with the general pattern of utilization within the population as a whole. In such circumstances, using empirical spending patterns to infer needs factors is problematic, as the models developed will perpetuate the implied inequity. At the opposite end of the spectrum to unmet need is the possibility of 'supplier-induced demand', leading to higher utilization among groups with especially high access to health care. Unmet need and supplier-induced demand have been the subject of great concern, especially in England, where the econometric methods in use are designed specifically to minimize the impact of supply factors on capitation (Carr-Hill et al. 1994). Recent proposals for Scotland (Scottish Executive Health Department 1999) offer an alternative perspective, using similar methods.

Whether a factor is included in a capitation scheme may be determined by the policy context. This consideration is especially important in relation to provider costs. In England, the tradition has been to assume that health plans are unable to control general input prices caused by local economic factors, and so some adjustment to local capitation is made for such variation using general wage data and land prices. However, every effort is made to avoid using health-sector prices as the basis for adjusting capitation, as these can be influenced by local health plan policy. In contrast, the risk-adjustment scheme in the Netherlands uses five categories of 'urbanization', for which the capitation sum can vary, say, from −11 per cent (rural) to +18 per cent (heavily urban) in specialist health care (Ziekenfondsraad 1999). No attempt is made to determine whether some of the observed variation in costs might be caused by variation in supply. The assumption appears to be that health plans are unable to control such variation in costs and must, therefore, be appropriately reimbursed. Such issues have been the subject of strong debate within competitive health care markets (such as Belgium, Germany and the Netherlands), where the extent to which plans can control the supply of local physicians and provider prices is disputed (van de Ven et al. 1994; DULBEA/KUL 1997).

It is also desirable to avoid using needs factors that may be vulnerable to manipulation by the recipient agencies or that create perverse incentives. For example, many studies have found that a history of previous inpatient utilization is a good predictor of current utilization (van Vliet and van de Ven 1993; Andersson et al. 2000). However, previous utilization may often be ruled out as a suitable capitation factor because it is considered vulnerable to manipulation by providers and may create an incentive for providers to offer more care than is strictly necessary, to distort reports of diagnosis or to indulge in other gaming activity to attract higher capitation in the future. Indeed, in the extreme case in which past expenditure is used as a crude predictor of future expenditure, the system of financing might effectively revert to one of full retrospective reimbursement.

The selection of factors to be included in calculating health care capitation has been highly complex and controversial for at least six reasons.

- Relevant data are often lacking.
- Research evidence on appropriate needs factors is sparse, dated or ambiguous.
- Establishing the independence of a particular needs factor from other needs factors (that is, handling covariance between needs factors) is very difficult.

- Disentangling legitimate health care needs factors from other policy and supply influences on utilization is very difficult.
- Empirically identifying the health care costs associated with a proven needs factor is often difficult.
- The plans receiving devolved budgets often feel they have a clear idea about which needs factors will favour their plan and will thus seek to influence the choice of needs factors through the political process.

Once needs factors have been identified – in whatever fashion – weights must be attached that reflect their relative influence on the need to spend. Risk-adjustment processes use two broad approaches to setting capitation: a matrix approach based on individual-level data and an index approach based on aggregate data. Under the matrix approach, one or more dimensions of need (such as age, sex, ethnic origin or disability status) are used to create a grid of capitation sums, in which each entry represents the expected annual health care costs of a citizen with the associated characteristics. Thus the matrix might comprise, say, eight age categories, two sex categories, three employment status categories and two disability status categories, giving rise in its unadulterated form to $8 \times 2 \times 3 \times 2 = 96$ cells – and capitation needs to be estimated for each.

Several schemes use a matrix approach based on age alone (France) or age and sex (Germany and Switzerland) (Files and Murray 1995; Beck 1998; Haut Comité de la Santé Publique 1999). At the other extreme, perhaps the apotheosis of the matrix approach is represented by the matrix of capitation developed in Stockholm County and proposed for use at a national level in Sweden (Diderichsen *et al.* 1997; Andersson *et al.* 2000). This extends the familiar age and sex capitation to include such variables as marital status, housing tenure and employment status as well as previous health care utilization. It is made possible by the comprehensive personal record of social circumstances and health care utilization maintained for all residents of Sweden. For purposes of empirical estimation, the matrix approach usually requires a substantial database of individual-level data for which all the relevant needs factors are recorded. The usual technique is then to estimate cell entries using conventional regression techniques, in which each cell is effectively represented by a dummy variable. For allocation purposes, the method requires universal and reliable recording of individual-level data among health care plans.

Estimating every cell entry is not always necessary, and statistical or judgemental methods can be used to reduce the number of cells used within the matrix. For example, in the Netherlands, age (19 categories), sex (2), urbanization (5) and employment and disability status (5) are used as the basis for capitation sums, implying the need to estimate $19 \times 2 \times 5 \times 5 = 950$ cells. In practice, the problem is reduced by setting a rudimentary matrix of capitation sums for age and sex ($19 \times 2 = 38$ cells). It is then assumed that the impact of urbanization and employment and disability status is independent of age and sex. The dimension of the problem is therefore reduced considerably by assuming that the same 'urbanization' factor applies to all citizens in rural areas, regardless of age and sex. This means that just 5 urbanization and 5 employment and disability factors need to be defined, in addition to the

38 age and sex cells (Ziekenfondsraad 1999). In effect, the regression problem has been reduced to one of estimating $38 + 5 + 5 = 48$ parameters (rather than 950). An alternative approach to reducing the dimension of the matrix problem is to combine adjacent cells that either are very sparse or vary little. This method is used in Stockholm County (Diderichsen *et al.* 1997; Andersson *et al.* 2000).

Because of the limitations associated with individual-level data, many risk-adjustment schemes use more aggregate data relating to the plan as a whole. Under the index approach, aggregate measures of the characteristics of a plan's population are combined to create an index that seeks to indicate the aggregate spending needs of the associated population. An example is Belgium's risk-adjustment scheme, which uses a series of indices based on such factors as demography, mortality, population density, proportion unemployed, proportion disabled and housing quality (DULBEA/KUL 1997; Schokkaert and van de Voorde 2000). The use of the index approach opens up the potential for an enormous increase in the data that can be used as the basis for capitation. In particular, where plans are based on geographical entities, aggregate population census data become available as the basis for setting expenditure targets.

However, a new problem emerges when such aggregate data are relied on to set capitation, in the form of the ecological fallacy (Selvin 1958). This is the possibility of identifying a relationship between a putative needs factor and health care expenditure at the aggregate level that does not hold at the individual level (the focus of capitation methods). This is because aggregate-level expenditure data may reflect both individual needs (legitimate factors) and supply considerations (illegitimate factors); disentangling the two using aggregate data poses profound methodological difficulties. Most analysts seem to have been aware of the potential for this problem, but they have often been constrained by data limitations. England's approach to identifying needs factors, using small areas with populations of about 10,000, appears to be the most technically advanced in this respect, and has been tested – although not always implemented – in Finland, Northern Ireland, Scotland and Spain (Carr-Hill *et al.* 1994; Häkkinen *et al.* 1996; Department of Health and Social Services 1997; Rico 1997; Scottish Executive Health Department 1999).

Several schemes use a hybrid approach. Preliminary capitation is based on a rudimentary matrix (based, say, on age and sex). The entire matrix is then adjusted by an index specific to each plan. This method is used in England, Northern Ireland, Scotland and Wales, where rudimentary capitation is set based on age (and sometimes sex) to which is applied a further adjustment based on an index of local population characteristics (Department of Health and Social Services 1997; NHS Executive 1997; Welsh Office 1998; Scottish Executive Health Department 1999). The method is also applied in Finland (Ministry of Social Affairs and Health 1996) and Italy (Mapelli 1998).

Given the data limitations of most systems, the personal (or plan-wide) factors on which any risk adjustment is to be based should in principle incorporate only those characteristics that are universally recorded (across all plans receiving funds), consistent, verifiable, free from perverse incentives, not vulnerable to manipulation and consistent with confidentiality requirements and plausible determinants of service needs. In practice, this severely limits the choice of variables, as limited information that conforms to such criteria is available on the joint characteristics of individuals. A further consideration is that capitation sums should in principle be updated regularly to reflect the rapid changes in health care technology and public preferences. However, this seems to have been considered unnecessary (or beyond technical capacity) in many systems.

The discussion implies that complex statistical and econometric considerations might surround the development of capitation based on empirical data. In principle, the methods used should be able to accommodate serious data limitations, to distinguish between legitimate and illegitimate sources of variation in utilization and to offer results that are statistically robust and readily implemented as a capitation formula. Use of the index approach can introduce the additional problem of the ecological fallacy. Although these methodological issues have been widely recognized, there have been few serious attempts to address them, and most current methods use fairly rudimentary statistical methods.

Findings

In this section, we summarize our findings for the 20 individual resource allocation schemes under scrutiny. Table 11.2 summarizes the resource allocation scheme, the plans to which financing is to be devolved, the needs factors used at an individual level, the needs factors defined at an aggregate level and any other notable features of the scheme.

Of the schemes surveyed, only Austria, Greece, Ireland and Luxembourg have no element of capitation. In Austria, citizens are assigned to a plan based on the sector of employment. Each plan must be self-financing, so premium levels vary depending on the risk profile of insured members. Greece also has employment-based insurance, subsidized in part by the national government, apparently based on historical accident and political judgement (Mossialos 1999). Ireland is unusual in having a basic health care system funded by taxation topped up by an extensively used private insurance sector (Kennedy 1996). This makes using capitation methods in the public sector difficult, as it is not easy to identify the level of private coverage in each of the eight health boards. The reimbursement of the public-sector regions is therefore based on activity (such as diagnosis-related groups). Although nominally using a system of social insurance with nine sickness funds, in practice Luxembourg pools the associated financing and therefore has no resource allocation problem of the type confronted by larger countries (Kerr 1999).

Capitation systems are largely based on empirical data and rely predominantly on analysing existing patterns of health care utilization. Exceptions include Spain, with no risk adjustment (Consejo de Politica Fiscal y Financiera 1998), Norway, where empirical results are moderated by political judgement (van den Noord *et al.* 1998), and Italy (Mapelli 1998), Portugal (Ministério da Sáude 1998) and Scotland (Scottish Executive Health Department 1999), which use indices of morbidity and mortality needs adjusters, without direct reference to the link with utilization.

Table 11.2 Description of the resource allocation schemes in 20 western European countries

Country	Scheme	Plans	Capitation: individual level	Capitation: plan level	Other factors
Austria	National insurance scheme	About 20 sickness funds (employment-based)	Not applicable	Not applicable	No risk-pooling between funds
Belgium	National Institute for Sickness and Disability Insurance risk-adjustment scheme	100 sickness funds (competitive)		Age, sex, unemployment, disability, mortality, urbanization	
Denmark	Local government financing system	16 regional councils (geography)	Age	Age, children of single parents	Local tax base
Finland	State subsidy system	452 municipalities (geography)	Age, disability	Archipelago, remoteness	Local tax base
England	Resource allocation formulae	100 health authorities (geography)	Age	Mortality, morbidity, unemployment, elderly people living alone, ethnic origin, socioeconomic status	Cost variation
France	Regional resource allocation	25 regions (geography)	Age		Phased implementation
Germany	Federal Insurance Office risk-adjustment scheme	Sickness funds (employment-based and competitive)	Age, sex		Fund's income base
Greece	National insurance scheme	About 40 sickness funds	Not applicable	Not applicable	Based on historical accident and political choice
Ireland	Regional resource allocation	8 health boards	Not applicable	Not applicable	Services funded based on diagnosis-related groups
Italy	Regional resource allocation system	21 regional governments (geography)	Age, sex	Mortality	One-third based on historical expenditure

Luxembourg	Union of Sickness Funds	9 sickness funds (employment)	Not applicable	Not applicable	Full risk-pooling
Netherlands	Central Sickness Fund Board risk-adjustment scheme	26 sickness funds (competitive)	Age, sex, welfare or disability status	Urbanization	Fund's income base
Northern Ireland	Health board allocation formula	4 health boards (geography)	Age, sex	Mortality, elderly living alone, welfare status, low birth weight	Rural cost adjustment
Norway	Local government financing system	19 county governments (geography)	Age, sex	Mortality, elderly living alone, marital status	Local tax base 50% based on diagnosis-related groups
Portugal	Regional health authority financing system	5 regional health authorities	Age	Relative 'burden of illness': diabetes, hypertension, tuberculosis, AIDS	84.5% based on historical expenditure
Scotland	Health authority revenue allocation scheme	15 health boards (geography)	Age, sex	Mortality	Rural costs
Spain	Regional resource allocation system	7 comunidades autónomas (regions) (geography)			Cross-boundary flows, declining population adjustment
Sweden	Stockholm County hospital resource allocation formula	9 health care authorities (geography)	Age, living alone, employment status, housing tenure, previous inpatient diagnosis		Phased implementation
Switzerland	Federal Association of Sickness Funds risk-adjustment scheme	Sickness funds (competitive)	Age, sex, region		Fund's income base
Wales	Health authority allocation formula	5 health authorities (geography)	Age, sex	Mortality	Cost adjustment for sparse population

Few systems adjust for 'unmet' need, although the issue of 'supplier-induced demand' has been the subject of some concern and has been central to the methods adopted in England (Carr-Hill *et al.* 1994). Although this has been a source of concern in other countries, there has been little practical effort to address the issue. An exception is Belgium, where there has been a considerable debate over whether to retain physician supply in the regression equations used to distribute funds to health plans (Schokkaert *et al.* 1998). The outcome has been that it has been excluded, meaning that health plans are not compensated for variation in physician supply available to their beneficiaries, even though the plans may have no control over the consequent variation in utilization.

Table 11.2 indicates the needs factors used for capitation at an individual level (corresponding to the matrix approach) and at the plan level (reflecting the index approach), confirming the widespread use of hybrid methods. In general, the schemes used within competitive markets use simpler methods and have been less adventurous than the population schemes, often basing risk adjustment on age and sex alone. This may reflect the lack of data on which capitation can be based or may result from the more complex political and legal environment within which the scheme must operate. Many of the geographically based schemes have been far more adventurous. They have sought, using a variety of methods, to link spending needs to a wide variety of social and demographic variables. The choice of needs factors appears to have been influenced more by availability of data than by compelling evidence of a link with needs for health care expenditure. Although a factor might be included in a capitation formula, it may not necessarily play an especially strong role in influencing the allocation of funds. The types of factors include demography, employment and disability status, geographical location, morbidity and mortality and social factors.

Demography. Only one scheme – that of Spain – fails to consider demographic factors in the form of age and (usually) sex groups. The crude per-capita allocation used in Spain seems to arise because securing a consensus more sensitive to needs is politically impossible (Consejo de Politica Fiscal y Financiera 1998).

Employment and disability status. Several mechanisms (for example, in the Netherlands and Northern Ireland) use a statutory measure of employment and/or disability status, such as social security categories, as the basis for adjusting risk. These indicators have the advantage that they are universally recorded and are regularly updated. Their principal disadvantages are that they are not specifically designed to capture variation in health care needs and that they are vulnerable to systematic misrecording or manipulation. Furthermore, they are weakest within the population for which risk adjustment is most important – those of pensionable age.

Geographical location. Geography may substantially influence expenditure for three reasons: variation in need (not captured by other factors), variation in the extent to which need is expressed (in the form of utilization) and variation in local health care supply and policy. Disentangling these sources of variation in health care costs is a profound problem that has rarely been seriously addressed. The typical approach, such as in the Netherlands, is to include all observed variation in local expenditure in the capitation formulae, although supply may cause some of the variation. Some public-sector schemes, such as those in Finland and the United Kingdom, adjust for the putative higher costs of delivering some services in rural areas using a variety of methods. England's system adjusts quite markedly for differences in input prices between the London area and the rest of the country (NHS Executive 1997).

Morbidity and mortality. Mortality rates (crude and standardized) are used in several schemes, such as in Belgium, Italy, Northern Ireland, Norway, Scotland and Wales. Morbidity is included explicitly in Portugal's scheme, and elsewhere is incorporated using statutory measures of permanent disability, such as those in use in Belgium, Finland and the Netherlands. The Northern Ireland formula for acute care includes a measure of low birth weight in infants. Measures of previous health care utilization or diagnosis of the type much used in the United States have rarely been used (Ash *et al.* 1989; Clark *et al.* 1995; Ellis *et al.* 1996; Fowles *et al.* 1996; Weiner 1996). The two main reasons for this appear to be a lack of suitable linked data and the fear of the perverse incentives (and potential for gaming) the use of such data introduce. Sweden is considering adopting a separate set of capitation sums for people who have previously experienced a hospital admission within a 'costly diagnosis group' (Andersson *et al.* 2000).

Social factors. Numerous social factors can be found in risk-adjustment schemes, their use being predominantly opportunistic – that is, usually based on data availability rather than a direct link to health care needs. Examples include:

- unemployment (Belgium, the Netherlands and Stockholm County);
- welfare status (the Netherlands and Northern Ireland);
- marital status (Norway and Stockholm County);
- family structure (France and Norway);
- housing quality (Belgium);
- housing tenure (Stockholm County);
- social class (Stockholm County);
- cohabitation (Northern Ireland and Stockholm County);
- income (Finland).

Although most schemes use an element of capitation, the extent to which it influences budgets varies substantially between countries. Norway makes the limited influence of the capitation scheme explicit by allocating 50 per cent of the budget according to previous activity as measured by diagnosis-related groups. This scheme has the explicit objective of seeking to encourage activity to reduce waiting lists. Many countries dampen budget expenditure prospectively by allowing budgets to be influenced by past spending levels. In England, a complicated 'pace of change' rule limits the speed at which health plans are expected to move towards capitation targets; in Italy and Portugal, regional budgets are a weighted average of past expenditure and capitated target.

Furthermore, the budgets set under a capitation scheme might be only indicative. For example, in the Scandinavian systems, local governments have some autonomy to vary expenditure from the capitated budget, financing the balance from local sources (local taxes or co-payments). Under competitive insurance systems, insurers are usually free to vary premiums from the assumed national level to finance variation in expenditure from the capitated budget.

Conclusions

Within health care systems of all types, the overarching objective of cost containment and a policy of devolved responsibility have placed an increasingly strong burden on strategic methods of allocating resources. Capitation has emerged as the favoured policy response in virtually all schemes. Significant exceptions are Ireland, where the strong private-sector presence makes public-sector capitation methods problematic, and Greece, where political considerations predominate. In general, however, there is a remarkable degree of unanimity that the need to set prospective budgets based on equitable criteria leads to the use of capitation methods in resource allocation.

Nevertheless, the focus of a capitation scheme is influenced somewhat by the health care system it seeks to serve. For example, systems of competitive insurance markets must focus on individuals. Their main objective is to minimize the potential for cream-skimming and the associated failure of the insurance market. The treatment of area-level effects on capitation (such as variation in input prices) is highly problematic within such schemes, as inadequately handling this may induce insurers to withdraw from offering coverage to entire areas, the crudest form of cream-skimming. Approaches to this are still in their infancy. The preoccupation with cream-skimming and the lack of alternative data may make using data on prior utilization attractive as a basis for adjusting risk in such settings. These data are very important indicators of future expenditure and are being implemented in the United States Medicare scheme (Health Care Financing Administration 1999). The potentially adverse consequences of using such data may be outweighed by the consequent reduction in cream-skimming opportunities.

Systems with captive insurance markets tend to be concerned more with demonstrating equitable treatment and avoiding perverse incentives at a population level. Thus, using data on prior utilization has been considered inappropriate, as it might adversely affect provider behaviour. There is, however, less need to be constrained to using individual-level data. The use of aggregate-level data opens up a richer source of information but has led to the use of quite elaborate statistical methods that may require careful audit.

The resource allocation systems in use have largely been chosen based on expediency, most notably in being strongly conditioned by the nature of the data available to policy-makers. Thus, many schemes have been constrained to the use of crude capitation adjustments for age and sex, in the full knowledge that such data are woefully inadequate but that they are all that are available and are better than nothing (Beck 2000). Given the very large sums of money redirected by strategic schemes for resource allocation, we have been surprised at the lack of investment in new data sources and think that there is a strong case for making such investment if the equity and efficiency objectives underlying capitation are genuinely considered important.

If suitable data were available, the matrix approach to setting capitation based on individual-level data, as epitomized in the Stockholm County model, is the most methodologically satisfactory method of setting capitation sums because it minimizes the ecological problem associated with the use of more aggregate data, although caution is still needed in accommodating potential supply effects (Carr-Hill et al. 2000). Imminent developments in information technology may lead to rapid increases in the availability of individual-level data, and policy-makers should be ready to take the opportunity they offer and, if possible, to influence the form they take. The main task confronting designers of data systems based on individual-level information is to develop objective indications of health status that can be used as sensitive indicators of expenditure needs. To date, most systems for inferring chronic diagnosis have been based on prior utilization and the attendant danger of introducing perverse incentives.

Variation in the cost of providing a standard level of service has been a concern in several of the schemes surveyed. The methods adopted have, on the whole, been rather rough and ready and have addressed major sources of cost variation, such as extreme remoteness. There appear to have been few satisfactory attempts to distinguish between legitimate and illegitimate sources of cost variation. This area of research may benefit from some fundamental conceptual study.

Fundamental to examining the suitability of a particular scheme is the issue of who carries the responsibility and who bears the risk for variation in expenditure from assumed resource allocation. Although many of the schemes examined appear very rudimentary, they are serving financing systems in which the budget holder does not necessarily bear a great deal of risk. This is often because – in one form or another – the central authority in practice bears a large part of the financial risk, for example by partly reimbursing excessive spending, by renegotiating budgets or by 'carving out' certain costly patients or procedures (Ettner et al. 2000). Alternatively, the health plan may be able to meet excessive spending by varying premiums or local tax rates. The capitation system cannot be considered in isolation from the risk-sharing arrangements in place, and there is scope for more research on how the two interact.

The financial risk a plan faces may be influenced by several factors, including:

- the use of historical expenditure as well as capitation as a basis for setting budgets, such as in Portugal;
- the use of other resource allocation mechanisms alongside capitation, such as the waiting list initiative in England or the federal hospital support programme in Switzerland;
- the willingness of the central authority to renegotiate budgets retrospectively, such as in Italy and Spain;
- the ability of the plans to vary their own sources of financing, including premiums or local taxes, such as in Scandinavia (taxes) and Switzerland (premiums);
- the extent to which the financing is designated for specific services;

- the ability of the plans to accumulate or run down reserves;
- the ability of the plans to vary the benefits on offer or the associated co-payments, such as in Finland; and
- more generally, the sanctions associated with overspending (ranging from the managerial imperative of meeting budget constraints in the United Kingdom to the virtual absence of sanctions found in France).

European health care systems are very diverse in all these dimensions, leading to variation in the priority attached to developing sensitive and robust capitation.

Thus, the financing system may influence the nature of the chosen resource allocation scheme and of any capitation methods adopted. For example, the magnitude of the private sector clearly influences the resource allocation methods used in Ireland and may be important in other schemes in which, for example, user charges form an important element of revenue. However, systems of financing and methods of resource allocation are not necessarily linked. Among the countries we surveyed, other influences, such as the availability of data, political preferences, risk-management arrangements and historical accident, seem to be just as influential in causing the variation reported.

Developing resource allocation mechanisms in general, and capitation methods in particular, requires reconciling several objectives, including:

- furthering society's objectives for health care;
- seeking to make resource allocation as sensitive as possible to legitimate health needs;
- seeking to make resource allocation as independent as possible from illegitimate factors;
- maximizing the availability of good-quality data on which the resource allocations can be based;
- minimizing the dysfunctional incentives introduced by the resource allocation mechanism;
- integrating systems of risk-sharing with resource allocation;
- designing health care systems that are impervious to the limitations of resource allocation schemes; and
- minimizing the costs of administering the resource allocation scheme.

Successfully addressing these issues is demanding and envisaging any system that satisfactorily reconciles them all is difficult. The schemes reviewed here offer a wide spectrum of experience and lessons. None can in any sense be held up as a model, and the most appropriate approach is likely to depend heavily on the institutional framework within which the resource allocation takes place. Nevertheless, we believe that the accumulated experience across European countries offers valuable lessons for policy-makers operating in almost all systems of health care financing.

Note

1 We thank more than 40 correspondents in 24 countries for their assistance in preparing this chapter. The chapter was greatly improved by the comments of the participants

at the European Observatory on Health Care Systems Workshop on Funding Health Care: Options for Europe (held in Venice, Italy in December 1999 and supported by the Veneto Region), especially René Christensen, Unto Häkkinen, Julian Le Grand and the organizers from the Observatory. We also thank the participants at the 1999 Spanish Health Economics Association meeting and a seminar at the University of Bergen.

References

Andersson, P-Å., Varde, E. and Diderichsen, F. (2000) Modelling of resource allocation to health care authorities in Stockholm County, *Health Care Management Science*, 3(2): 141–9.

Ash, A., Porell, F., Gruenberg, L., Sawitz, E. and Beiser, A. (1989) Adjusting Medicare payments using prior utilization data, *Health Care Financing Review*, 10(4): 17–29.

Beck, K. (1998) Competition under a regime of imperfect risk adjustment: the Swiss experience, *Sozial- und Präventivmedizin*, 43: 7–8.

Beck, K. (2000) Growing importance of capitation in Switzerland, *Health Care Management Science*, 3(2): 111–19.

Brown, L.D. and Amelung, V.E. (1999) 'Manacled competition': market reforms in German health care, *Health Affairs*, 18(3): 76–91.

Carr-Hill, R.A., Sheldon, T.A., Smith, P. *et al.* (1994) Allocating resources to health authorities: development of methods for small area analysis of use of inpatient services, *British Medical Journal*, 309: 1046–9.

Carr-Hill, R.A., Rice, N. and Smith, P. (2000) Towards locally based resource allocation in the NHS, in P. Smith (ed.) *Reforming Markets in Health Care: An Economic Perspective*. Buckingham: Open University Press.

Clark, D.O., von Korff, M., Saunders, K., Baluch, W.M. and Simon, G.E. (1995) A chronic disease score with empirically derived weights, *Medical Care*, 33(8): 783–95.

Consejo de Politica Fiscal y Financiera (Council on Fiscal and Financial Policy) (1998) Financiación de los servicios de sanidad en el periodo 1998–2001 [Financing of health services, 1998–2001], *Revista de Administración Sanitaria*, 11(6): 125–51.

Department of Health and Social Services (1997) *Allocation of Resources for the Northern Ireland Health and Personal Social Services: A Second Report from the Capitation Formula Review Group*. Belfast: Department of Health and Social Services.

Diderichsen, F., Varde, E. and Whitehead, M. (1997) Resource allocation to health authorities: the quest for an equitable formula in Britain and Sweden, *British Medical Journal*, 315: 875–8.

DULBEA/KUL (1997) *Dépenses normatives des organismes assureurs de soins de santé dans le cadre de l'instauration de la responsabilité financiére* [*Expenditure of Health Care Insurers within the Framework of the Introduction of Financial Responsibility*]. Brussels: DULBEA, Université Libre de Bruxelles.

Ellis, R.P., Pope, G.C., Iezzoni, L. *et al.* (1996) Diagnosis-based risk adjustment for Medicare capitation payments, *Health Care Financing Review*, 17(3): 101–28.

Emery, D.W., Fawson, C. and Herzberg, R.Q. (1997) The political economy of capitated managed care, *American Journal of Managed Care*, 3(3): 397–416.

Ettner, S.L., Frank, R.G., Mark, T. and Smith, M.W. (2000) Risk adjustment of capitation payments to behavioural health care carve-outs: how well do existing methodologies account for psychiatric disability?, *Health Care Management Science*, 3(2): 159–69.

Files, A. and Murray, M. (1995) German risk structure compensation: enhancing equity and effectiveness, *Inquiry*, 32: 300–9.

Fowles, J.B., Weiner, J.P., Knutson, D. *et al.* (1996) Taking health status into account when setting capitation rates: a comparison of risk-adjustment methods, *Journal of the American Medical Association*, 276(16): 1316–21.

Giacomini, M., Luft, H.S. and Robinson, J.C. (1995) Risk adjusting community rated health plan premiums: a survey of risk assessment literature and policy applications, *Annual Review of Public Health*, 16: 401–30.

Häkkinen, U., Mikkola, H., Nordberg, M. and Salonen, M. (1996) *Tutkimus kuntien terveyspalveluiden valtionosuuksien perusteista [A Study on the Foundations of the State Subsidies for Municipal Health Services]*. Helsinki: Sisäasiainministeriö (Ministry of the Interior).

Haut Comité de la Santé Publique (High Committee on Public Health) (1999) *Allocation régionale des ressources et réduction des inégalités de santé [Regional Allocation of Resources and Reducing Inequality in Health]*. Paris: Haut Comité de la Santé Publique.

Health Care Financing Administration (1999) *Medicare + Choice Rates 2000: 45 Day Notice*. Washington, DC: Health Care Financing Administration.

Hoffmeyer, U. and McCarthy, T. (eds) (1994) *Financing Health Care*. Dordrecht: Kluwer Academic.

Hutchison, B., Hurley, J., Reid, R. *et al.* (1999) *Capitation Formulae for Integrated Health Systems: A Policy Synthesis*. Hamilton: Centre for Health Economics and Policy Analysis, McMaster University.

Kennedy, A. (1996) Private health insurance in Ireland: the advent of a competitive market and a risk equalisation scheme, in Alliance Nationale des Mutualités Chrétiennes (ed.) *Risk Structure Compensation*. Brussels: Alliance Nationale des Mutualités Chrétiennes.

Kerr, E. (1999) *Health Care Systems in Transition: Luxembourg*. Copenhagen: European Observatory on Health Care Systems.

Mapelli, V. (1998) *L'allocazione delle risorse nel Servizio Sanitario Nazionale [Resource Allocation in Italy's National Health Service]*. Rome: Commissione Tecnica per la Spesa Pubblica, Ministero del Tesoro, del Bilancio e della Programmazione Economica (Ministry of Treasury, Budget and Economic Planning).

McCarthy, T., Davies, K., Gaisford, J. and Hoffmeyer, U. (1995) *Risk-adjustment and its Implications for Efficiency and Equity in Health Care Systems*. Basle: Pharmaceutical Partners for Better Healthcare.

Ministério da Sáude (Ministry of Health) (1998) *Orçamento do SNS para 1999 (Orçamento Ordinário) – Critérios de Financiamento [Portugal's National Health Service Budget for 1999 – Financing Criteria]*. Lisbon: Ministério da Sáude.

Ministry of Social Affairs and Health (1996) *The Health Care System in Finland*. Helsinki: Ministry of Social Affairs and Health.

Mossialos, E. (1999) Health care and cost containment in Greece, in E. Mossialos and J. Le Grand (eds) *Health Care and Cost Containment in the European Union*. Aldershot: Ashgate.

Mossialos, E. and Le Grand, J. (eds) (1999) *Health Care and Cost Containment in the European Union*. Aldershot: Ashgate.

Newhouse, J.P. (1994) Patients at risk: health reform and risk adjustment, *Health Affairs* (*Millwood*), 13(1): 135–46.

Newhouse, J.P. (1996) Reimbursing health plans and health providers: efficiency in production versus selection, *Journal of Economic Literature*, 34: 1236–63.

Newhouse, J.P. (1998) Risk adjustment: where are we now?, *Inquiry*, 35: 122–31.

NHS Executive (1997) *HCHS Revenue Resource Allocation to Health Authorities: Weighted Capitation Formulas*. Leeds: NHS Executive.

Oliver, A.J. (1999) *Risk Adjusting Health Care Resource Allocations: Theory and Practice in the United Kingdom, the Netherlands and Germany*. London: Office of Health Economics.

Rattso, J. (ed.) (1998) *Fiscal Federalism and State-Local Finance*. Cheltenham: Edward Elgar.

Rice, N. and Smith, P. (1999) *Approaches to Capitation and Risk Adjustment in Health Care: An International Survey.* York: Centre for Health Economics, University of York.

Rice, N. and Smith, P.C. (2000) Capitation and risk adjustment in health care, *Health Care Management Science*, 3(2): 73–5.

Rico, A. (1997) *Descentralización y reforma sanitaria en España [Decentralization and Reform of Health Care in Spain].* Madrid: Centro de Estudios Avanzados en Ciencias Sociales (Center for Advanced Study in the Social Sciences).

Schokkaert, E. and van de Voorde, C. (2000) Risk adjustment and the fear of markets: the case of Belgium, *Health Care Management Science*, 3(2): 121–30.

Schokkaert, E.G., Dhaene, G. and van de Voorde, C. (1998) Risk adjustment and the trade-off between efficiency and risk selection: an application of the theory of fair compensation, *Health Economics*, 7: 465–80.

Scottish Executive Health Department (1999) *Fair Shares for All.* Edinburgh: Scottish Executive Health Department.

Selvin, H.C. (1958) Durkheim's 'suicide' and problems of empirical research, *American Journal of Sociology*, 63: 607–19.

Swartz, K. (1998) The view from here: risk selection and Medicare + Choice: beware, *Inquiry*, 35: 101–3.

van Barneveld, E.M., van Vliet, R.C.J.A. and van de Ven, W.P.M.M. (1996) Mandatory high-risk pooling: an approach to reducing incentives for cream skimming, *Inquiry*, 33: 133–43.

van de Ven, W.P.M.M. and Ellis, R. (2000) Risk adjustment in competitive health plan markets, in J.P. Newhouse and A.J. Culyer (eds) *Handbook of Health Economics.* Amsterdam: North-Holland.

van de Ven, W.P.M.M, van Vliet, R.C., van Barneveld, E.M. and Lamers, L.M. (1994) Risk-adjusted capitation: recent experiences in the Netherlands, *Health Affairs*, 13(5): 120–36.

van den Noord, P., Hagen, T. and Iversen, T. (1998) *The Norwegian Health Care System*, Economics Department Working Papers No. 198. Paris: Organisation for Economic Co-operation and Development.

van Vliet, R.C.J.A. and van de Ven, W.P.M.M. (1993) Capitation payments based on prior hospitalizations, *Health Economics*, 2: 177–88.

Weiner, J.P. (1996) Risk-adjusted Medicare capitation rates using ambulatory and in-patient diagnoses, *Health Care Financing Review*, 17(4): 77–100.

Welsh Office (1998) *Allocation of Health Authority Discretionary Resources in Wales (1998).* Cardiff: Welsh Office.

Ziekenfondsraad (Dutch Health Insurance Council) (1999) *Budgettering Ziekenfondswet 1999 [Budgeting of Sickness Funds in the Netherlands, 1999].* Amstelveend: Ziekenfondsraad.

chapter twelve

Funding health care in Europe: weighing up the options

Elias Mossialos and Anna Dixon

Introduction

The chapters in this book have analysed the advantages and disadvantages of different methods of funding health care and how they are implemented in different countries. In this chapter, we synthesize the evidence and evaluate different funding systems against a set of policy objectives.[1] Equity and efficiency are perhaps the most important of these. They are highly contentious concepts and their meanings are debated extensively elsewhere (Le Grand 1991a; Light 1992; Culyer and Wagstaff 1993). Here we simply assess the different funding systems against the following objectives.

- Is the funding system progressive (vertically equitable)?
- Is the funding system horizontally equitable?
- Does funding result in redistribution?
- How does the funding system affect coverage and access to health care?
- How does the funding system affect cost containment?
- How does the funding system affect the wider economy?
- How does the funding system affect allocative efficiency and technical efficiency?

The first four of these are related to equity and the last three to efficiency. In dealing with the question of redistribution, we examine the combined effect of progressivity and the incidence of public spending on health care. We also examine to what extent health care funding systems are path dependent – that is, whether 'history matters', whether today's choices are limited by what has gone before (Putnam *et al.* 1993).

The evidence about how revenue collection mechanisms affect public policy objectives is by no means exhaustive. For example, the impact on equity of access is difficult to measure, hence the evidence is scarce. There is some evidence on how different funding mechanisms affect cost containment. However, any possible links between revenue collection and allocative and technical efficiency are less easy to determine. Indeed, to the extent that these are more a function of purchasing than revenue collection, the links may not exist at all. However, certain methods of collection may have indirect implications for allocative and technical efficiency resulting from their associated market structure of pooling and purchasing.

This chapter synthesizes material presented in the previous chapters with additional evidence from the national and international literature. Because most health care systems are funded from a mixture of sources, the relative importance of these sources also affects the overall impact.

Is the funding system progressive (vertically equitable)?

To answer this question, we need to examine who pays and how much. In determining who pays, there is an important difference between statutory or formal incidence and economic or effective incidence. Statutory incidence refers to the legal responsibility for the payment; for example, both the employer and employee for social health insurance contributions or the consumers for value-added tax. Economic incidence measures where the burden of payment actually falls: prices, wages or profit – or often a combination of all three. Empirical evidence conflicts as to the true economic incidence of different payments.

Generally, vertical equity is concerned with the extent to which the system is progressive (affluent people pay proportionately more), proportional (both affluent and poor people pay equal proportions) or regressive (affluent people pay proportionately less). A variety of indices have been developed to measure vertical equity, the most common of which is the Kakwani Progressivity Index (Kakwani 1977). It measures the extent to which funding systems depart from proportionality (= 0), with positive values indicating progressivity and negative values regressivity.

Taxation

Taxation is more than simply a means of raising revenue. It has a normative and political component in so far as it reflects a society's understanding of a reasonable and equitable distribution of the tax burden (Ervik 1998). Where general taxation funds health care, the effect on equity of the welfare state in general versus health care in particular often cannot be distinguished. Some of the empirical evidence presented on taxation, therefore, draws on wider literature on the welfare state.

An analysis of the progressivity of health care financing in OECD (Organisation for Economic Co-operation and Development) countries using data from the 1980s and early 1990s (Wagstaff *et al.* 1999)[2] found that direct taxes were progressive in all countries, whereas indirect taxes were regressive in all countries except Spain (in 1980).[3] In the countries in which taxes fund most health care, the mix of direct and indirect taxes renders overall taxation mildly progressive (between 0.04 and 0.06 on the Kakwani Progressivity Index).

The progressivity of income taxation depends on two factors: the number of marginal tax bands and the rate of each band. In Europe, reforms of the tax systems in the 1980s focused on broadening the tax base and treating different sources of income more equally. These measures would have reduced any negative impact on the wider economy and the burden on particular sources of income. However, these reforms were combined with a reduction in the number of tax bands and a lowering of marginal tax rates, both of which reduce progressivity. Research using household micro-data sets from the Luxembourg Income Study analysed inequality before and after income tax among households in Australia, Canada, France, Germany, the Netherlands, Sweden, Switzerland, the United Kingdom and the United States. Income tax appears to be progressive in each of the countries studied, with income being transferred from the 20 per cent of the population with the highest incomes to the other quintiles. In Australia, Canada, Germany, the Netherlands and the United Kingdom, income is transferred from the most affluent 40 per cent to the least affluent 60 per cent of the population (Zandvakili 1994).[4] Data for central and eastern Europe and the former Soviet Union are more difficult to obtain. Personal income tax rates at the level of the average wage in 1997 were 10 per cent in the Czech Republic, 18 per cent in Poland and 25 per cent in Estonia. Income transfer in these countries plays an important role in reducing poverty in each stage of the life cycle. Data suggest that, of the people with an income under the poverty line before income transfers, more than 80 per cent are lifted above the poverty line by transfers in the Czech Republic and Slovakia and about 50 per cent in Hungary and Poland. This compares with less than 30 per cent in the United States (Kangas 2000).

Indirect taxes on goods and services are usually charged as a percentage of the price; consumption patterns, therefore, determine the distribution of the burden of payment. Data for the United Kingdom show that households in the bottom income decile pay 32 per cent of gross income in indirect taxes compared with 11 per cent for the top income decile (Glennerster 1997). From a health point of view, the imposition of high indirect taxes on products harmful to health is justified to reduce consumption of these products. Some people argue against further increasing taxes on cigarettes – on income distributional grounds – because taxes constitute a larger proportion of income of poor people than affluent people (Manning *et al.* 1989). Research on the relative price elasticity of demand for cigarettes shows that low-income consumers are more price responsive and are therefore more likely to give up smoking (Townsend *et al.* 1994). However, the greater consumption among low-income groups of such products as cigarettes and alcohol keep indirect taxes regressive on average.

Local taxes are generally less progressive than national taxes, as they are more often proportional, although progressive local income taxes are feasible. Wagstaff *et al.* (1999) show that the income taxation by national governments in Denmark, Finland, Sweden and Switzerland is more progressive (higher Kakwani Progressivity Index) than the taxes levied by lower levels of government. Following a major economic recession in Finland during the early 1990s, the progressivity of local income taxes declined because the average rate increased and because tax rates rose most in the least affluent municipalities (Klavus and Häkkinen 1998). In addition, increased user charges further reduced progressivity during this period.

Social health insurance

Social health insurance originated in compensation schemes set up to cover loss of income during times of ill health. As a result contributions were, and still are, proportional to income. Unlike taxation systems, the objective of income redistribution has not been of major concern in their design, and data on the progressivity of compulsory social health insurance schemes are, therefore, also more limited. Social health insurance can be more regressive because it only levies contributions on earned income. Income from investments and savings which are exempt from contributions are higher among those with high incomes.

Wagstaff *et al.* (1999) found social health insurance to be regressive in Germany, the Netherlands and Spain (in 1980).[5] In each case part of the population (determined by income in Germany and the Netherlands, and civil servant status in Spain) opt out of the statutory health insurance system. About 12 per cent of the population in Germany choose to remain in the statutory system or to purchase private health insurance (self-employed people are excluded from the statutory scheme, as are permanent public employees). Nine per cent of the population are covered by private health insurance. In the Netherlands, 31 per cent of the population is required to opt out. This results in a concentration of people on lower incomes and higher risk[6] in the statutory health insurance schemes and consequently higher contribution rates. To address this problem, a levy placed on the private insurers in the Netherlands was used to subsidize the statutory insurance funds (Wagstaff and van Doorslaer 1997). This has been subject to legal challenge and it is not clear whether it will be allowed to continue.

In contrast the Netherlands, contributions to the AWBZ (universal public insurance for long-term care and long-stay treatment) are marginally progressive. Wagstaff and van Doorslaer (1997) attempted to determine the source of progressivity in the AWBZ system. Under the first simulation, removing the income ceiling (above which contributions are not levied) made the system significantly more progressive. Removing exemptions from contributions (which exist for pensioners and other groups) would make the distribution more regressive (Wagstaff and van Doorslaer 1997). This provides empirical support for the logical assertion that upper-income ceilings render social health insurance more regressive, whereas exemptions for low-income groups or minimum thresholds increase progressivity. Germany combines a proportional income contribution with a ceiling above which income is exempt. The introduction of a 10 per cent contribution rate for those on incomes below €322 per month in Germany in 1999 is likely to have increased the regressivity of financing (see Chapter 3). Where there is no income ceiling and no exemption or opting out of the social insurance scheme, such as in France, the progressivity of social health insurance contributions and taxation do not appear to differ systematically.

Introducing insurer competition in the Netherlands appears to have had very little effect on progressivity. The burden on middle-income groups has increased slightly and declined slightly for high-income groups; for the low-income groups, the reforms have been neutral (Müller *et al.* 2000).

Private health insurance

Data on the characteristics of subscribers to all types of private health insurance in the European Union show a concentration of high-income individuals (see Chapter 6). In Germany, where the decision to leave the statutory scheme is voluntary for those on high incomes, the take-up of private health insurance still varies substantially according to age, place of residence,[7] gender and employment. In France, where as many as 85 per cent of the population have supplementary insurance, people with lower incomes, non-French citizens and people aged 20–24 years or over 70 years are all less likely to be covered by supplementary health insurance.

Wagstaff *et al.* (1999) found private health insurance to be regressive where it was the major source of coverage – in Switzerland (before 1996) and the United States. Private health insurance was also found to be regressive in France, Ireland and Spain, proportional to income in Finland and progressive in Denmark, Germany, Italy, the Netherlands, Portugal and the United Kingdom (Wagstaff *et al.* 1999). Where private health insurance was progressive, this applied within the group of those with private health insurance and may not necessarily contribute to the overall progressivity of the system. It can be argued that encouraging people with high incomes to purchase supplementary or complementary health insurance will increase the progressivity of the financing system, as the rich will pay a greater proportion than those on low incomes (providing that this is not done using tax subsidies). However, in some countries, private health insurance skews the provision of services to favour affluent people (see Chapter 6).

Medical savings accounts

Medical savings accounts do not pool funds or risks and thus do not redistribute between rich and poor or healthy and sick. Medical savings accounts act solely as a personal savings account: distributing resources over an individual's life cycle from periods of good health to periods of ill health. Accounts are individual and there are no transfers between households with high and low income. In Singapore, the problems faced by low-income households in financing health services led to the establishment of a public fund, Medifund, to finance the costs of health care for poor people.

Medical savings accounts were introduced in the United States under the Health Insurance Portability and Availability Act of 1996. Several incentives were introduced for people to save – tax-free interest on savings, tax deduction on contributions to the medical savings account and allowing the money to be used for other purposes on retirement, death or disability. This means that medical savings accounts benefit high-rate taxpayers, those with surplus income to save and those with a low risk of ill health. Thus, in the United States, where medical savings accounts operate in parallel with traditional private health insurance, they may concentrate higher risks in the regular health insurance market, increase premiums and increase the number of uninsured people (Jefferson 1999). Other studies have also shown that the appeal of high-deductible plans to younger and healthier workers can split the insurance market. Premiums for traditional plans would rise, forcing more people to forego insurance coverage (Moon *et al.* 1996). Empirical evaluation of the effect of medical savings accounts in the United States is limited, as fewer accounts have been established than expected – only 50,172 accounts had been established by June 1998, well below the cap of 600,000 set in the initial legislation (Jefferson 1999). However, it seems that they will contribute to the regressivity of the financing system.

Out-of-pocket payments

User charges have been justified on the grounds that they improve efficiency, equity and quality. Equity benefits can only be achieved if revenue is targeted at poor and underserved people and an effective exemption scheme is implemented. Both industrialized and developing countries have had great difficulty in achieving equitable systems of formal charging. The additional income often paves the way for tax cuts, which typically benefit more affluent people.

User charges fall more heavily on high users of health care services – that is, ill people – and can be highly regressive because ill health and low income are correlated. According to Wagstaff *et al.* (1999) direct payments are highly regressive, showing negative values between –0.4 and 0 on the Kakwani Progressivity Index. These contribute significantly to the overall regressivity of financing particularly in countries where direct payments account for a high proportion of the financing mix (such as Portugal, Switzerland and the USA). A study of out-of-pocket payments in Croatia showed that the lowest income quartile paid 5 per cent of income in co-payments versus 0.6 per cent of income for the highest income quartile. Combined with other direct payments, including informal payments, the financing becomes even more regressive – those on a low income pay 17.3 per cent of income versus 2.9 per cent of income for the highest income group (Mastilica and Bozikov 1999).

Is the funding system horizontally equitable?

Treating individuals at the same income level differently gives rise to horizontal inequity. In other words, horizontal equity requires that people with the same income and wealth pay the same (Wagstaff *et al.* 1993).

Taxation

Collecting and spending taxes locally may create regional inequity if there is no national system of redistribution. For example, data from Switzerland, where federal and cantonal taxes account for 25 per cent of total health expenditure (in 1997), show large variation in the burden of taxation in different cantons. If 100 represents the national average, the lowest tax burden is in Zug (55.5) and the highest in Jura (135.3) (Swiss Federal Statistical Office 2000). However, national revenues may be used to equalize resources between regions. For example, in Sweden, in addition to local taxation, the population pays national taxes and contributions, which are then used to subsidize less affluent regions.

In a complementary analysis to the study of progressivity of health care funding, van Doorslaer et al. (1999) assessed the extent of horizontal equity of different funding sources. Differential treatment has the greatest impact in Portugal, with different tax rules applying to wage earners and self-employed people. Tax rates vary geographically in Denmark and Sweden and thus there are significant horizontal inequities.

Social health insurance

Horizontal equity would be violated in social health insurance systems if:

- different sickness funds apply different contribution rates;
- certain occupational groups or regions have concentrations of people with low incomes or high risks; and
- membership of funds is determined by location or occupation.

In the Netherlands, sickness funds' activities were limited within regional boundaries from 1964 until the implementation of the 1988 Dekker Committee proposals to allow insurers to offer insurance throughout the country. All funds have now opted to extend coverage to the entire country. Before 1996, Germany's social health insurance system was partly segmented according to occupation. For this reason, contribution rates differed greatly between the sickness funds, with high-risk occupational groups subject to the highest rates. One motivation for the Health Care Structure Act of 1993 was to reduce contribution rate differences by allowing choice of fund and by redistributing contributions among funds (Busse 2000). Thus, in 1994, 27 per cent of all members paid a contribution rate differing by more than 1 per cent from the average. This fell to only 7 per cent of all members in 1999 following enactment of the 1993 legislation (Busse 2000). Thus, competitive social health insurance systems such as in the Netherlands and Germany have lower measures of horizontal inequities than social health insurance systems with geographically and/or occupationally defined funds such as in Austria.

Private health insurance

Premiums for individual private health insurance are usually risk rated based on the actuarial risk of becoming ill or needing health care. Risk-rated premiums are unrelated to income, so two people with the same income are likely to be paying different premiums. For example, a person who has a family history of disease pays a high premium; another who has no family history of disease nor any pre-existing condition pays a low premium. Thus, risk rated pools violate horizontal equity. However, evidence from France suggests that horizontal equity does not seem to be an issue in access to supplementary health insurance (Bocognano *et al.* 2000).

Out-of-pocket payments

Many countries apply exemptions to overcome some of the equity problems associated with user charges. If these are related to income or means tested, then they may reduce the regressivity of payments. However, if exemptions are based on factors other than income, such as age or disease, they may result in horizontal inequity. Horizontal inequity arising from out-of-pocket payments is in part due to variations in the utilization of health care at a given income level. Variations in utilization within any income level (which to some extent reflect the incidence of ill health) are, however, likely to be random. Inequities may also result from different choices. For example, the choice to buy supplementary insurance to cover co-payments in France. However, the distribution of supplementary insurance coverage is related to income (Chapter 6) and therefore variations between income levels (vertical equity) are likely to be greater than variations within a given income level. Levels of co-payment also vary between geographic areas (municipalities in Finland, local sickness funds in Germany), by occupational status (sickness funds in Austria) and by type of employment (e.g. salaried versus self-employed in Belgium, France and the Netherlands) (van Doorslaer *et al.* 1999).

Does funding result in redistribution?

The redistributive effect depends on both the progressivity of revenue collection (discussed above) and the incidence of public spending. Accounting for both factors may produce a different picture compared with analysing only one factor. These are two separate issues, but the combination raises interesting policy questions. For example, a proportional system must distribute benefits unequally to obtain the same redistributive effect as a progressive system (Ervik 1998). If more revenue could be generated through a less progressive system of collection but public spending disproportionately benefited low-income people, the net effect might be better for those on a low income than a case in which collection is more progressive but less is collected and public spending does not benefit those on a low income as much. In some countries, it is difficult to disentangle the redistributive effect of health care spending from overall public spending that may also aim at redistribution. Indeed, because health care is usually delivered as an in-kind rather than cash benefit, its incidence is hard to measure.

Gaining a complete picture of the redistributive effect of a system requires a longitudinal perspective. If a system is analysed at one point in time, this fails to account for the life-cycle (inter-temporal) redistribution between periods of wealth (or health) to periods of relative poverty (or ill health). Most studies of redistributive effect are cross-sectional, focusing on one point in time. Longitudinal studies of the welfare state generally show a redistribution from 'lifetime richest' to 'lifetime poorest', but the redistribution is relatively flat. To this extent, the welfare state is more of a savings bank than a Robin Hood-style redistribution (Hills 1995). Here, we limit the analysis to taxation and social health insurance.

Taxation

A study of the redistributive effect of tax and benefit systems in eight countries showed that, in the early 1990s, Sweden redistributed most, reducing income inequality by 50 per cent. The United States redistributed least, reducing inequality in income by less than 20 per cent. Of the European countries in the study, the United Kingdom redistributed least, reducing income inequality by 25 per cent. Denmark and Germany reduced income inequality by more than 40 per cent. The study concluded, however, that social transfers accounted for most of the redistributive effect rather than taxation (Ervik 1998). This suggests less progressive tax systems are being combined with targeted benefits.

A study of the effect of taxes and benefits on household incomes in 1998–99 in the United Kingdom shows that the final income of those in the bottom quintile of original income averaged 300 per cent of original income versus 69 per cent for the top quintile. Again, this was mostly the result of public spending and not taxation. In fact, the study indicates that the tax system was slightly regressive because of indirect taxes, with the bottom quintile paying 40 per cent of gross income in tax and the top quintile paying only 36 per cent of gross income (Commission on Taxation and Citizenship 2000).

There have been some attempts to measure health care utilization by income groups to ascertain the distribution of in-kind benefits. Le Grand (1978) specifically investigated the redistributive effect of the UK NHS, analysing the distribution of benefits among different income groups. Le Grand (1982) argued that whereas cash benefits were highly redistributive, going largely to poor people, services in kind were different, benefiting the more articulate middle class. He found that the distribution of health care benefits disproportionally favoured the higher income groups when adjusted for need.

The redistributive effect of taxation for long-term care in the United Kingdom is profound both between men and women and between low-income and high-income groups. A shift from long-term care funded by taxes or social insurance to private long-term care insurance would adversely affect women and low-income groups. Simulations have shown that such a switch would be regressive, with the lower-income deciles losing as much as £16,000 and most people in the upper-income deciles benefiting (Burchardt *et al.* 1996).

Social health insurance

Germany's statutory health insurance system illustrates three types of interpersonal redistribution.

1 The renunciation of experience rating implies a considerable volume of *ex-ante* vertical and horizontal redistribution, because individual health risks vary widely.
2 The scope of interpersonal redistribution is increased because:
   - dependants are insured at no extra cost – they are implicitly included in calculating contribution rates and benefits, suggesting some income redistribution from single people and couples to people in large families; and
   - all insured people are equally entitled to health care services, which are not related to the length or amount of previous contributions.
3 Inter-generational redistribution occurs between employed and retired people. This is likely to increase as the proportion of elderly people in the population grows and life expectancy rises. It has been estimated that payments to social health insurance will exceed the present value of the lifetime benefits for all cohorts born after the 1960/1970 cohorts (Hinrichs 1997).

Lutz and Schneider (1998) further analysed the redistributive effect of social health insurance using data from 1990. They found that contributions did not facilitate income equalization efficiently and that the tax-transfer system should be used instead to obtain the goal of income redistribution (Lutz and Schneider 1998). Schmahl (1998) reached the same conclusions, arguing that using insurance contributions linked to earnings to achieve interpersonal redistribution has negative economic effects and that redistribution should instead be achieved through general public budgets.

In Germany, interpersonal redistribution takes place between recipients at different earning levels because family members who have no earnings are insured at no extra cost, as are spouses under long-term care insurance. Longitudinally, this results in inter-temporal or life-cycle redistribution. When the health insurance system was established, the family structure and life cycle was more uniform, so that coverage for dependants without additional contributions did not affect the equity of the system (Lutz and Schneider 1998). However, the long-term care insurance established much more recently perpetuates the marriage-centred nature of social welfare (Scheiwe 1997). One redistributive effect of social health insurance is from single households to families with children (Hinrichs 1995). These subsidies of families with children mean that private health insurance is especially attractive for single people and double-income couples; conversely, it explains why people with children who are eligible to opt out of the statutory system choose to remain in it (Busse 2000).

There is also significant redistribution between the working population and pensioners, who only pay half the contribution on pension income. As the dependency ratio increases, inter-generational redistribution increases. Calculations suggest that, without the subsidies to pensioners and dependants, the average contribution rate could have been reduced by one-half in 1988 (Hinrichs 1995).

How does the funding system affect coverage and access to health care?

The system of revenue collection may affect both access to insurance coverage and access to health care services. Countries in which private health insurance is the sole form of coverage for much of the population have the most extreme differences in access to insurance coverage. In the United States, for example, 17 per cent of the non-elderly population are eligible for Medicaid and 71 per cent have private insurance coverage, which leaves 12 per cent of the population uninsured. Over half of uninsured people are either self-employed or working in firms with fewer than 25 employees (Kaiser Family Foundation 2000). Access to insurance is determined by several factors: formal employment, the size of the employer and the status of the employer (public or private sector), any pre-existing condition and the ability of an individual to afford the insurance premium. The right to benefit from private insurance coverage is determined by income in Ireland, Germany and the Netherlands and is available to civil servants in Germany and Spain.

Private long-term care insurance displays many of the features of private health insurance but is further exacerbated by the fact that up to one-third of people in their sixties (the age at which most policies are taken out) report mobility or health problems. Thus, many people would be excluded or face high premiums (Burchardt *et al.* 1996). Such problems can be overcome if the policy is purchased at a younger age, but young people have too little information on the prevalence of risk to assess their need for insurance.

Coverage is not necessarily universal in social health insurance systems; rather, eligibility may be limited to certain income groups or occupational groups or may depend on contributions made. However, in western Europe, coverage through a publicly funded health care system is virtually universal in most countries except Germany and the Netherlands. The introduction of competition in social health insurance systems has increased the risk borne by the insurer and has therefore introduced the possibility of (covert) cream-skimming.[8] However, analysis of current sickness fund data suggests that the risk-adjustment formula with integrated diagnostic cost groups may be sufficient to prevent risk selection (Müller *et al.* 2000).

Low- and middle-income countries have been attempting to achieve universal coverage by extending coverage to groups such as self-employed people and low-income workers. Another challenge is extending coverage to elderly, unemployed and disabled people. Many countries in central and eastern Europe and the former Soviet Union enshrined a universal right to health care in the constitution. Thus, social health insurance was required to provide coverage for the whole population from the outset. This has been much more difficult to achieve in practice. In the countries that have introduced social health insurance, the state covers the contributions of the non-employed population through taxation. This population is eligible for the same benefits as employed people, thus guaranteeing equity of access. If this is not the case, in countries with limited formal employment, the usual result is an explicitly inequitable arrangement. The social health insurance system has a pool of lower risks, higher-income beneficiaries and has more highly paid providers. Systems funded by general tax revenue are often a poor system for poor people. As wage-related contributions are not sufficient to provide universal benefits, the funds rely on subsidies from government revenue to cover deficits. Informal payments cover the 'deficits' at the provider level.

In some countries, social health insurance operates as a parallel system, whereby people in certain occupations receive care superior to that offered to the rest of the population funded through taxation. Insurance funds may be exclusive: members of insurance funds cannot access national health service facilities or coverage may be duplicated, providing for services also covered by the statutory system (double coverage). In Portugal, for example, occupational insurance funds cover 25 per cent of the population, allowing members access to private physicians, more rapid access to hospital services and certain services not available from the national health service (Dixon and Mossialos 2000).

Even if access to services is universal in theory, practice may present other barriers. Studies of health care utilization reveal skewed distributions relative to need: high-income groups utilize services more than low-income groups, which have greater need (Wagstaff *et al.* 1993). There may be several barriers to utilization – both financial and non-financial – and reasons why some groups are more proactive in seeking care or offered additional services. Gaining access to services in kind could be costly, both in time and in earnings foregone. Many poor people can afford the time less than affluent people and are less able to push for good service (Le Grand 1982).

Systems of universal coverage with user charges negatively affect equity of access, deterring both necessary and unnecessary utilization, especially among lower-income groups. Growing evidence from the United States and Europe shows that user charges deter access to health care services. Research from the United States suggests that cost-sharing can deter the utilization of appropriate health services and affect those on low incomes disproportionately. Furthermore, user charges were linked to poorer health outcomes on several indicators (Newhouse and the Insurance Experiment Group 1993). Additional research in Europe confirms the deterrent effect of charging. Research in France shows that socioeconomic groups differ more in physician consultations and purchase of medicines than in access to hospital care. This may be because the first two are not fully reimbursed (Jourdain 2000). Research in Sweden using data from the 1990s shows the re-emergence of inequality in utilization favouring affluent people following major increases in user charges (Whitehead *et al.* 1997). Elofsson *et al.* (1998) have shown that user charges hinder financially and psychosocially disadvantaged groups seeking care in the Stockholm area. Those who assessed their financial situation as being poor were ten times more likely to forego care as those who assessed their financial situation as being good. In Denmark, despite an overall increase in demand for dental care, household income has been positively related to the probability of obtaining regular dental care, with utilization being higher at higher incomes (Schwarz 1996).

The more significant role of out-of-pocket funding in the United States is reflected in the results of another international survey into the affordability of care. Eighteen per cent of people in the United States reported having difficulty paying medical bills compared with just 3 per cent in the United Kingdom and 5 per cent in Canada. Twelve per cent of people in Australia and 15 per cent in New Zealand reported not having filled a prescription because they could not afford it. In the United States, financial problems and lack of access to health care are most prevalent among uninsured people (Donelan et al. 1999). User charges, whether from high co-payments or lack of insurance, reduce ability to afford health care and appear to heighten anxiety and result in foregoing services.

Nevertheless, user charges have some appeal for low- and middle-income countries as a way of mobilizing additional revenue: first, because establishing prepayment health funding is difficult in a dire economic environment and, second, because of the pre-existing informal payments. In these countries, the revenue base for employment-related contributions or taxation is extremely limited because unemployment is high, a high proportion of labour is in agriculture, self-employed or informal and the informal economy is large. Charging, therefore, is one of the few ways of mobilizing any revenue at all. However, substantial evidence indicates that fees disproportionately affect the rural poor.

There is much less evidence on how informal payments affect utilization because obtaining information is difficult. However, where these are required *ex-ante* (in some countries in both western and eastern Europe), patients who cannot afford the payments either cannot obtain treatment or access the same level of services or have to wait longer for it. In addition to the financial barrier imposed by fees, patients in some countries are further deterred by the uncertainty about prices caused by informal payments (Mills et al. 2001). There is no evidence as to whether official fees affect equity more strongly than informal payments.

The direct effect of user charges on health is more difficult to measure, and few studies provide relevant evidence. After charges for eye tests were introduced in the United Kingdom, 19 per cent fewer patients were identified as requiring treatment or follow-up for potentially blinding glaucoma (Laidlaw et al. 1994). These charges may thus increase the prevalence of preventable blindness. Theoretically, if the deterrent effect was directed at reducing the utilization of so-called frivolous services, then the differential access to non-cost-effective services would not result in inequity in health. However, there is evidence that user charges deter the utilization of cost-effective services and therefore adversely affect health.

How does the funding system affect cost containment?

Total health care expenditure in OECD countries is lower on average in systems predominantly funded through general taxation (OECD 2000). There are several possible hypotheses as to why this is the case, although the evidence is limited. Here, we focus on the differences between predominantly tax-funded systems and social health insurance systems. We examine in turn the importance of greater transparency, less political interference, greater linkage between contributions and benefits and the multiple purchasers in social health insurance systems.

The first hypothesis is that the higher levels of transparency under social health insurance weaken resistance to contribution increases compared with tax increases. A survey of European Union countries found that most people in social health insurance systems thought that the government should spend the same amount as is currently spent on health care (Mossialos 1998). Interestingly, people in countries with local tax financing of health care also thought spending was about right. The countries in which most respondents thought that the government should spend more were Greece, Ireland, Portugal and the United Kingdom, which rely on tax funding at the national level (Mossialos 1998). These countries are among those in which public expenditure on health care as a percentage of gross domestic product is low.

The public will accept increases in insurance contributions if the health care provided in return is perceived as efficacious and efficient; in Germany, increasing contributions are more readily accepted than curtailing benefits, such as exclusions and co-payments (Hinrichs 1995). Nevertheless, the evidence of higher public resistance to tax increases and the associated political opposition to tax-and-spend policies is weak. Careful analysis of public opinion suggests that more of the population supports increased taxes when this is linked to increased spending (Mossialos and King 1999; Commission on Taxation and Citizenship 2000).

A second argument is that social health insurance revenue is earmarked and, therefore, not subject to political interference. In Belgium, where health care is financed about equally from taxation and social health insurance contributions, the deviation of average annual growth rates was greater for revenue from government sources than from non-government sources (Nonneman and van Doorslaer 1994). In other words, annual government spending on health care fluctuated more than insurance-based revenue. Nonneman and van Doorslaer (1994) argue that the financial strains on the health care system result from the 'whimsical nature of governments', depending on the good fortune of political coalition and the changing mood of the bodies governing the country. Consequently, relying more on funding from general taxation than on payroll contributions is likely to make revenue less stable.

The third explanation is that the insurees raise their demands to maximize the return on the contributions they make (Hinrichs 1995). Under general taxation, the money paid and the benefits received are not directly related, whereas under social health insurance the link is still explicit.[9]

Finally, higher levels of spending under social health insurance may be linked to the organization of purchasing and payment of providers. It is argued that monopsony purchasing power, often a feature of tax-financed systems, is responsible for the tight control of expenditure. This could also be the case with some social health insurance systems organized around a single fund that could exercise similar leverage over providers. However, there is little evidence of whether monopsony power works in practice. Purchasing within social health insurance systems has traditionally been based on reimbursement, whereas tax-funded systems have had more widespread use of global budgets and capitation. The recent trend in social health insurance has been to introduce global budgets, either for the health sector as a whole, as in France, or for sectors. However, these budgets only contain costs if they are fixed, with the budget holder bearing deficits (see Chapter 4).

How does the funding system affect the wider economy?

Job mobility and labour market flexibility

In contrast to, for instance, general taxation, occupationally related insurance – both social and private – may give rise to job lock, which can create inefficiency in the wider economy. According to economists who advocate a free market in labour, reduced mobility negatively affects the economy as a whole because workers do not take the jobs in which they would be most productive for fear of losing health insurance coverage. Others argue that investment in labour and skill development means that a long-term employee is more valuable than a new recruit; thus, reducing job mobility allows firms to reap the benefits of firm-specific human capital investment (Gruber 1998). The extent of job lock is difficult to measure because isolating confounding variables is difficult. For example, are people who are less healthy less mobile for that reason rather than because of anything to do with the funding system?

The problem of job lock has been hotly debated, especially where insurance is occupationally determined. Much of the literature focuses on the United States, where 90 per cent of the people who are privately insured have employment-related plans. There is more limited research available on Germany, where membership of a sickness fund was occupationally determined for some of the population until 1996.

In the United States, most small employers are less able to provide comprehensive and affordable coverage than most large employers, including many public-sector employers. This may limit the relative ability of small employers to recruit the best suited personnel. Entrepreneurs and new market entrants may be less able to attract employees, reducing the potential of the skill mix in the labour force and having negative macroeconomic effects. This was an explicit motivation for the health care reform proposals put forward by President Clinton: 'Worker mobility is one of the most important values in an entrepreneurial society, where most jobs are created by small businesses. The present health care system is a big brake on that' (quoted in Holtz-Eakin 1994: 157). In the United States, many workers are reluctant to move jobs because of fear of losing insurance coverage. Workers may decide to remain in a job because they fear that they would be liable for large costs or be uninsurable because of pre-existing conditions, be subject to a probationary period for new coverage, lose credits towards deductibles and co-payments, have a more restricted choice of insurer or be unable to use their established health care provider under the new plan, especially under managed-care programmes (Gruber 1998).

Between 11 and 30 per cent of individuals in the United States reported that they or a family member remained in a job at some time because they did not wish to lose the health insurance coverage the employer offered (General Accounting Office 1995). Other estimates suggest that people in the United States who have employer-provided insurance have 25–30 per cent lower mobility than the average among the general population (Gruber 1998).

In Germany, social health insurance is portable, since the benefits are the same regardless of sickness fund, but contribution rates differ between funds. Thus, people who change jobs still get the same benefits but at a different price. People in Germany who are free to choose private health insurance because they exceed a certain income threshold have portable coverage and varying prices. Before the choice of insurer was expanded in 1996, employment or geographical location determined membership of insurance fund for about half the population (Busse 2000). Job movement would be expected to be lower among this group, who may have hesitated to change job because it may have necessitated a change in fund (potentially with a higher contribution rate). Although isolating the effect of health insurance from other variables in the job market is difficult, evidence suggests that the health insurance system does not interfere strongly in the labour market. Health insurance systems, therefore, should not be judged only by their secondary effects on labour mobility but mainly by their primary effects: access to health care and the efficiency of the provision of health insurance (Holtz-Eakin 1994).

Impact on labour costs and international competitiveness

A widely held view is that rising payroll taxes or social insurance contributions are linked to falling employment (OECD 1994). It is argued that increasing employment requires reducing labour costs. However, studies in the United States show no or little effect of employer-provided insurance benefits on employment (Gruber and Krueger 1991; Gruber 1998). Studies modelling the effect on labour for different levels of contribution rates in Germany have found that employment is not sensitive to the health insurance contribution portion of the wage bill. Thus, Bauer and Riphahn (1998) conclude that unemployment cannot be reduced by reducing the contribution rates and correspondingly reducing social insurance benefits.

If expanding benefits increases labour costs and this is considered problematic, one option is to increase the employee contribution but not the employer contribution. This is effectively a wage cut, and its acceptability would depend on whether workers valued the additional benefit enough to accept lower wages (Summers 1989). Such a policy cannot realistically be tested in most European countries, as corporate bargaining prevents reducing wages. Nevertheless, in Germany, for example, employers feared that an insurance-based model for long-term care would increase non-wage-labour costs, and workers therefore agreed to work an extra day per year instead of reducing pay (Evers 1996). Despite the power of the trade union movement in Germany, a compromise was reached that one paid holiday should be abolished – to be determined by each *Land*[10] (Schneider 1999).

Industrialists based in the United States have argued against the introduction of mandated employer-provided insurance, because high labour costs reduce international competitiveness. However, economists based in the United States argue that private health insurance costs do not affect competitiveness under the present health system. They argue that private health insurance costs do not raise overall labour costs but simply change the composition of labour costs from wages to benefits. There is no knock-on effect on prices; the ability to sell products overseas, therefore, remains unaffected (Glied 1997).

Nevertheless, the potential negative impact on industry was one of the justifications for diversifying funding sources from an employee social insurance contribution to an income tax under the Juppé Plan in France. Social insurance contributions were believed to inhibit job creation: international comparisons have shown that employment growth in France lags behind other OECD countries (OECD 1994). Other options for reducing the cost of labour, such as reducing the minimum wage, were rejected because of public opposition (Clasen 1997). In Germany, introducing insurance competition and espousing the objective of reducing contribution rates was somewhat motivated by a need to re-establish economic competitiveness and reduce the burden on industry following reunification. Finally, in the United Kingdom, tax funding has been justified as contributing to the international competitiveness of the economy (Department of Health 2000).

How does the funding system affect allocative efficiency and technical efficiency?

How resources are allocated, what mix of inputs is used and what service outputs are obtained may significantly affect health, but the method of funding and allocative or technical efficiency are not clearly linked conceptually. These are more a function of purchasing than collection, resulting from the market structure of pooling and purchasing. As has been noted, the links between efficiency and funding mechanisms cannot be supported either by theory or empirical evidence (Jonsson and Musgrove 1997).

Allocative efficiency

There are at least three ways of looking at allocative efficiency: allocation between health care and other sectors of the economy; how money is allocated to different sectors within the health care system, such as between acute care and preventive services; and how resources are allocated to specific clinical services, such as which drugs to reimburse and how much. Allocative efficiency is difficult to measure because data are limited and there are methodological problems. Analysis of expenditure by sector can indicate the allocative efficiency of the health care system. However, the analysis depends largely on judgements about the relative value and effectiveness of different sectors; notably, allocative efficiency does not indicate the output achieved, which depends largely on the cost and mix of inputs (technical efficiency) and the boundaries between sectors, which are often poorly defined. Determining the extent to which this allocation improves population health relies on detailed data on outcomes, which are not forthcoming.

Data from the OECD (2000) and the National Forum on Health (Canada) (1998) have shown that the relative size of the ambulatory and acute sectors varies between countries but does not systematically differ according to the predominant source of funding. In most health care systems, the pharmaceutical sector has grown faster than any other sector. However, aggregate data do not clearly show whether the growth in pharmaceuticals has substituted for other expenditure. For example, did the increase in drug expenditure reduce admissions and lengths of stay in inpatient settings or did it just reflect waste and increased profit for drug companies?

Aday *et al.* (1998) provide evidence that the United States fails to achieve allocative efficiency compared with other industrialized countries. The problems identified with the 'market-maximized' model of health care, of which voluntary private health insurance is an element, were substantial underinvestment in selected preventive services, many ineffective and inappropriate health care procedures and a focus on procedure-oriented care. However, generalization should be avoided, because the United States is an outlier both in how much it spends on health care and how it finances health care.

Technical efficiency

Health care payers are increasingly concerned about securing the most bang for their buck or, in the language of economic theory, achieving technical efficiency. Unit costs are thereby minimized by maximizing the output from any given bundle of resources. Conceptually, technical efficiency and the method of funding are not systematically linked. Can any association be observed in practice?

Technical efficiency is driven by purchasing. General taxation and payroll taxation do not necessarily integrate collection and purchasing. With private health insurance in a competitive market, however, collection, pooling and purchasing are usually integrated within the same organization; this method of collection, therefore, influences the efficiency of purchasing. In addition, historical links between funding methods and specific organizational arrangements of purchasers and providers may account for some variation in technical efficiency.

An analysis of the ratio of nurses to physicians in OECD countries suggests that the supply of physicians primarily determines the mix of inputs. Where the supply of physicians exceeds the optimal demand, they substitute for nurses. The mix of generalist and specialist physicians varies. In five of the twelve European Union countries for which there are data, the numbers of general practitioners and specialists are nearly equal (OECD 2000). The source of funding is not related to this variation.

Some tax-funded systems have achieved successful cost-reducing substitution, especially for drugs (Department of Health 2000). However, policies to control prices and promote the utilization of generics are more related to incentives for prescribers, pharmacists and patients than to the method of funding health care.

Furthermore, the mix of technological inputs varies between countries (Banta 1995). Variation in the diffusion of big-ticket technologies reflects limits on the purchasing of equipment or reimbursement policies for tests or treatment, not the source of funding. The price of inputs is also important in determining the extent of technical efficiency. Physicians and nurses in the countries with the highest expenditure on health care (the United States, Switzerland and Canada) receive more than the average income for all countries and less than the average in the countries with the lowest expenditure (Sweden, Japan and the United Kingdom). In the countries where physicians receive the highest income in relation to average income, they are traditionally paid fees for services (National Forum on Health (Canada) 1998). Thus, the method of provider payment rather than the method of health care funding appears to determine the variation.

Administrative efficiency, as measured by the costs of administration as a proportion of total expenditure on health care, appears to be related to the type and organization of the funding method. Administration costs appear to be positively associated (higher) with privatization (for-profit insurers), competition (additional costs of marketing), decentralization and the number of collection agents (duplication of the administrative function with no economies of scale) (OECD 2000). Competitive for-profit insurance companies have the additional costs of underwriting, profit and marketing (see Chapter 6).

To what extent are funding mechanisms path dependent?

In addition to analysing the effects of funding systems, it is important to understand the context in which funding systems operate in order to implement change. In this section, we analyse the impact of historical factors on the development of funding systems in Europe highlighting both the constraints on and opportunities for change. Drawing on the ideas of the new-institutionalism school of economics, we examine the evidence supporting the idea that institutions limit the scope of feasible change and that the decisions taken when a policy is first introduced affect future development (Bonoli 2000). In other words, 'particular policies create particular institutional environments; they sustain particular sets of interests which in turn tend to sustain them' (Freeman and Moran 2000: 45). Historical analysis of established health care systems has shown considerable continuity (Fuchs

1976; Korpi 2001). We briefly examine whether this assertion is valid with particular reference to central and eastern Europe, long-term care insurance in Germany and the NHS in the United Kingdom.

Under communism, most countries in central and eastern Europe adopted the system of universal free health care first established in post-revolutionary Russia. The adoption of Soviet-style health care was less a matter of choice than ideological necessity for these countries.[11] For instance, in Czechoslovakia, the government initially continued with an insurance-based system after the Second World War. Even when the Communists seized power in 1948, the system was rolled out under the National Insurance Act of 1948 to cover all citizens under a single national insurance fund (Kaser 1976). It was not until 1951 that a System of Unified State Health Care was introduced modelled on the system of health care in the Soviet Union (Jaros and Kalina 1998).

After communism fell, many central and eastern European countries and the Baltic states were quick to re-establish systems of social health insurance similar to those that existed before 1945. The original establishment of social health insurance in these countries was strongly influenced by the Bismarck system of social insurance, first established in Germany in 1883, which was widely adopted throughout the Austro-Hungarian Empire and retained after its demise (Schroetter 1923). In Czechoslovakia, for example, between 1919 and 1924, health insurance was gradually expanded to cover all wage-earners, about one-third of the population (Jaros and Kalina 1998). By the 1920s, several hundred funds competed for clients and contracted with private physicians and public hospitals for services. The original law was amended in Hungary, but the essential elements were retained: state responsibility for the indigent population not able to provide for themselves and individual responsibility for everyone else, with insurance provision through occupationally based funds for employed people (de Dobrovits 1925). Thus the reversion to a model of social health insurance in these countries appears to be broadly 'path dependent'.

More recently, the introduction of long-term care insurance in Germany can be seen as path dependent, as it adopted and modified the pre-existing model of funding already in use for health insurance. Political consensus existed on the need to establish some basic guarantee for long-term care coverage, but the political disagreement centred on how to fund it. The proposed solutions reflected the political ideology of the parties that voted in favour of them. The model ultimately chosen was a public insurance plan in line with the traditional model of welfare in Germany that received support from a broad majority of the Christian Democrats and Social Democrats. Long-term care insurance breaks somewhat with the traditional employment links of insured risks, as care risks are not closely connected with the inability to work. However, it follows the historical tradition of social insurance in Germany. Path dependence meant that change remained mainly within the parameters of the institutional framework set up as long ago as the nineteenth century and that the main path of development has been smooth adaptation, minor change at the micro-level of single types of provision with no overhaul (Scheiwe 1997).

Historical analysis also shows that there are opportunities to deviate from historical patterns when a radical break with the past is possible (Freeman and Moran 2000). This applies to the establishment of the NHS in the United Kingdom. The Labour Party came to power in a landslide victory in July 1945 following the end of the Second World War, during which public opinion had shifted to the left (Holland and Stewart 1998) and consensus grew around the need for widening the role of national government (Addison 1975). The National Health Service Act came into force on 5 July 1948. The social and political changes wrought by the upheaval of the Second World War provided a window of opportunity (Kingdon 1984) for a major reform of the welfare state that included the establishment of the NHS.

Subsequent attempts to modify radically the funding of health care in the United Kingdom have been thwarted, which suggests that significant breaks with the past are rare and that incremental change is more usual. The Conservative Party in the United Kingdom, which took power in the general election of 1979, promoted individual responsibility and a minimum role for the state. Despite strong ideological grounds favouring a radical change to a system of funding health care based on insurance, strong public opposition forced a retreat. Political fallout from widespread suspicion of an impending attack on the popular tax-funded NHS led swiftly to Margaret Thatcher's public assurance that 'the NHS is safe in our hands'. Early in 1988, Thatcher took the decision to concentrate on reforming the structure rather than the financing of the NHS (Thatcher 1993).

Factors other than history influence the development of models of funding, such as political and technical factors. Such issues as whether the public and powerful interest groups support the policy and whether it is consistent with the dominant values and beliefs of a society are important. The political feasibility of a funding system may also depend on the wider political context: the stability and legitimacy of government and levels of corruption. Moreover, the nature of the policy-making process can have a significant influence on the development and implementation of policies; for example, whether the policy-making process is consensual or non-consensual or built around single-party rule or multi-party coalitions (Immergut 1992).

Technical issues, such as whether institutions exist with appropriately trained and skilled staff for policy formulation, management and administration, or whether appropriate infrastructures such as information and telecommunication systems and financial institutions are in place, influence the development of systems of health care funding. These issues merit a comprehensive analysis, which has not been attempted in this book. However, political and technical factors should be taken into account in any policy debate on reforming health care funding.

Conclusions

This book compiles both theoretical and empirical evidence on how different methods of raising revenue for health care affect public policy objectives. It also presents comparative examples to illustrate the historical development of health care funding. International comparison may contribute to a better understanding of how funding mechanisms are implemented. However, there are significant limitations to the relevance and transferability of lessons across countries. Contextual factors such as the social, economic and political environment as well as the constraints of history play a major role in how policies are realized and function in practice. These factors are highlighted throughout the book so that experiences can be interpreted within a particular context.

Most health care systems in Europe are funded from a mix of sources, including taxation, social health insurance, private health insurance and out-of-pocket payments. Nevertheless, taxation and social health insurance dominate as methods of funding in nearly all European countries and private health insurance still plays a minor role. Three clusters of countries can be identified in western Europe – those predominantly funded by taxes, those predominantly funded by social health insurance and those with mixed system. Three clusters can also be identified in countries in central and eastern Europe and the former Soviet Union – those predominantly funded by taxes, those predominantly funded by social health insurance and those predominantly funded from out-of-pocket payments (both official and informal), where the prepaid sources of revenue have declined substantially and, in some cases, largely collapsed.

Several issues have emerged from the analysis related to how funding methods affect progressivity, horizontal equity, redistribution, equity of access and coverage, cost containment, the wider economy and allocative and technical efficiency. In theory, collecting health care revenue from general taxation or social health insurance can be associated with improved equity, better cost control, economies of scale and the creation of monopsony purchasing power over providers. However, there is no clear causal relation between the source of funds and other objectives, such as improvements in allocative or technical efficiency. Moreover, apart from equity in financing, the evidence base to support conclusions related to these other objectives is weak.

The available evidence on how different revenue sources affect equity shows that taxation and social health insurance are more progressive than private health insurance and out-of-pocket payments, which are both highly regressive. Equity of access is greater when health care is funded through taxation or social health insurance than when funded from private health insurance or out-of-pocket payments. User charges are a blunt policy instrument deterring both necessary and 'frivolous' utilization and disproportionately affect poor people.

The success of cost containment as measured by the growth rate of health care expenditure is not affected by whether the system is funded mainly through taxation or social health insurance. However, expenditure may be able to be capped if these systems of funding are organized with a single funding pool. Because an explicit political decision is required to set the level of funding for health care, tax-funded systems are theoretically better able to contain costs than systems funded by social health insurance. However, this does not necessarily improve resource allocation. Caps can be imposed on social health insurance systems, although this requires state regulation, which may be resisted by those who hold power in the social health insurance funds.

Private health insurance is associated with high spending because of the extra costs of administration, marketing and profit margins, especially where there are for-profit competitive insurance providers. The motivations of the insurers or third parties greatly affect the incentives to contain costs. Private health insurers are interested in maximizing profit, which provides incentives to maximize revenue (charging high premiums) and minimize expenditure, including cream-skimming, reviewing utilization to eliminate unnecessary procedures and excluding expensive treatments from benefits. The motivations of the state in tax-funded systems are very different and affected by political motivations such as getting re-elected, although cost control is usually a part of this.

It has been argued that excessive labour costs associated with social health insurance may reduce the international competitiveness of a country's economy. Job lock, associated with occupationally based insurance, may lead to inefficiency in the economy by reducing labour market flexibility, but evidence of this is mixed.

Social health insurance may affect the economy and labour market more than taxation because contributions are levied on wages and employers are liable for part of the contribution. Evidence from the United States shows that private health insurance provided by employers reduces job mobility. However, evidence from Germany, when membership of sickness funds was limited by occupation, suggests that job lock was not significant.

The evidence on the link between funding and allocative and technical efficiency is weak. Nevertheless, private health insurance, medical savings accounts and user charges cost more to administer. Moreover, these systems of collecting revenue also influence how resources are allocated. Apart from the managed-care techniques many private insurers have introduced, these collection mechanisms tend to allocate resources through market forces, usually driven by observed consumer demand.

Historical factors influence the development of health care systems, as do political and technical factors. Mechanisms of funding health care appear to be broadly path dependent in terms of the broad direction of change. However, external factors such as strong economic pressures, shifts in political ideology, changes in social values or major external events may create impetus for a major departure from historical trends.

Methods of generating revenue do not operate in a vacuum but depend on the context in which they are applied. Whatever the method of raising revenue, the economic circumstances significantly influence the ability of a country to mobilize resources for health care. The economic climate in central and eastern Europe and the former Soviet Union has left most countries with significant difficulty in raising revenue to meet health care expenditure. Informal payments are widespread and the major challenge remains how to (re)establish official payment mechanisms in the context of negative or low economic growth. Spending on health care has an opportunity cost, and other sectors may take priority in times of economic contraction. Clearly, in a situation of conflict, military priorities may well consume most of a country's resources and may negatively affect productivity through infrastructural damage and human loss. The reliance on resources generated and managed by government is particularly vulnerable to pressure – both internal and external – on government expenditure. During periods of high unemployment, methods relying on wage-related contributions will suffer. Changes in the labour market generally suggest that the shift towards short-term, part-time and flexible working arrangements and the trend to take early retirement are eroding the traditional basis for social insurance eligibility, especially discriminating against women. Demographic changes and changes in household structure affect the supply of informal care, which may increase the demand for formal health and long-term care services. Changes in social values may also influence decision-making. However, at least in western Europe, public support for public funding of health services still appears to be widespread.

The fact that most funding systems are mixed in practice means that evaluating a system's performance based on the sources of funding is difficult. The key to improving policy outcome is to weigh up the advantages and disadvantages of each funding method carefully and to relate the discussion to the specific national context.

Notes

1 Evaluation has been defined as 'the systematic assessment of the operation and/or the outcomes of a program or policy, compared to a set of explicit or implicit standards as a means of contributing to the improvement of a program or policy' (Weiss 1998: 4).

2 The results of the ECuity Project are extensively referenced in this book, as it is one of the few pieces of comparative empirical research to examine equity in financing. The ECuity Project first published its results in 1992, using data collected in the 1980s from household and family expenditure surveys and from family income and budget surveys, and was subsequently updated using data from the late 1980s and early 1990s (Wagstaff and van Doorslaer 1992; Wagstaff *et al.* 1999). The reader should be aware of several methodological concerns. First, the comparability and validity of the data – the purposes of the surveys differ, the demographic unit may be defined differently and income is often underestimated in such surveys, especially where there is a significant grey economy. Second, the basis of the calculations – the same equivalence scale was used for all countries despite the difference in household composition, and the Gini coefficient was used as the measure of income inequality but no sensitivity analysis of the use of other coefficients was presented. Finally, the results of the two studies are not directly comparable, and the differences between studies have not been tested for statistical significance (Wagstaff *et al.* 1999).

3 The positive value (indicating progressivity) for Spain in 1980 may result from differential and higher value-added tax rates on luxury goods.

4 There are a number of methodological limitations associated with the comparison of progressivity and income redistribution cross-nationally. Such analyses should therefore be interpreted with caution. First, ranking of countries according to the overall level of income inequality needs to take account of the relative importance of inequality at different points on the income scale. Second, such analyses will be sensitive to the equivalence scale used. Third, and specifically relating to the Luxembourg Income Study datasets, they do not provide an explanation of policy. Finally, they are strongly cash-income oriented and ignore the distribution of in-kind benefits (Atkinson *et al.* 1994; Mabbett and Bolderson 1999). That is why, when discussing the overall redistributive effect of funding systems for health care, we also examine the incidence of benefits-in-kind.

5 Spain has subsequently shifted its funding base and now relies on taxation as the main source of funding health care.
6 This is especially true in Germany, where high-risk individuals with high incomes are likely to choose to remain in the public system because private health insurance premiums are high.
7 Differences between eastern and western Germany are partly an economic effect with regional inequity in wealth between these areas.
8 Under social health insurance, insurers are legally obliged to accept anyone applying for insurance. Any risk selection by the insurers is, therefore, unlikely to result in individuals being denied insurance in general.
9 People enrolled in social insurance schemes perceive that contributions and benefits are directly linked. However, the link between contributions and benefits has been weakened, since coverage is extended to the non-employed population.
10 No agreement was reached in Saxony and employees, therefore, pay the entire premium (1.35% of earned income) (Schneider 1999; Wahner-Roedler et al. 1999).
11 The only significant deviation from a Soviet-style health service in the communist bloc was Yugoslavia, where health centres and hospitals were 'self-managed': unconstrained by the centrally planned norms that dominated health services in other countries (Kunitz 1979).

References

Aday, L.A., Begley, C.E., Lairson, D.R. and Slater, C.H. (1998) *Evaluating the Healthcare System: Effectiveness, Efficiency and Equity.* Chicago, IL: Health Administration Press.

Addison, P. (1975) *The Road to 1945: British Politics and the Second World War.* London: Cape.

Atkinson, A., Rainwater, L. and Smeeding, T. (1994) *Income Distribution in OECD Countries: The Evidence from the Luxembourg Income Study (LIS).* Luxembourg: LIS.

Banta, D. (1995) *An Approach to the Social Control of Hospital Technologies,* Current Concerns SHS Paper No. 10. Geneva: World Health Organization.

Bauer, T. and Riphahn, R.T. (1998) *Employment Effects of Payroll Taxes – An Empirical Test for Germany,* Bonn: Institute for the Study of Labor (IZA).
http://www.iza.org/publications/discussion_paper/dp11.pdf (accessed 5 March 2001).

Bocognano, A., Couffinhal, A., Dumesnil, S. and Grignon, M. (2000) Which coverage for whom? Equity of access to health insurance in France, paper presented to the European Public Health Association Congress, Paris, 14–16 December.
http://www.credes.fr/En_ligne/ WorkingPaper/pdf/euphaac.pdf (accessed 5 March 2001).

Bonoli, G. (2000) *The Politics of Pension Reform: Institutions and Policy Change in Western Europe.* Cambridge: Cambridge University Press.

Burchardt, T., Hills, J. and Joseph Rowntree Foundation (1996) *Private Welfare Insurance and Social Security: Pushing the Boundaries.* York: York Publishing Services for the Joseph Rowntree Foundation.

Busse, R. (2000) *Health Care Systems in Transition: Germany.* Copenhagen: European Observatory on Health Care Systems.

Clasen, J. (ed.) (1997) *Social Insurance in Europe.* Bristol: Policy Press.

Commission on Taxation and Citizenship (2000) *Paying for Progress: A New Politics of Tax for Public Spending.* London: Fabian Society.

Culyer, A.J. and Wagstaff, A. (1993) Equity and equality in health and health care, *Journal of Health Economics,* 12: 431–57.

de Dobrovits, A. (1925) *Public Health Services in Hungary*. Geneva: League of Nations, Health Organization.

Department of Health (2000) *The NHS Plan: A Plan for Investment, a Plan for Reform*. London: The Stationery Office.

Dixon, A. and Mossialos, E. (2000) Has the Portuguese NHS achieved its objectives of equity and efficiency?, *International Social Security Review*, 53(4): 49–78.

Donelan, K., Blendon, R.J., Schoen, C., Davis, K. and Binns, K. (1999) The cost of health system change: public discontent in five nations, *Health Affairs*, 18(3): 206–16.

Elofsson, S., Unden, A.L. and Krakau, I. (1998) Patient charges – a hindrance to financially and psychosocially disadvantaged groups seeking care, *Social Science and Medicine*, 46(10): 1375–80.

Ervik, R. (1998) *The Redistributive Aim of Social Policy: A Comparative Analysis of Taxes, Tax Expenditure Transfers and Direct Transfers in Eight Countries*. New York: Syracuse University Press.

Evers, A. (1996) The new long term care insurance in Germany: characteristics, consequences and perspectives, in T. Harding, B. Meredith and G. Wistow (eds) *Options for Long Term Care: Economic, Social and Ethical Choices*. London: HMSO.

Freeman, R. and Moran, M. (2000) Reforming health care in Europe, in M. Ferrera and M. Rhodes (eds) *Recasting European Welfare States*. London: Frank Cass.

Fuchs, V.R. (1976) From Bismarck to Woodcock: the 'irrational' pursuit of national health insurance, *Journal of Law and Economics*, 19(2): 347–59.

General Accounting Office (1995) *General Insurance Portability: Reform Could Ensure Continued Coverage for up to 25 Million Americans*. Washington, DC: US General Accounting Office.

Glennerster, H. (1997) *Paying for Welfare: Towards 2000*, 3rd edn. Englewood Cliffs, NJ: Prentice-Hall.

Glied, S. (1997) *Chronic Condition: Why Health Reform Fails*. Cambridge, MA: Harvard University Press.

Gruber, J. (1998) *Health Insurance and the Labor Market*, Cambridge, MA: National Bureau of Economic Research, Inc. http://www.nber.org/papers/w6762.pdf (accessed 5 March 2001).

Gruber, J. and Krueger, A.B. (1991) The incidence of mandated employer-provided insurance: lessons from workers' compensation insurance, in D. Bradford (ed.) *Tax Policy and the Economy*. Cambridge, MA: MIT Press.

Hills, J. (1995) Funding the welfare state, *Oxford Review of Economic Policy*, 11(3): 27–43.

Hinrichs, K. (1995) The impact of German health insurance reforms on redistribution and the culture of solidarity, *Journal of Health Politics, Policy and Law*, 20(3): 653–87, 689–94.

Hinrichs, K. (1997) *Social Insurances and the Culture of Solidarity: The Moral Infrastructure of Interpersonal Redistributions – with Special Reference to the German Health Care System*. Bremen: Centre for Social Policy Research, University of Bremen.

Holland, W.W. and Stewart, S. (1998) *Public Health: The Vision and the Challenge*. London: Nuffield Trust.

Holtz-Eakin, D. (1994) Health insurance provision and labor market efficiency in the United States and Germany, in R.M. Blank (ed.) *Social Protection Versus Economic Flexibility: Is there a Trade-off?* Chicago: University of Chicago Press.

Immergut, E.M. (1992) *Health Politics: Interests and Institutions in Western Europe*. Cambridge: Cambridge University Press.

Jaros, J. and Kalina, K. (1998) *Czech Health Care System: Delivery and Financing*. Paris: Organisation for Economic Co-operation and Development.

Jefferson, R.T. (1999) Medical savings accounts: windfalls for the healthy, wealthy and wise, *Catholic University Law Review*, 48(3): 685–723.

Jonsson, B. and Musgrove, P. (1997) Government financing of health care, in G.J. Schieber (ed.) *Innovations in Health Care Financing: Proceedings of a World Bank Conference*, 10–11 March 1997. Washington, DC: World Bank.

Jourdain, A. (2000) Equity of a health system, *European Journal of Public Health*, 10(2): 138–42.

Kaiser Family Foundation (2000) *State Reforms of Small Group Health Insurance*, Menlo Park, CA: Kaiser Family Foundation.
http://www.kff.org/content/archive/1315/state. html (accessed 5 March 2001).

Kakwani, N.C. (1977) Measurement of tax progressivity: an international comparison, *Economic Journal*, 87(March): 71–80.

Kangas, O. (2000) *Social Policy in Settled and Transitional Countries: A Comparison of Institutions and their Consequences*, Helsinki: Ministry of Social Affairs and Health.
http://www.vn.fi/stm/english/tao/publicat/tandem/kangas/olli.htm (accessed 5 March 2001).

Kaser, M. (1976) *Health Care in the Soviet Union and Eastern Europe*. London: Croom Helm.

Kingdon, J.W. (1984) *Agendas, Alternatives, and Public Policies*. Boston, MA: Little, Brown.

Klavus, J. and Häkkinen, U. (1998) Micro-level analysis of distributional changes in health care financing in Finland, *Journal of Health Services Research and Policy*, 3(1): 23–30.

Korpi, W. (2001) Contentious institutions: an augmented rational-actor analysis of the origins and path dependency of welfare state institutions in the western countries, *Rationality and Society*, 13(2): 235–83.

Kunitz, S.J. (1979) Health care and workers' self-management in Yugoslavia, *International Journal of Health Services*, 9(3): 521–37.

Laidlaw, D.A., Bloom, P.A., Hughes, A.O., Sparrow, J.M. and Marmion, V.J. (1994) The sight test fee: effect on opthalmology referrals and rate of glaucoma detection, *British Medical Journal*, 309: 634–6.

Le Grand, J. (1978) The distribution of public expenditure: the case of health care, *Economica*, 45: 125–42.

Le Grand, J. (1982) *The Strategy of Equality: Redistribution and the Social Services*. London: Allen & Unwin.

Le Grand, J. (1991a) *Equity and Choice: An Essay in Applied Economics and Philosophy*. London: HarperCollins Academic.

Le Grand, J. (1991b) The distribution of health care revisited: a commentary on Wagstaff, van Doorslaer and Paci, and O'Donnell and Propper, *Journal of Health Economics*, 10(2): 239–45.

Light, D.W. (1992) Equity and efficiency in health care, *Social Science and Medicine*, 35(4): 465–9.

Lutz, P.F. and Schneider, U. (1998) Der soziale Ausgleich in der gesetzlichen Krankenversicherung [Income redistribution under Germany's statutory health insurance scheme], *Jahrbücher für Nationalökonomie und Statistik*, 217(6): 718–40.

Mabbett, D. and Bolderson, H. (1999) Theories and methods in comparative social policy, in J. Clasen (ed.) *Comparative Social Policy: Concepts, Theories and Methods*. Oxford: Blackwell.

Manning, W.G., Keeler, E.B., Newhouse, J.P., Sloss, E.M. and Wasserman, J. (1989) The taxes of sin. Do smokers and drinkers pay their way?, *Journal of the American Medical Association*, 261(11): 1604–9.

Mastilica, M. and Bozikov, J. (1999) Out-of-pocket payments for health care in Croatia: implications for equity, *Croatian Medical Journal*, 40(2): 152–9.

Mills, A., Bennett, S. and Russell, S. (2001) *The Challenge of Health Sector Reform: What Must Governments Do?* Hampshire: Palgrave.

Moon, M., Nichols, L.M. and Wall, S. (1996) *Medical Savings Accounts: A Policy Analysis*, Washington, DC: Urban Institute. http://www.urban.org/pubs/HINSURE/MSA.htm (accessed 5 March 2001).

Mossialos, E. (1998) *Citizens and Health Systems: Main Results from a Eurobarometer Survey*. Brussels: European Commission, Directorate-General for Employment, Industrial Relations and Social Affairs.

Mossialos, E. and King, D. (1999) Citizens and rationing: analysis of a European survey, *Health Policy*, 49(1–2): 75–135.

Müller, R., Braun, B. and Gress, S. (2000). *Allokative und distributive Effekte von Wettbewerbselementen und Probleme ihrer Implementation in einem sozialen Gesundheitswesen am Beispiel der Erfahrungen in den Niederlanden [Allocative and Distributional Effect of Competition and Problems with its Implementation in a Social Health Care System, the Example of the Netherlands]*. Bremen: University of Bremen.

National Forum on Health (Canada) (1998). *Striking a Balance: Health Care Systems in Canada and Elsewhere*. Québec: Editions MultiMondes.

Newhouse, J.P. and the Insurance Experiment Group (1993) *Free for All? Lessons from the RAND Health Insurance Experiment*. Cambridge, MA: Harvard University Press.

Nonneman, W. and van Doorslaer, E. (1994) The role of the sickness funds in the Belgian health care market, *Social Science and Medicine*, 39(10): 1483–95.

OECD (1994) *The OECD Jobs Study Evidence and Explanation. II. The Adjustment Potential of the Labour Markets*. Paris: Organisation for Economic Co-operation and Development.

OECD (2000) *OECD Health Data 2000: A Comparative Analysis of 29 Countries*. Paris: Organisation for Economic Co-operation and Development.

Putnam, R.D., Leonardi, R. and Nanetti, R. (1993) *Making Democracy Work: Civic Traditions in Modern Italy*. Princeton, NJ: Princeton University Press.

Scheiwe, K. (1997) *New Demands for Social Protection – Changing Family Structures, Women's Roles and Institutional Responses. The Case of the German Long-term Care Insurance*. Mannheim: Mannheimer Zentrum für Europäische Sozialforschung (Mannheim Centre for European Social Research).

Schmahl, W. (1998) Financing social security in Germany: proposals for changing its structure and some possible effects, in S.W. Black (ed.) *Globalization, Technological Change and Labor Markets*. Dordrecht: Kluwer Academic.

Schneider, U. (1999) Germany's social long-term care insurance: design, implementation and evaluation, *International Social Security Review*, 52(2): 31–74.

Schroetter, H. (1923) *Public Health Services in Austria*. Geneva: League of Nations, Health Organization.

Schwarz, E. (1996) Changes in utilization and cost sharing within the Danish National Health Insurance dental program, 1975–90, *Acta Odontologica Scandinavica*, 54(1): 29–35.

Summers, L. (1989) Some simple economics of mandated benefits, *American Economic Review*, 79(2): 177–83.

Swiss Federal Statistical Office (2000) *Burden of Taxation*, Neuchâtel: Swiss Federal Statistical Office. http://www.statistik.admin.ch/stat_ch/ber18/eu1803.htm (accessed 5 March 2001).

Thatcher, M. (1993) *The Downing Street Years*. London: HarperCollins.

Townsend, J., Roderick, P. and Cooper, J. (1994) Cigarette smoking by socioeconomic group, sex, and age: effects of price, income, and health publicity, *British Medical Journal*, 309(6959): 923–7.

Van Doorslaer, E., Wagstaff, A., van der Burg, H. *et al.* (1999) The redistributive effect of health care finance in twelve OECD countries, *Journal of Health Economics*, 18(3): 291–314.

Wagstaff, A. and van Doorslaer, E. (1992) Equity in the finance of health care: some international comparisons, *Journal of Health Economics*, 11(4): 361–87.

Wagstaff, A. and van Doorslaer, E. (1997) Progressivity, horizontal equity and reranking in health care finance: a decomposition analysis for the Netherlands, *Journal of Health Economics*, 16(5): 499–516.

Wagstaff, A., Rutten, F. and van Doorslaer, E. (eds) (1993) *Equity in the Finance and Delivery of Health Care: An International Perspective*. Oxford: Oxford University Press.

Wagstaff, A., van Doorslaer, E., van der Burg, H. *et al.* (1999) Equity in the finance of health care: some further international comparisons, *Journal of Health Economics*, 18: 263–90.

Wahner-Roedler, D.L., Knuth, P. and Juchems, R.H. (1999) The German *Pflegeversicherung* (long-term care insurance), *Mayo Clinic Proceedings*, 74(2): 196–200.

Weiss, C.H. (1998) *Evaluation*. Englewood Cliffs, NJ: Prentice-Hall.

Whitehead, M., Evandrou, M., Haglund, B. and Diderichsen, F. (1997) As the health divide widens in Sweden and Britain, what's happening to access to care?, *British Medical Journal*, 315(7114): 1006–9.

Zandvakili, S. (1994) Income distribution and redistribution through taxation: an international comparison, *Empirical Economics*, 19: 473–91.

Index

Page numbers in *italics* refer to tables and figures